W9-DHX-673

Study Guide to Accompany
Linton, Matteson, and Maebius:

INTRODUCTORY NURSING CARE OF ADULTS

Written by:

Nancy K. Maebius, Ph.D., R.N.

Instructor
The Health Institute of San Antonio
San Antonio, Texas

W. B. SAUNDERS COMPANY
A Division of Harcourt Brace & Company
Philadelphia London Toronto
Montreal Sydney Tokyo

1999 2000

W. B. SAUNDERS COMPANY
A Division of Harcourt Brace & Company
The Curtis Center
Independence Square West
Philadelphia, Pennsylvania 19106

Study Guide to Accompany Linton, Matteson, and Maebius:
Introductory Nursing Care of Adults, by Nancy K. Maebius

ISBN 0-7216-3318-8

Printed in the United States of America

Last digit is the print number: 9   8   7   6   5

Preface

This Study Guide, written by Nancy K. Maebius, is designed to help you obtain the most benefit from your textbook, *Introductory Nursing Care of Adults*. The textbook gives current and comprehensive coverage of medical-surgical nursing care, gerontological nursing, and basic information about psychiatric-mental health nursing. This Study Guide will help you, the student, learn vocabulary, identify and master the most important content in the textbook, and help prepare you for examinations. Think of the Study Guide as your "friend," who checks your reading and makes sure you are identifying the most important ideas as you read.

VOCABULARY EXERCISES

One of the basic steps in studying that will help you learn and remember more is to develop a good understanding of the many new words dealing with anatomy and physiology, medical treatments and equipment, nursing assessments and interventions, and drugs. Each chapter in the textbook opens with a list of important vocabulary words with definitions. Each Study Guide chapter includes a matching exercise to check your understanding of the vocabulary.

OTHER LEARNING ACTIVITIES

The matching and completion Learning Activities emphasize the most important facts and ideas in the chapter. The questions in the Study Guide are closely coordinated with the textbook chapter. Questions cover the text material, plus tables, figures, and special features such as "Pharmacology Capsules" and "Nutrition Concepts."

You will be able to find the exact answers in the text to some questions. However, some questions require that you analyze, synthesize (put together), and evaluate the facts in the textbook. These questions are important because they will help you to apply the facts that you learn to real clinical situations.

MULTIPLE CHOICE QUESTIONS

Each chapter in the Study Guide concludes with a section of multiple choice questions. These questions cover content in any part of the chapter; by answering these questions you will test your own knowledge and can become more proficient and self confident in taking multiple choice examinations.

ANSWERS TO STUDY GUIDE QUESTIONS

Answers to all of the Study Guide questions are provided in the Instructor's Manual.

Acknowledgments

I greatly appreciate the strong support I received from two colleagues and close friends, Lea Ann Loftis and Beverly Halter, who helped in many areas of manuscript preparation for the Study Guide and Instructor's Manual, reviewing galley proofs and being available for listening and advising. Two fellow faculty members, Colette Strauss and Nathan Porter, were helpful in providing examples of student experiences and test questions; discussion with them about vocational nursing students was lively. In addition, Gaylynn Schilhab was very helpful with suggestions on Death and Dying. I would also like to thank my son, Andrew, and his two friends, Paulo Barker and Danny MacNelly, for support and assistance with writing distracters.

My husband, Jed, my son, Andrew, and my other children, Stephen, Brian, and Elizabeth have provided much humor, support, and love while these manuscripts were developed.

I am very grateful to Linda Weinerman, who took a very rough draft of many questions and transformed them into a logical, cohesive, edited set of questions. Also, Terri Wood was a terrific help in coordinating the many aspects of Study Guide and Instructor's Manual development. Finally, Ilze Rader was eager with encouragement, and thoughtful about letting me know when to "let go" and how to set priorities.

My vocational nursing students deserve special thanks. I am grateful to all of them for enthusiastically spending hours with me in class, asking and answering questions which were incorporated into the Study Guide and Instructor's Manual. It is wonderful to work with them and to watch them think and learn, and, in turn, to learn from them.

Nancy K. Maebius

Contents

UNIT 13: REPRODUCTIVE DISORDERS

UNIT 14: INTEGUMENTARY DISORDERS

UNIT 15: DISORDERS OF THE EYES, EARS, NOSE, AND THROAT

UNIT 16: MENTAL HEALTH AND ILLNESS

The Health Care System

OBJECTIVES

1. Describe the organization of the health care system in the United States.
2. Describe the components of the health care system that provide both outpatient and inpatient care.

LEARNING ACTIVITIES

I. Match the definition on the left with the most appropriate term on the right.

____ 1. Branch of the Department of Health and Human Services of the U.S. Government whose chief purpose is to provide better health services for the American people

____ 2. Health insurance program administered by the federal government that is funded by Social Security payments

____ 3. Program that provides health care services for needy, lower-income, and disabled individuals

____ 4. Health care organization that provides care and services through group practice and prepayment plans

____ 5. Act passed in 1965 to ensure that elderly persons have an adequate income and suitable housing, physical and mental health services, community services, and the opportunity to pursue meaningful activities

____ 6. System enacted under Medicare that reimburses hospitals for patient care based on their medical diagnoses

____ 7. Type of nursing home that provides rehabilitative care for people who need nursing care that consists of observation during illness, administration of medications and treatments, bowel or bladder retraining, and changing of sterile dressings

____ 8. Nursing homes that provide custodial care for people who are unable to care for themselves because of mental or physical infirmity

A. Medicaid

B. Intermediate Care Facility

C. Public Health Service

D. Diagnosis Related Group (DRG)

E. Medicare

F. Health Maintenance Organization (HMO)

G. Older Americans Act

H. Skilled Nursing Facility

II. Describe how the following 7 factors interfere with a comprehensive plan of health care in the United States.

1. Finance

2. Plan for health care

3. Emphasis

4. Standards

5. Consumer participation

6. Coordination

7. Communication

III. List the 3 primary branches of DHHS.

1.

2.

3.

IV. List 6 activities of the Public Health Service.

1.

2.

3.

4.

5.

6.

V. Components of the Health Care System: Match the descriptions on the left with the appropriate term on the right.

___ 1. Provides for patients who do not require hospitalization

___ 2. Settings include acute care hospitals, psychiatric hospitals, and extended care facilities

___ 3. Involves health promotion and disease prevention

___ 4. Settings include physician's offices, clinics, HMOs, day surgery, home health

A. Outpatient (ambulatory)

B. Inpatient

VI. Match the description on the left with the appropriate term on the right.
Comparisons between Medicare and Medicaid

Funding

___ 1. Monthly premium from paycheck; funds matched by federal government

___ 2. Federal, state and local taxes

A. Medicare

B. Medicaid

Eligibility

___ 3. Needy, low-income, and disabled persons and their dependent children younger than 65 years

___ 4. All persons older than 65 years plus disabled persons younger than 65 who qualify for Social Security benefits

How Administered

___ 5. Federal government

___ 6. Both federal and state governments

VII. Choose the most appropriate answer.

1. Which are examples of outpatient care?
   A. hospital operating rooms
   B. acute care hospitals
   C. physician's offices
   D. extended care facilities

2. HMOs provide health care and services:
   A. through group practice
   B. through solo practice
   C. to all older Americans
   D. to all disabled (physically and mentally challenged) persons

3. In recent years, the number of older adults admitted to the hospital has:
   A. decreased
   B. stayed the same
   C. stabilized
   D. increased

4. Of all people over age 65, how many are admitted to the hospital each year?
   A. one in five
   B. one in ten
   C. one in fifty
   D. one in one hundred

5. Which system classifies patients according to the medical diagnosis so that hospitals receive a fixed payment based on the patient's diagnosis?
   A. HMOs
   B. DRGs
   C. ABGs
   D. TPNs

6. Physicians are now discharging patients as early as possible in order to:
   A. improve care, because Medicare pays the hospitals more if patients leave earlier
   B. improve care, because Medicare pays only a fixed fee no matter how long the length of stay
   C. reduce costs, because hospitals only receive a fixed amount of money from Medicare
   D. reduce costs, because hospitals receive more money if patients stay in the hospital longer

7. A person who needs rehabilitative care and who has the potential to regain function would go to:
   A. a SNF (skilled nursing facility)
   B. an ICF (intermediate care facility)
   C. a hospital
   D. an ambulatory care center

The Leadership Role of the Nurse

1. Differentiate leadership from management.
2. Describe leadership styles and management theories.
3. Discuss the leadership process.
4. Describe the role of the licensed vocational nurse as a team leader.
5. Discuss leadership issues in relation to safe health care.

LEARNING ACTIVITIES

I. Match the definition on the left with the most appropriate term on the right.

____ 1. Guidance or showing the way to others; "inspiration"

____ 2. Effective use of selected methods to achieve the goals; "perspiration"

____ 3. Authoritarian, directive, or bureaucratic types of leadership

____ 4. Achievement of goals through participation by all group members

____ 5. Nondirective type of leadership

____ 6. Management by autocratic rule with little participation in decision making by workers

____ 7. Democratic style of management with some participation in decision making by workers

____ 8. Management with full participation in decision making by workers

A. Autocratic Leadership

B. Theory X

C. Laissez-faire Leadership

D. Democratic Leadership

E. Theory Y

F. Leadership

G. Theory Z

H. Management

II. Choose the most appropriate answer.

1. Guidance of others, or showing them the way, is an example of:
   A. management
   B. demonstration
   C. leadership
   D. democracy

2. Three basic types of leadership are autocratic, democratic, and:
   A. authoritarian
   B. sympathetic
   C. empathetic
   D. laissez-faire

3. Individuals who achieve their goals by setting objectives and having them carried out without input or suggestions from others are individuals who display what style of leadership?
   A. democratic
   B. autocratic
   C. laissez-faire
   D. cooperative

4. Individuals who make decisions based on group consensus display what style of leadership?
   A. democratic
   B. autocratic
   C. laissez-faire
   D. authoritarian

5. Individuals who lead by suggestion rather than by domination exhibit what style of leadership?
   A. autocratic
   B. laissez-faire
   C. authoritarian
   D. democratic

6. Individuals who provide little or no leadership exhibit what style of leadership?
   A. democratic
   B. autocratic
   C. authoritarian
   D. laissez-faire

7. A focus on participative management based on mutual trust and loyalty reflects which type of management?
   A. theory X
   B. theory Y
   C. theory Z
   D. laissez-faire

8. Deciding in advance what needs to be done and how to do it is:
   A. coordinating
   B. directing
   C. planning
   D. controlling

9. The process of selecting one course of action from alternatives is:
   A. coordinating
   B. decision making
   C. directing
   D. evaluating

10. Once the problem is identified, the next step in decision making involves:
    A. choosing the most desirable solution
    B. evaluating the best response
    C. coordinating the representative ideas
    D. evaluating the solution

11. Once the best solution for solving the problem is determined, the next step in decision making is to:
    A. plan the action
    B. diagnose the action
    C. evaluate the action
    D. implement the action

12. The final step in the decision making process is:
    A. planning
    B. implementation
    C. evaluation
    D. diagnosis

13. The second step in the management process is:
    A. directing
    B. coordinating
    C. controlling
    D. organizing

14. The next step, after planning and organizing, is:
    A. directing
    B. coordinating
    C. controlling
    D. evaluating

15. In making assignments, an attempt should be made to match the skills of the personnel with:
    A. patient personalities
    B. nursing needs
    C. patient needs
    D. nursing personalities

16. When making assignments for patient care, which approach encourages cooperation and tends to get more work done?
    A. ordering that a task be done
    B. requesting that a task be done
    C. delegating tasks to more than one person
    D. asking to see the staffing plan

17. The pulling together of various activities in order to achieve a goal is:
    A. directing
    B. planning
    C. organizing
    D. coordinating

18. Controlling is basically a form of:
    A. evaluation
    B. assessment
    C. planning
    D. implementation

19. Protection of the patient's confidentiality is stated in the:
    A. Joint Commission of Accreditation Act
    B. Social Security Act
    C. Patient's Bill of Rights
    D. Right to Privacy Act

III. Following are characteristics of people in their work environment. Mark an "X" after the characteristic if it refers to the theory X classical management theory, and a "Y" if it refers to the theory Y classical management theory.

1. Work with others to do the job well ___

2. Care about what they are doing ___

3. Find no pleasure in work ___

4. Constantly striving to grow ___

5. Naturally lazy and prefer to do nothing ___

6. Work mainly for the money ___

7. Do not want to think for themselves ___

8. Mature and responsible ___

9. Self-directed ___

10. Work only because they fear being fired ___

11. Childlike and like being told what to do ___

12. Work for rewards other than money ___

13. Active and enjoy setting their own goals ___

14. Not capable of making decisions for themselves ___

15. Productive because of their own personal goals ___

IV. Match the Process step on the left with Methods to Accomplish on the right.
   Steps in the Decision Making Process

____ 1. Identify the problem

____ 2. Explore possible solutions

____ 3. Choose most desirable action

____ 4. Implement action

____ 5. Evaluate results

A. Determine whether action is realistic and can accomplish organization goals

B. Involve others and brainstorm

C. Communicate decision to others

D. Use audits and verbal feedback

E. Find out who, how, when, why

V. Match the characteristics of leadership styles on the left with the leadership styles on the right. The terms on the right may be used more than once.

____ 1. Decision making by the leader and group together

____ 2. Decision making by the group or by no one

____ 3. Shared responsibility

____ 4. Leader assumes responsibility

____ 5. Decision making by the leader

____ 6. Leadership by suggestion rather than by domination

A. Authoritarian

B. Democratic

C. Laissez-faire

The Nurse-Patient Relationship

OBJECTIVES

1. Define holistic view of nursing.
2. Define the concept of *self*.
3. Discuss the use of self in the practice of nursing.
4. Compare the meaning of the terms *patient* and *client*.
5. List commonly held expectations of patients and families.
6. Describe guidelines for nurse-patient relationships.

LEARNING ACTIVITIES

I. Match the definition on the left with the most appropriate term on the right.

____	1. Process involving understanding and action	A. Holism
____	2. Listening to others in order to perceive their feelings and the meaning of their words	B. Caring
		C. Empathy
____	3. Responding to others with genuineness, warmth, sensitivity and self-disclosure	D. Understanding
		E. Patient
____	4. Viewing people as whole individuals	F. Self
____	5. One's personhood	G. Client
____	6. Person for whom the nurse provides care; denotes a feeling of doing to or for the person	H. Action
____	7. Person with whom a nurse has a feeling of partnership or working with someone	
____	8. Identifying with and understanding another person's situation, feelings, and motives	

II. Match the definition on the left with the most appropriate term on the right.

____	1. Principles or standards shared by members of a society that determine what is desirable or worthwhile	A. Attitudes
		B. Values
____	2. Convictions or opinions	C. Beliefs
____	3. Feelings toward persons or things	

III. List 6 characteristics the nurse must have to assume the helper role.

1.   4.

2.   5.

3.   6.

IV. Choose the most appropriate answer.

1. The ability to be open and honest about one's feelings is characteristic of:
   A. self-image
   B. self-esteem
   C. self-disclosure
   D. self-trust

2. Exchanging ideas, beliefs, thoughts, and feelings between two or more people is:
   A. organization
   B. caring
   C. delegation
   D. communication

3. An active process that involves trying to understand what is being said is:
   A. listening
   B. talking
   C. explaining
   D. delegating

4. Understanding another's feelings and becoming immersed in the situation is:
   A. empathy
   B. helping
   C. sympathy
   D. apathy

5. A view of human health that considers biologic, psychological, social, and cultural components is:
   A. anthropology
   B. holistic health
   C. folk medicine
   D. pathology

V. List 3 benefits of touch in a nurse-patient relationship.

1.

2.

3.

VI. List 3 benefits of giving a bedridden client a back rub before surgery.

1.

2.

3.

VII. Fill in the blank.

Communication involves a message, a sender, and a _____.

VIII. List 2 types of communication behavior.

1.   2.

IX. List 7 examples of nonverbal communication.

1.   5.

2.   6.

3.   7.

4.

X. Fill in the blank.

Observation is to nonverbal language as listening is to _____.

XI. List 4 behaviors that may help the nurse initiate a therapeutic interaction:

1.

2.

3.

4.

XII. Indicate by an X in the appropriate column whether the description refers to a helping person or a friend.

	Helping Person	Friend
1. Does not share personal information		
2. Responsible to client		
3. Sexual overtones or a sexual relationship may develop		
4. Both individuals express feelings, attitudes, and opinions		
5. Attitude is nonjudgmental		
6. Relationship is goal directed		
7. Individuals meet each other's needs		
8. Relationship is time limited		
9. Objective of relationship is to meet client's needs		
10. Relationship may continue		
11. No plan involved		
12. Discourages any sexual overtones in relationship		

XIII. Match the examples of communication techniques on the left with the proper label on the right. Answers may be used more than once.

_____ 1. Fight urge to fill quiet periods with conversation.

_____ 2. Leave time for the client to think and respond.

_____ 3. "You say you're feeling better since your brother has returned?"

_____ 4. Review the subject matter that the client has just discussed.

_____ 5. "I hear you say you're concerned about your son."

_____ 6. "Do you mean sad when you say upset?"

A. Reflecting

B. Clarification

C. Silence

D. Restating

E. Summarizing

CHAPTER

4

Cultural Aspects of Nursing Care

OBJECTIVES

1. Describe cultural concepts related to nursing and health care.
2. Identify health habits and beliefs of major ethnic groups in the United States.
3. Explain cultural influences on interactions of patients and families with the health care system.
4. Discuss cultural influences and implications for nursing care.

LEARNING ACTIVITIES

I. Match the definition on the left with the most appropriate term on the right.

___ 1. A group of individuals within a culture whose members share different beliefs, values, and attitudes from those of the dominant culture

___ 2. The existence of many cultures in a society

___ 3. Arts, beliefs, customs, institutions, and all other products of human work and thought of a group at a particular time

_A_ 4. The process of learning to be part of a culture

A. Cultural diversity

B. Enculturation

C. Subculture

D. Culture

II. Choose the most appropriate answer.

1. The ideas, beliefs, values, and attitudes that a group of people possess represent:
   A. race
   B. religion
   C. ethnicity
   D. culture

2. The effort of many immigrants to assimilate into society is known as:
   A. salad bowl
   B. melting pot
   C. cultural diversity
   D. true ethnicity

3. The way in which new arrivals seek to maintain individual differences while acclimating to new surroundings is termed:
   A. melting pot
   B. salad bowl
   C. cultural diversity
   D. true ethnicity

4. The Latinos are examples of a:
   A. salad bowl
   B. melting pot
   C. subculture
   D. democracy

5. What percentage of households in the United States are single-parent families?
   A. Less than 1%
   B. 10%
   C. 20%
   D. 50%

6. People who claim that illness is a result of punishment for a sin that an individual has committed believe in:
   A. divine punishment
   B. corporal punishment
   C. legal punishment
   D. ethnic punishment

7. People who believe that health and illness are influenced by four humors that regulate body function believe in:
   A. divine punishment theory
   B. cultural diversity theory
   C. salad bowl theory
   D. hot and cold theory

8. Culture shock associated with hospitalization occurs in three stages. They include asking questions, being disenchanted, and:
   A. generalization
   B. denial
   C. adaptation
   D. bargaining

9. The majority of nursing home residents are:
   A. white women
   B. black women
   C. white men
   D. black men

10. Which group may believe that all health and illnesses are controlled by God?
    A. White Americans
    B. Latinos
    C. French
    D. Germans

III. List the 3 basic characteristics of all cultures:

1. Culture is _____

2. Culture is _____

3. Culture is _____

IV. List 3 examples of cultural symbols.

1.

2.

3.

V. Match the healers on the left with the ethnic group that may be likely to use them on the right. Answers may be used more than once.

____ 1. Spiritualists

____ 2. Curanderos

____ 3. Root doctors

____ 4. Medicine men

____ 5. Herbalists

____ 6. Acupuncturists

A. Asian

B. Native American

C. Latino

D. African American

Health and Illness

OBJECTIVES

1. Describe the health-illness continuum.
2. Discuss traditional and current views of health and illness.
3. List Maslow's five basic human needs.
4. Explain the four levels of adaptability to stress.
5. Discuss concepts related to health promotion, disease, prevention, and health maintenance.
6. Define acute and chronic illness.
7. Discuss illness behavior and the impact of illness on the family.
8. Describe nursing measures for health promotion, health maintenance, and illness.

LEARNING ACTIVITIES

I. Match the definition on the left with the most appropriate term on the right.

B   1. Systems within the body   A. Health

C   2. Systems outside the body   B. Internal environment

D   3. Biologic and/or psychophysiologic malfunction   C. External environment

          D. Disease

A   4. Physical, mental, and social well-being

II. Choose the most appropriate answer.

1. Fluctuation along the health-illness continuum is influenced by which of the following factors?
   A. absolute health
   B. absolute illness
   C. education and intelligence
   D. personal and environmental

2. The ability to function well physically and mentally and to express the full range of one's potential within the environment is a definition of:
   A. wellness
   B. well-being
   C. health
   D. esteem

3. A biologic or psychophysiologic malfunction is a definition of:
   A. disease
   B. illness
   C. stress
   D. anxiety

4. Personal, interpersonal, and cultural reactions to disease refer to:
   A. homeostasis
   B. illness
   C. stress
   D. anxiety

5. Oxygen, food, and safety are examples of:
   A. psychological needs
   B. physiologic needs
   C. emotional needs
   D. affectional needs

6. Sensual-sexual and affectional-emotional needs are:
   A. physiologic needs
   B. safety needs
   C. libidinal needs
   D. mobility needs

7. Security, approval, and care are examples of:
   A. physiologic needs
   B. safety needs
   C. environmental needs
   D. affectional-emotional needs

8. The highest level of Maslow's hierarchy is:
   A. love and belonging
   B. self-esteem
   C. physiologic needs
   D. self-actualization

9. The most fundamental needs that sustain life are:
   A. physiologic needs
   B. safety needs
   C. belonging needs
   D. self-esteem needs

10. Mental or emotional pressure is a definition of:
    A. anxiety
    B. fear
    C. stress
    D. illness

11. Which is included as one of the top ten major stressors?
    A. death of a close family member
    B. marriage of a child
    C. celebration of 25th wedding anniversary
    D. first employee evaluation

12. Areas in which most people seek control even while they are sick include:
    A. their work environment
    B. their play environment
    C. treatments and procedures
    D. their local adaptation syndrome

13. Wound healing and inflammation are examples of:
    A. general adaptation syndrome
    B. local adaptation syndrome
    C. negative feedback response
    D. counter-current response

14. A physiologic response of the whole body to stress is an example of:
    A. local adaptation syndrome
    B. general adaptation syndrome
    C. total adaptation syndrome
    D. absolute adaptation syndrome

15. Increased hormone levels, heart rate, and oxygen intake are components of the:
    A. resistance stage
    B. exhaustion stage
    C. alarm reaction stage
    D. local adaptation stage

16. Adaptation to the stressor occurs in the:
    A. resistance stage
    B. alarm stage
    C. exhaustion stage
    D. initial stage

17. With a long-term stressor such as a chronic physical or mental illness, the individual enters the third stage of adaptation, or the:
    A. alarm stage
    B. exhaustion stage
    C. resistance stage
    D. local adaptation stage

18. Cold hands and feet and tensed muscles are signs or symptoms of:
    A. withdrawal
    B. depression
    C. adaptation
    D. stress

19. Slowed speech, inability to concentrate, and hesitant speech may be signs of:
    A. stress
    B. adaptation
    C. depression
    D. alarm

20. Behavioral or cognitive activities used to deal with stress are:
    A. feedback behaviors
    B. coping behaviors
    C. depressive behaviors
    D. automatic behaviors

21. Maintaining stability of the internal environment is a definition of:
    A. diffusion
    B. fluctuation
    C. osmosis
    D. homeostasis

22. Mammograms, Pap smears, and tests to detect glaucoma are activities undertaken for what type of prevention?
    A. tertiary
    B. final
    C. secondary
    D. primary

23. Rehabilitation and management of an illness after the condition has stabilized and no further healing is expected are activities undertaken for what type of prevention?
    A. primary
    B. final
    C. tertiary
    D. secondary

24. When the goal is to maintain an individual at the highest level of function and to prevent further disability after the condition has stabilized, the prevention is called:
    A. secondary
    B. primary
    C. final
    D. tertiary

25. An illness or disease that has a relatively rapid onset and short duration is said to be:
    A. chronic
    B. acute
    C. disabling
    D. emergency

26. Permanent impairments or disabilities, requiring long-term rehabilitation and treatment, are said to be:
    A. disabling
    B . challenging
    C. chronic
    D. acute

27. Which factor does NOT influence the effect of illness on the family?
    A. role of family member affected by illness
    B. seriousness and duration of illness
    C. social and cultural customs of family
    D. usual diet of family members

28. Nursing interventions to increase adaptability in the elderly should be geared toward helping older clients to:
    A. use past successful coping mechanisms to deal with new stressors
    B. assess their strengths and weaknesses in dealing with new stressors
    C. develop new coping mechanisms to deal with new stressors
    D. learn new methods of dealing with stressors

29. Biofeedback, meditation, and imagery are examples of measures that patients may use to help:
    A. encourage exercise
    B. increase appetite
    C. relieve stress
    D. promote bowel regularity

30. Tasks for chronically ill individuals include:
    A. ignoring disease
    B. preventing and managing crises
    C. curing disease
    D. promoting social isolation

31. A biologic and/or psychophysiologic malfunction is:
    A. fight or flight response
    B. stress
    C. adaptability
    D. disease

32. Mental or emotional pressure resulting from internal or external causes is:
    A. stress
    B. illness
    C. disease
    D. adaptability

33. Any behavioral or cognitive activity used to deal with stress is:
    A. illness
    B. disease
    C. prevention
    D. coping

34. Activities directed toward maintaining or enhancing well-being as a protection against illness are:
    A. health adapation
    B. health promotion
    C. prevention of illness
    D. homeostasis measures

35. A deviation from a healthy state that may occur in the form of an acute episode or as a series of long-term chronic events is:
    A. illness
    B. anxiety
    C. coping
    D. stress

36. Health and illness are:
    A. absolute, unchanging states of being
    B. unconditional states of being
    C. relative, ever-changing states of being
    D. homeostasis measures

III. List the 5 levels of human needs in Maslow's hierarchy.

1.

2.

3.

4.

5.

IV. Maslow's Hierarchy—Match the needs on the left with the correct level on the right.

____ 1. Oxygen, fluid, nutrition, temperature, elimination, shelter, rest, and sex

____ 2. Security, protection from harm, freedom from anxiety and fear

____ 3. Feeling loved by family and friends, and accepted by peers and community

____ 4. Feeling good about oneself and feeling that others hold one in high regard

____ 5. Self-fulfillment; able to problem-solve, accept criticism from others, self-confidence, maturity, and eager to acquire new knowledge

A. Self-esteem

B. Safety

C. Physiologic

D. Self-actualization

E. Love and belonging

V. List the 3 stages of the general adaptation syndrome.

1.

2.

3.

VI. Fill in the blank.

The alarm reaction that helps the body defend against stressors is the _____.

VII. List 3 goals of the Healthy People 2000 document.

1.

2.

3.

VIII. Match Henderson's 14 components of basic nursing care on the left with Maslow's hierarchy of human needs on the right.

___ 1. Communicate with others in expressing emotions, needs, fears, and opinion.

___ 2. Select suitable clothing—dress and undress.

___ 3. Play or participate in various forms of recreation.

___ 4. Avoid dangers in the environment and avoid injuring others.

___ 5. Move and maintain desirable posture.

___ 6. Eat and drink adequately.

___ 7. Worship according to one's faith.

___ 8. Keep the body clean and well-groomed and protect the integument.

___ 9. Maintain body temperature within the normal range by adjusting clothing and modifying the environment.

___ 10. Learn, discover, or satisfy curiosity.

___ 11. Sleep and rest.

___ 12. Breathe normally.

___ 13. Work in such a way that there is a sense of accomplishment

___ 14. Eliminate body wastes.

A. Physiologic needs

B. Safety and security needs

C. Love and belonging needs

D. Self-esteem and self-actualization needs

IX. Match the statements on the left with the correct method of increasing adaptability on the right.

___ 1. "What is your worst possible stressor, and how does this present stress compare with the worst?"

___ 2. "What ways have you coped with stress in the past that have been successful for you?"

___ 3. "What kinds of things do you do when you are stressed?" "Do you eat more or less?"

___ 4. "Whom do you turn to when you are feeling stressed?"

A. Assess past methods of dealing with stress

B. Assess internal coping strategies

C. Determine external coping strategies

D. Assess the degree of stress

X.   Match the descriptions on the left with traditional or current view on the right.

____   1. Emphasis is on maintenance of health and prevention of disease

____   2. Health and illness are separate entities

____   3. Focus is on crisis management of disease

____   4. Health and illness are relative and ever-changing

A. Traditional view

B. Current view

XI.   Match the descriptions on the left with internal or external stressors on the right. Answers may be used more than once.

____   1. Conflictual relations

____   2. Inability to relate

____   3. Perception of threat from events

____   4. Loss of relationship

____   5. Economic inadequacies

____   6. Ethnic, religious, or national differences

____   7. Intrapsychic conflict

____   8. Noxious stimuli

____   9. Climatic extremes

____   10. Boredom

A. Internal

B. External

XII.   Match the examples of stressors on the left with the source of stress on the right. Answers may be used more than once.

____   1. Prejudice based on nationality, race, or creed

____   2. Repressive social system

____   3. Overexertion or other imposed strains on body system; infections or allergens; physical trauma, e.g., surgery, accident; nutritional deficiency

____   4. Feeling angry while fearing the consequences of expressing it

____   5. Observing an angry person; illness of a loved one

____   6. Unemployment, poor diet, poor housing, little recreation

____   7. Language barrier

____   8. Death of a loved one

____   9. Belief that life is impossible without the help and love of a significant other

____   10. Rain, clouds, little sun

A. Internal, physical

B. Internal, psychological

C. External, psychological

D. External, socioeconomic

Introductory Nursing Care of Adults

XIII. Match each example on the left with the correct coping strategy on the right.

_____ 1. Mental and verbal preparation for an event or practice of coping strategies

_____ 2. Aggressive seeking of information, anger, refusal of treatments

_____ 3. Unwillingness or inability to talk about events, going on as if nothing has happened

_____ 4. Stoicism, showing no feelings

_____ 5. Seeking out family, friends, or others in similar situations

_____ 6. Verbally placing responsibility for situation on self

_____ 7. Praying, reading of religious material, seeking out clergy or religious guidance

_____ 8. Making plans, verbally outlining what will be done next

_____ 9. Speaking of how situation has fostered growth

_____ 10. Discussing situations or coping that has occurred

A. Distancing or denial

B. Accepting responsibility

C. Self-control

D. Positive reappraisal

E. Problem solving

F. Event rehearsal

G. Event review

H. Faith

I. Social support

J. Confrontation

XIV. Maslow's Hierarchy

Your patient is a 45-year-old male who has been admitted to the hospital with pneumonia. As you are conducting your admission interview, you find out the following:

_____ 1. He has recently separated from his wife and three children.

_____ 2. He is afraid to jog due to crime in neighborhood.

_____ 3. He states that he feels like he will never amount to anything.

_____ 4. He eats fast foods, drinks a lot of coffee.

_____ 5. He states he does not feel very positive about himself right now.

_____ 6. His parents live 300 miles away; he has few close friends in town.

Indicate for each finding (1 through 10) the appropriate level of needs to which it relates in Maslow's hierarchy (A through D).

A. Physiologic needs

B. Safety and security

C. Love and belonging

D. Self-esteem and self-actualization

XV. Match the definition on the left with the most appropriate term on the right.

_____ 1. Health promoting behaviors used to prevent or delay the onset of illness

_____ 2. A physical and emotional state always present in individuals that is intensified when an internal or external environment change or threat occurs to which they must respond

_____ 3. Illness or disease that has a relatively rapid onset and a short duration

_____ 4. Any behavioral or cognitive activity used to deal with stress

_____ 5. Prevention of disease with an emphasis on screening for diseases already present in the body so that early diagnosis and treatment can be carried out

_____ 6. Permanent impairment or disabilities that require long-term rehabilitation and medical or nursing treatment

_____ 7. A tendency of biologic systems to maintain stability of the internal environment while continuously adjusting to changes necessary for survival

_____ 8. Rehabilitation and management of illness after the condition has stabilized and no further healing is expected

A. Acute illness

B. Chronic illness

C. Coping

D. Homeostasis

E. Primary prevention

F. Secondary prevention

G. Stress

H. Tertiary prevention

CHAPTER

6

Developmental Processes

OBJECTIVES

1. List the developmental tasks for successful adulthood.
2. Identify the health problems specific to the adult age groups.
3. Discuss the health care needs of young, middle-aged, and older adults.

LEARNING ACTIVITIES

I. Match the definition on the left with the most appropriate term on the right.

___ 1. The functional capabilities of various organ systems in the body

___ 2. The behavioral capacity of a person to adapt to changing environmental demands

___ 3. The roles and habits of a person in relation to other members of society

A. Social age

B. Biologic age

C. Psychological age

II. Match the definition on the left with the most appropriate developmental stage on the right. Answers may be used more than once.

___ 1. A time when many adjustments must be made to physiologic, psychological, and social changes

___ 2. 45 to 65 years of age

___ 3. Over the age of 65

___ 4. A time when persons earn most of their money, pay most of the taxes, and have most of the power in business and government

___ 5. A time when physical growth ends, and social expectations begin

___ 6. 20 to 45 years of age

A. Young adulthood

B. Middle age

C. Old age

III. Match the characteristics on the left with the most appropriate developmental stage on the right. Answers may be used more than once.

____ 1. Earn most of money

____ 2. Retirement

____ 3. Marriage, childbearing and work

____ 4. Settling down to job and raising a family

____ 5. Decreased short-term memory

____ 6. Pay most of taxes

A. Young adulthood

B. Middle age

C. Old age

IV. Match the developmental tasks on the left with the developmental stage on the right. Answers may be used more than once.

____ 1. Give time and resources to the community

____ 2. Focus on marriage, childbearing, and work

____ 3. Learn to combine new dependency needs with the continuing need for independence

____ 4. Adjust to decreasing physical strength and health changes

____ 5. Establish independence from parental home and financial aid

____ 6. Accept role reversal with aging parents

____ 7. Adjust to loss of physical strength, illness, and the approach of one's death

____ 8. Accept self and stabilize self-concept

____ 9. Become established in a vocation or profession

____ 10. Maintain emotional satisfaction in relationships with spouse, children, grandchildren, and other living relatives

A. Young adulthood

B. Middle age

C. Old age

V. Match the health problems on the left with the most appropriate developmental stage on the right. Answers may be used more than once.

____ 1. Benign or malignant prostate enlargement

____ 2. Respiratory disease causing absence from work among women

____ 3. Anxiety or depression

____ 4. Difficulties with pregnancy

____ 5. Smoking, alcohol and drug abuse

____ 6. Injuries a frequent cause of absence from work among men

____ 7. Chronic illness a major cause of death

____ 8. Vehicular accidents and suicide

____ 9. Breast cancer common in women

____ 10. Stress related to managing a household

A. Young adulthood

B. Middle age

C. Old age

VI. List 6 factors to be included in a physical examination for persons in their twenties (some factors may apply to women or men only).

1.

2.

3.

4.

5.

6.

VII. Match the health problems on the left with the most appropriate developmental age on the right. Answers may be used more than once.

____ 1. Complications of pregnancy

____ 2. Peptic ulcer

____ 3. Vehicular accidents

____ 4. Arthritis

____ 5. Obesity

____ 6. Prostate enlargement

____ 7. Accidental falls

____ 8. Emphysema

____ 9. HIV infection

____ 10. Alcoholism

A. Young adulthood

B. Middle age

C. Old age

VIII. Choose the most appropriate answer.

1. Establishing independence from parental home and financial aid is a developmental task of the:
   A. Middle-aged adult
   B. Older adult
   C. Young adult
   D. Teenager

2. A baseline mammogram is recommended for women at age:
   A. 20
   B. 25
   C. 45
   D. 35

3. Health promotion for persons in their thirties includes:
   A. effective parenting, stress management
   B. yearly blood pressure screening
   C. influenza vaccinations
   D. yearly mammograms

The Older Patient

OBJECTIVES

1. Define the terms *aging, elderly, geriatrics, gerontology,* and *gerontological nurse.*
2. Describe the roles of the gerontological nurse.
3. Compare the myths and stereotypes of the aging population with current statistical trends.
4. Describe biologic and physiologic factors associated with aging.
5. Explain psychosocial factors associated with aging.
6. Describe modifications needed for activities of daily living.
7. Identify various groups of drugs that need modification because of changes brought about by aging.

LEARNING ACTIVITIES

I. Match the characteristics on the left with the correct theory of aging on the right. Answers may be used more than once.

____ 1. Based on the belief that aging is the natural and expected result of a purposeful sequence of events

____ 2. Based on the belief that the rate of aging is directly related to the organism's rate of living

____ 3. Damage accumulates over time, resulting in cellular, molecular, and organ malfunction

____ 4. Immunologic theory

____ 5. Wear and tear theory

A. Error theory

B. Programming theory

II. Match the characteristics of aging on the left with the system affected on the right. Answers may be used more than once.

____   1. Arterial oxygen values of 70–80 mm Hg

____   2. Atrophy and weakening of the respiratory muscles

____   3. Chronic cerebral tissue hypoxia

____   4. Alterations in pulmonary circulation

____   5. Altered learning

____   6. Decreased conduction speed in the brain

____   7. Diminished activity of enzymes associated with synaptic transmission

____   8. Loss of elastic tissue around alveoli

____   9. Decreased diffusion across the alveolar-capillary membrane

____ 10. Calcification of costal cartilage

A. Nervous system

B. Respiratory system

III. Match the biologic and physiologic factors on the left with the direction of change on the right. Answers may be used more than once.

____   1. Ability to perform prolonged strenuous work

____   2. Exertional dyspnea

____   3. Arterial oxygen values

____   4. Sound judgment

____   5. Creativity

____   6. Loss of brain neurons

____   7. Functional ability of brain

____   8. Decreased conduction speed associated with synaptic transmission

____   9. Diminished activity of enzymes associated with synaptic transmission

____ 10. Impeded short-term memory

A. Decreases with aging

B. Increases with aging

C. Does not change

IV. Match the characteristics of aging on the left with the system affected on the right. Answers may be used more than once.

___ 1. Impaired acid-base balance

___ 2. Decreased oxygenation of heart cells

___ 3. Increased extracellular fluid

___ 4. Murmur develops

___ 5. Decreased stroke volume

___ 6. Cerebral blood flow maintained

___ 7. Increased residual volume

___ 8. Increased resistance to blood flow

___ 9. Decreased muscle tone of ureters, bladder, and urethra

___ 10. Inelasticity of vessel walls

A. Cardiovascular system

B. Renal system

V. Match the areas of age-related physiologic change on the left with the direction of change on the right. Answers may be used more than once.

___ 1. Lean muscle mass

___ 2. Renal function

___ 3. Serum albumin

___ 4. Body fat

___ 5. Body water

___ 6. Hepatic blood flow

A. Increased

B. Decreased

VI. Match the drugs on the left with adverse drug reactions in older persons on the right. (Some adverse reactions may be used more than once.)

DRUG (EXAMPLE)

___ 1. Analgesics (Aspirin)

___ 2. Antibiotics (Streptomycin)

___ 3. Anticoagulants (Warfarin)

___ 4. Antidepressants (Amitriptyline-Elavil)

___ 5. Antihypertensives (Verapamil)

___ 6. Antiparkinsonians (Levodopa)

___ 7. Antipsychotics (Haloperidol-Haldol)

___ 8. Diuretics (Diuril)

___ 9. Sedative/hypnotics (Flurazepam)

ADVERSE REACTION

A. Hypokalemia

B. Drowsiness

C. Confusion/Sedation

D. Hypotension

E. Bleeding or hemorrhage

F. Nephrotoxicity

G. Extrapyramidal symptoms; dystonia

Introductory Nursing Care of Adults

VII. Choose the most appropriate answer.

1. The study of aging is called:
   A. geriatrics
   B. ageism
   C. gerontology
   D. pulmonology

2. The biomedical science of old age is called:
   A. geriatrics
   B. gerontology
   C. pediatrics
   D. ageism

3. Which system shows only slight decline with age?
   A. renal system
   B. central nervous system
   C. respiratory system
   D. cardiovascular system

4. A frequent concern of the aged is:
   A. long-term memory loss
   B. creativity loss
   C. short-term memory loss
   D. judgment loss

NEUROLOGIC SYSTEM

5. Neurologic features that show age-related changes include:
   A. size of the brain, oxygenation function, and emotions
   B. personality, cardiac output, and excretion of drugs
   C. elasticity of cells, vision changes, and gastric secretions
   D. temperature regulation, pain perception, and tactile sensation

6. In order to compensate for neurologic changes, the aged individual may:
   A. avoid temperature extremes and accomplish tasks at a slower pace
   B. wear warm clothes and exert extra effort to get tasks accomplished
   C. wear hats and concentrate for longer periods of time
   D. check blood pressure frequently

RESPIRATORY SYSTEM

7. Kyphosis, vertebral loss of calcium, and calcification of costal cartilage result in:
   A. increased anteroposterior chest diameter and increased vital capacity
   B. increased anteroposterior chest diameter and decreased vital capacity
   C. decreased anteroposterior chest diameter and increased vital capacity
   D. decreased anteroposterior chest diameter and decreased vital capacity

8. By the age of 70, arterial oxygen values have decreased to approximately:
   A. 20–30 mm Hg
   B. 40–50 mm Hg
   C. 90–100 mm Hg
   D. 70–80 mm Hg

9. A reduction in cardiac output in the aged results in:
   A. increased pulmonary blood flow
   B. decreased elastic tissue around the alveoli
   C. decreased pulmonary blood flow
   D. increased elastic tissue around the alveoli

10. With increasing age, alveolar dead space:
    A. decreases
    B. increases
    C. fills up
    D. collapses

11. A frequent respiratory complaint with the aged is:
    A. orthostatic hypotension
    B. inability to breathe
    C. increased respirations
    D. exertional dyspnea

12. Epithelial atrophy in the lungs results in:
    A. increased ciliary action and decreased movement of pulmonary secretions
    B. decreased ciliary action and decreased movement of pulmonary secretions
    C. decreased lung expansion and decreased muscle tone
    D. increased lung expansion and decreased muscle tone

13. Respiratory assessment data for the aged should include:
    A. auscultation of lungs and measurement of chest diameter
    B. measurement of chest diameter and pulmonary function tests
    C. baseline resting and exertional respiratory rate and pulmonary function tests
    D. baseline resting and exertional respiratory rate and drug history

14. Standard components of respiratory care for the older adult include:
    A. cough and deep breathing exercises and range of motion exercises to facilitate lung expansion
    B. frequent ambulation and auscultation of lungs
    C. intake and output and postural drainage exercises
    D. deep breathing exercises and positioning to facilitate lung expansion and gas exchange

CARDIOVASCULAR SYSTEM

15. In the absence of cardiovascular disease, heart size:
    A. remains unchanged or slightly decreases
    B. increases markedly
    C. decreases markedly
    D. remains unchanged or slightly increases

16. With increasing age, a person's reduced tolerance for physical work may be due to the decreased:
    A. size of the brain
    B. capacity of heart cells to utilize oxygen
    C. size of the heart
    D. resistance to blood flow in many organs

17. An average blood pressure for a 70-year-old person is:
    A. 170/100
    B. 150/90
    C. 120/80
    D. 110/90

18. Reduced cardiac output in the elderly is due to:
    A. decreased heart rate and decreased stroke volume
    B. decreased heart rate and decreased cerebral blood flow
    C. increased heart rate and increased stroke volume
    D. increased heart rate and increased cerebral blood flow

RENAL SYSTEM

19. Which changes occur in aging kidneys?
    A. decreased renal function, decreased cell mass, and decreased extracellular fluid
    B. decreased renal function, increased cell mass, and increased extracellular fluid
    C. decreased renal function, decreased cell mass, and increased extracellular fluid
    D. increased renal function, decreased cell mass, and increased extracellular fluid

INTEGUMENTARY SYSTEM

20. One of the first signs of aging of the skin is:
    A. infection
    B. thickening
    C. elasticity
    D. wrinkles

21. An age change that occurs due to loss of oils in the skin is:
    A. infection
    B. itching
    C. wrinkles
    D. elasticity

22. The nails in most older persons tend to become:
    A. blue and thinner
    B. red and thicker
    C. yellow and thicker
    D. clear and thinner

GASTROINTESTINAL SYSTEM

23. Which symptoms are suggestive of possible gastrointestinal system illness?
    A. decreased appetite, decreased thirst, unexplained weight gain
    B. increased appetite, excessive thirst, change in bowel movements
    C. decreased appetite, excessive thirst, change in bowel movements
    D. increased appetite, decreased thirst, intestinal motility

MUSCULOSKELETAL SYSTEM

24. The leading cause of disability in old age is:
    A. infection
    B. hemorrhage
    C. fever
    D. arthritis

25. The curvature of the thoracic spine that causes a bent-over appearance in some older adults is:
    A. kyphosis
    B. arthritis
    C. myelitis
    D. presbycusis

SENSORY SYSTERM

26. The term for hearing loss associated with age is:
    A. tinnitus
    B. ototoxicity
    C. presbyopia
    D. presbycusis

27. What percentage of older adults are hearing impaired?
    A. 10%
    B. 50%
    C. 25%
    D. 75%

28. The type of hearing loss most easily treated is:
    A. sensorinerual
    B. tinnitus
    C. conduction
    D. ototoxicity

29. The type of hearing loss that results from exposure to loud noises, disease, and certain drugs is:
    A. conduction
    B. ototoxicity
    C. infection
    D. sensorineural

30. The clouding or opacity of the transparent lens of the eye is:
    A. macular degeneration
    B. cataract
    C. glaucoma
    D. conjunctivitis

31. Presbyopia is corrected by:
    A. laser surgery
    B. reading glasses or bifocal lenses
    C. treatment with antibiotics
    D. eye patches

32. The leading cause of blindness in this country is:
    A. glaucoma
    B. presbyopia
    C. cataract
    D. conjunctivitis

PSYCHOSOCIAL FACTORS IN AGING

33. What percentage of the aged is unable to function independently and fails to maintain or sustain a sense of well-being?
    A. 15%
    B. 25%
    C. 50%
    D. 75%

34. The optimal psychological, social, and biologic adaptation achieved at some point during the midlife years (45–65 years of age) is:
    A. self-actualization
    B. self-esteem
    C. maturity
    D. adaptation

35. The developmental challenge in old age is to:
    A. develop close relations with other people to learn and experience love
    B. find a vocation or hobby where the individual can help others or in some way contribute to society
    C. establish trusting relationships with other people
    D. review life and gain a feeling of accomplishment or fulfillment

36. Two thirds of the suicides among older people are due to depression resulting from:
    A. infection
    B. loss
    C. medication
    D. denial

37. For effective gerontological care, the crucial denominator in deciding care needs is the:
    A. medical diagnosis
    B. functional assessment
    C. activities of daily living
    D. community resources

DRUG THERAPY AND AGED ADULTS

38. With aging, there is:
    A. decreased lean body mass, decreased body water content, decreased fat
    B. increased lean body mass, decreased body water content, decreased fat
    C. increased lean body mass, increased body water content, decreased fat
    D. decreased lean body mass, decreased body water content, increased fat

39. A highly fat soluble drug may result in:
    A. shorter storage of drug before excretion
    B. higher blood concentrations of the drug
    C. lower blood concentrations of the drug
    D. longer storage of drug before excretion

40. Decreased liver size, reduced blood flow through the liver, and reduced liver enzyme activity affect the:
    A. storage of drugs
    B. tissue sensitivity of drugs
    C. inactivation of drugs
    D. absorption of drugs

VIII. Match the definition on the left with the most appropriate term on the right.

_____ 1. The study of aging

_____ 2. The process of growing older or more mature

_____ 3. An annoying ringing or buzzing in the ear

_____ 4. A health service that incorporates basic nursing methods and specialized knowledge about the aged to increase healthy behaviors in the aged; minimize and compensate for health-related losses and impairments of aging; provide comfort and sustenance through the distressing and debilitating events of aging; and facilitate the diagnosis, care, and treatment of disease in the aged

_____ 5. Clouding or opacity of the normally transparent lens within the eye; causes blurred vision and objects to take on a yellowish hue

_____ 6. The term for hearing loss associated with old age

_____ 7. Old or advanced in years

_____ 8. A hearing impairment due to a blockage of the ear canal caused by excessive wax buildup, abnormal structures, or infection

_____ 9. Professional nurses and advanced level practitioners such as nurse practitioners, clinical specialists, and nurses holding national certification in the specialty of gerontological nursing

_____ 10. A process of systemic stereotyping and discrimination against people because of their age; usually directed against older people

_____ 11. A hearing impairment resulting from damage to the nerve centers within the brain as a result of exposure to loud noises, disease, and certain drugs

_____ 12. A visual impairment associated with older age in which the lens becomes more rigid and less able to change shape, resulting in a decreased ability to focus on near objects

_____ 13. Condition in which high pressure of the fluid in the eye causes damage to the optic nerve

A. Aged

B. Ageism

C. Aging

D. Cataract

E. Conduction deafness

F. Gerontologic nurse

G. Gerontologic nursing

H. Gerontology

I. Glaucoma

J. Presbycusis

K. Presbyopia

L. Sensorineural deafness

M. Tinnitus

The Nursing Process

OBJECTIVES

1. Describe the five components of the nursing process.
2. Explain the role of the licensed practical nurse or licensed vocational nurse in the nursing process.
3. Describe the proper documentation of the nursing process using a problem-oriented medical record format, nurses' notes, and flow sheets.

LEARNING ACTIVITIES

I. Match the term on the left with the most appropriate definition on the right.

___ 1. Physical examination that is a systematic, thorough way of obtaining objective data

___ 2. Method of record keeping that focuses on patient problems rather than on medical diagnoses

___ 3. Systematic, problem-solving approach to providing nursing care in an organized, scientific manner

___ 4. Tapping on the skin to assess the underlying tissues

___ 5. Method of physical examination that uses the sense of touch to assess various parts of the body

___ 6. Listening to sounds produced by the body, such as heart, lung, and intestinal sounds

___ 7. Purposeful observation or scrutiny of the person as a whole and then of each body system

___ 8. Actual or potential health problems derived from data gathered during the assessment of a patient or client

___ 9. Information reported by patients or family members

___ 10. Collection of data about the health status of a patient or client

___ 11. Information about the patient collected by the nurse or other members of the health care team

A. Auscultation

B. Objective data

C. Physical assessment

D. Nursing diagnosis

E. Problem-oriented medical record

F. Subjective data

G. Nursing process

H. Percussion

I. Inspection

J. Assessment

K. Palpation

II. Match the definition on the left with the most appropriate component of the nursing process on the right.

____ 1. Putting the plan into action

____ 2. Systematic collection of data relating to patient and their problems

____ 3. Assessing the effectiveness of the plan and changing the plan as indicated by current needs

____ 4. Choice of solutions

____ 5. Interpretation of the data for problem identification

A. Nursing diagnosis

B. Implementation

C. Evaluation

D. Assessment

E. Planning

III. Match the description on the left (objective data) with the problem on the right.

____ 1. A patient's disheveled appearance based on sight

____ 2. A patient's noisy and labored breathing based on hearing

____ 3. A fruity mouth odor based on smell

____ 4. Cold and clammy skin based on touch

A. Possible respiratory problems

B. Possible sign of diabetic acidosis

C. May indicate that patient is in shock

D. May indicate inability to carry out self-care activities at home

IV. Match each step on the left with the correct component of the nursing process on the right. Answers may be used more than once.

____ 1. Identify health problems or potential health problems

____ 2. Determine priorities from the list of nursing diagnoses

____ 3. Write nursing orders to direct care to meet the goals

____ 4. Physical examination, including height and weight, vital signs, and inspection of body systems

____ 5. Obtain information through a health history by direct questioning

____ 6. Provide data regarding the quality of care in a health care institution

____ 7. Focus is on the response of the whole person to the health problem

____ 8. Collection of data about the health status of the patient

____ 9. Actual performance of nursing interventions identified in the care plan

A. Assessment

B. Nursing diagnosis

C. Planning

D. Implementation

E. Evaluation

V.   Match each description relating to the health history on the left with the most appropriate system on the right. Answers may be used more than once.

____ 1. Kidney stones, oliguria, or polyuria

____ 2. Coldness, numbness and tingling of extremities; varicose veins

____ 3. Itching, excessive bruising, rash, or lesion

____ 4. Double vision, glaucoma or cataracts

____ 5. Diabetes, thyroid disease

____ 6. Seizure disorder, stroke, fainting, paralysis, nervousness

____ 7. Rectal conditions, hemorrhoids, fistula

____ 8. Menstrual pain, menopausal signs or symptoms

____ 9. Arthritis, gout, stiffness and swelling of joints; coordination problems

____ 10. Ulcer, jaundice, colitis

____ 11. Headache, dizziness, vertigo

____ 12. Heartburn; indigestion; nausea and vomiting

____ 13. Shortness of breath, cough, sputum, hemoptysis/coughing up blood

____ 14. Tinnitus

____ 15. Hypertension, coronary artery disease, cyanosis

____ 16. Allergies or hayfever; change in sense of smell

____ 17. Fatigue, weakness

____ 18. Toothache, difficulty swallowing

____ 19. Self-care ability, bathing, dressing, and toileting

____ 20. Asthma, emphysema, bronchitis, tuberculosis

____ 21. Fever, chills, night sweats

____ 22. Goiter

____ 23. Present weight, weight gain or loss

A. Gastrointestinal

B. Eyes

C. General overall health

D. Nose and sinuses

E. Respiratory

F. Skin

G. Functional assessment

H. Mouth and throat

I. Head

J. Cardiovascular

K. Peripheral vascular

L. Urinary system

M. Ears

N. Neck

O. Endocrine system

P. Female genital system

Q. Neurological

R. Musculoskeletal

VI.   Match the area or function examined on the left with the most appropriate category
or system on the right.

___   1. General appearance, skin, lymphatic drainage areas, nipple, axilla

___   2. Height, weight, vital signs

___   3. Facial expression, mood and affect, speech,
dress, personal hygiene, hair, and makeup

___   4. Gait, range of motion, no involuntary movement

___   5. Perianal area, anus, rectum, stool

___   6. Age, sex, level of consciousness, skin color,
facial features, no signs of acute distress

___   7. Cranial nerves, motor system (muscles, cer-
ebellar function), sensory system (pain, temperature, light touch, vibration, position),
reflexes (stretch or deep tendon reflexes, superficial reflexes)

___   8. Carotid artery pulse, jugular venous pulse,
jugular venous pressure, anterior chest inspection, rate and rhythm, heart sounds,
murmurs

___   9. Internal genitalia (cervix, vagina)

___ 10. Pulses, capillary refill, skin color and temperature, edema, pain

___ 11. Penis, scrotum, hernia, inguinal lymph nodes

___ 12. Inspection (size and contour of joint, skin and
tissues surrounding joint), palpation (temperature, muscles, and bony articulations of
joint), range of motion, muscle strength, functional assessment

___ 13. Stature, nutrition (normal weight for height
and body build), symmetry, posture, body
build (normal proportions), obvious physical
deformities

___ 14. Posterior chest (symmetric expansion, fremi-
tus [palpable vibration], lung fields, breath
sounds)

___ 15. Palpation (surface and deep areas, liver edge,
spleen, kidneys)

A. Musculoskeletal system

B. Abdomen

C. Thorax and lungs

D. Anus, rectum, and prostate

E. Physical appearance

F. Female genitalia

G. Breasts and regional lymphatics

H. Measurements

I. Male genitalia

J. Neurologic system

K. Heart and neck vessels

L. Body structure

M. Peripheral vascular system

N. Behavior

O. Mobility

VII. Match the description on the left with the correct SOAPIER component for charting on the right.

____ 1. How effective the plan or intervention was

____ 2. Why the patient has the problem

____ 3. What specific care is given

____ 4. What changes should be made in the original plan of care

____ 5. What the nurse observes about the patient

____ 6. How the intervention is to be carried out

____ 7. Information on how the patient perceives the problem.

A. Subjective

B. Objective

C. Assessment

D. Plan

E. Intervention

F. Evaluation

G. Revision

VIII. Match each description on the left with the correct component of SOAPE notes on the right.

____ 1. Turn from side to side every 2 hr. Get out of bed at least twice a day. Begin ambulating as tolerated.

____ 2. Turned q 2 hr. OOB twice a day; taking 6 small steps to and from bed. Decubitus ulcer healing; now 1.5 cm.

____ 3. Feels weak; does "not have the energy" to move around.

____ 4. Decubitus ulcer on sacrum related to immobility.

____ 5. Does not turn self in bed; 2 cm, stage 2 decubitus ulcer on sacrum.

A. S

B. O

C. A

D. P

E. E

IX. Choose the most appropriate answer.

1. The goal of the nursing process is to:
   A. obtain information through observation, physical examination, or diagnostic testing
   B. interview the patient or family in a goal-directed, orderly, and systematic way
   C. record objective data, writing exactly what is observed
   D. alleviate, minimize, or prevent real or potential health problems

2. The nursing process can be applied in any interaction that involves:
   A. a doctor and a nurse
   B. a nurse and a patient
   C. a nurse in a hospital setting
   D. a health care team

3. Choosing solutions is:
   A. planning
   B. assessment
   C. nursing diagnosis
   D. evaluation

Introductory Nursing Care of Adults

4. Putting the plan into action is:
   A. assessment
   B. planning
   C. evaluation
   D. implementation

5. The role of the LPN in relation to the planning phase of the nursing process is to:
   A. perform a complete physical assessment
   B. perform therapeutic nursing measures
   C. assist with the development of nursing care plans
   D. evaluate the nursing care given

6. The role of the LPN in relation to the evaluation phase of the nursing process is to:
   A. report observed outcomes and make necessary changes
   B. carry out the established plan of care
   C. collect data and take objective measurements of body functions
   D. develop nursing care plans

7. Information obtained through a health history by direct questioning of the patient or family members is:
   A. observation data
   B. subjective data
   C. objective data
   D. evaluative data

8. Data observed by the nurse or other members of the health care team are:
   A. historical
   B. perspective
   C. objective
   D. subjective

9. Information obtained through observation, physical examination, or diagnostic testing is:
   A. interview data
   B. objective data
   C. subjective data
   D. evaluative data

10. A systematic, thorough way of obtaining objective data is by:
    A. physical assessment
    B. subjective assessment
    C. intuitive assessment
    D. judgmental assessment

11. Four methods of physical examination include inspection, palpation, auscultation, and:
    A. interview
    B. observation
    C. percussion
    D. evaluation

12. The purposeful observation or scrutiny of the person as a whole and then of each body system is:
    A. palpation
    B. auscultation
    C. inspection
    D. percussion

13. Using the sense of touch to assess various parts of the body, helping to confirm things that are noted on inspection, is:
    A. auscultation
    B. percussion
    C. inspection
    D. palpation

14. In palpation, which body part is used to assess skin texture, moisture, and temperature, or the presence of swelling, lumps, masses, tenderness, or pain?
    A. palms of hands
    B. fingers
    C. wrist
    D. fingertips

15. Auscultation is carried out through the use of:
    A. fingertips
    B. stethoscopes
    C. hands
    D. thermometers

16. Tapping on the skin to assess the underlying tissues is called:
    A. palpation
    B. inspection
    C. percussion
    D. auscultation

17. A diagnosis used to identify the cause of a disease is:
    A. nursing diagnosis
    B. medical diagnosis
    C. assessment
    D. evaluation

18. The PES (Problem, Etiology, Signs and Symptoms) format helps to make the general nursing diagnosis:
    A. fit a broad classification of patient responses
    B. apply to a larger population
    C. fit a specific patient care problem
    D. applicable to any group of patients

Questions 19 to 24 refer to the following situation: An elderly woman has developed a 2-cm decubitus ulcer on her sacrum because she is bedridden and immobilized. Her specific nursing diagnosis is: Impaired skin integrity related to immobility as evidenced by 2-cm decubitus ulcer on sacrum.

19. The problem or nursing diagnosis is:
    A. Impaired skin integrity
    B. Immobility
    C. 2-cm decubitus ulcer on sacrum
    D. Alteration in activity

20. The etiology or cause is:
    A. impaired skin integrity
    B. 2-cm decubitus on sacrum
    C. immobility
    D. aging

21. The signs or symptoms are:
    A. immobility
    B. impaired skin integrity
    C. 2-cm decubitus ulcer on sacrum
    D. open wound

22. The goal is to:
    A. increase ambulation
    B. restore skin integrity
    C. increase immobility
    D. keep skin uncovered

23. The objective is:
    A. ambulation increased to twice a day
    B. decubitus ulcer over sacrum healed within 2 weeks
    C. patient remains on bedrest
    D. patient feels better

24. Appropriate nursing orders might include:
    A. keep off sacrum to promote healing
    B. heal decubitus ulcer over sacrum
    C. restore skin integrity
    D. keep patient on bedrest

25. The actual performance of the nursing interventions identified in the plan of care is:
    A. assessment
    B. nursing diagnosis
    C. evaluation
    D. implementation

26. An ongoing process in which the nurse determines what progress the patient has made in meeting the goals for care is:
    A. assessment
    B. planning
    C. evaluation
    D. implementation

27. An organization that requires systematic review of hospitals and other health care organizations is:
    A. Joint Commission on Accreditation of Healthcare Organizations (JCAHO)
    B. Medicare
    C. Medicaid
    D. ANA Standards of Care

28. What helps to achieve continuity of care because it provides for communication among caregivers as well as a record of the patient's progress?
    A. nursing orders
    B. documentation
    C. objectives
    D. evaluation

29. The POMR is a method of record keeping that focuses on:
    A. medical diagnoses
    B. patient problems
    C. medical treatments
    D. diagnostic tests

30. If an error in charting is made, the entry should be:
    A. erased, new entry entered, and initialed
    B. erased, "error" written in, and initialed
    C. crossed out, "error" written above, initialed
    D. crossed out, new entry written above, and initialed

31. SOAPIER stands for subjective and objective information, assessment, plan, intervention, evaluation, and:
    A. revision
    B. repetition
    C. renewal
    D. reassessment

32. The statement, "Does not turn self in bed; 2 cm, stage 2 decubitus ulcer on sacrum," refers to which component of SOAPIER charting?
    A. subjective information
    B. assessment
    C. plan
    D. objective information

33. The statement, "Turn from side to side every 2 hours. Get out of bed at least twice a day. Begin ambulating as tolerated," refers to which component of SOAPE charting?
    A. plan
    B. assessment
    C. evaluation
    D. objective information

Inflammation and Infection

OBJECTIVES

1. Explain the mechanisms of the protective structures of the body.
2. Describe the ways in which inflammatory changes act as bodily defense mechanisms.
3. Identify the signs and symptoms of inflammation.
4. Discuss the process of repair and healing.
5. Differentiate infection from inflammation.
6. Discuss the actions of commonly found infectious agents.
7. Describe the ways that infections are transmitted.
8. Identify the signs and symptoms of infection.
9. Compare community-acquired and nosocomial infections.
10. Discuss the nursing care of patients in isolation.
11. Discuss the nursing care of patients with infections.

LEARNING ACTIVITIES

I. Match the definition on the left with the most appropriate term on the right.

_C_ 1. One-celled organisms capable of producing disease that are usually spread by contaminated food and water

_H_ 2. Vegetable-like organisms that exist by feeding on organic matter and are capable of producing disease

_D_ 3. Several classifications of one-celled microorganisms that are capable of multiplying rapidly and causing illness

_A_ 4. Worms that are parasites found in the soil and water and are transmitted to humans from hand to mouth

_F_ 5. Microorganisms that cause illness by stimulating an antigen-antibody response in the tissues, producing inflammation and cell destruction

_B_ 6. Microorganisms that are usually transmitted to humans through flea and tick bites

_G_ 7. Part of the inflammatory process that causes an increase in white blood cells

_E_ 8. Gram-negative organisms usually causing infections in the respiratory tract

A. Helminths

B. Ricksettiae

C. Protozoa

D. Bacteria

E. Mycoplasmas

F. Viruses

G. Leukocytosis

H. Fungi

Introductory Nursing Care of Adults

II. Match the definition on the left with the most appropriate term on the right.

G___ 1. A series of cellular changes that signal the body's response to injury or infection

C___ 2. Hospital-acquired infections

B___ 3. Replacement of damaged cells by connective tissue and then eventually by scar tissue during the wound healing process

J___ 4. Infections that are acquired in day-to-day contact with the public

I___ 5. Limiting the spread of microorganisms, often called *clean technique*

H___ 6. Protection of severely compromised clients from other patients and health care workers

D___ 7. Elimination of microorganisms from any object that comes in contact with the patient, often called *sterile technique*

A___ 8. Replacement of damaged cells by cells of their own kind during the wound healing process

E___ 9. Isolation of infected patients from other patients and health care workers

E___ 10. Infections caused by the caregiving process

A. Repair

B. Regeneration

C. Nosocomial infections

D. Surgical asepsis

E. Iatrogenic infections

F. Isolation technique

G. Inflammation

H. Reverse isolation

I. Medical asepsis

J. Community-acquired infections

III. List 3 causes of inflammation.

1. Systemic inf : headace, musclease,

2.

3.

IV. List 4 observable signs of infection.

1.

2.

3.

4.

V. Match the definition on the left with the most appropriate term on the right.

___ 1. Tumor

___ 2. Dolor

___ 3. Calor

___ 4. Rubor

A. Heat

B. Swelling

C. Redness

D. Pain

VI.   List 4 actions that occur when the inflammation process is initiated.

1.

2.

3.

4.

VII.   List 5 signs of local inflammation.

1.

2.

3.

4.

5.

VIII.   List 5 signs of systemic inflammation.

1.

2.

3.

4.

5.

IX.   Match the signs of inflammation on the left with the most appropriate type of inflammation on the right. Answers may be used more than once.

____   1. Headache

____   2. Sweating

____   3. Loss of function

____   4. Fever

____   5. Pain

____   6. Redness

____   7. Heat

____   8. Chills

____   9. Muscle aches

____   10. Swelling

A. Local inflammation

B. Systemic inflammation

X. List 4 factors that influence the speed with which wound healing takes place.

1.

2.

3.

4.

XI. List 2 reasons why the healing process can be delayed in the elderly.

1.

2.

XII. List 7 infectious agents.

1.

2.

3.

4.

5.

6.

7.

XIII. Match the definition on the left with the most appropriate term on the right.

____	1. Round bacteria that cluster in groups of two	A. Anaerobes
____	2. Rod-shaped organisms that form spirals	B. Gram-positive bacteria
____	3. Chains of round bacteria	C. Bacilli
____	4. One-celled microorganisms that retain a violet-colored stain	D. Aerobes
		E. Spirochetes
____	5. Bacteria that do not grow in the presence of oxygen	F. Diplococci
____	6. Clusters of round bacteria	G. Streptococci
____	7. Rod-shaped organisms	H. Bacteria
____	8. Bacteria that grow in the presence of oxygen	I. Staphylococci
____	9. Round bacteria	J. Fusiform bacilli
____	10. Rod-shaped organisms with tapered ends	K. Gram-negative bacteria
____	11. One-celled microorganisms that can be decolorized and counterstained pink	L. Cocci
____	12. One-celled microorganisms capable of multiplying rapidly within a susceptible host	

XIV. Match each disease or infection on the left with the most appropriate causative agent on the right. Answers may be used more than once.

___	1. Malaria	A. Fungi
___	2. Hookworm infection	B. Protozoa
___	3. Pneumocystic pneumonia	C. Mycoplasmas
___	4. Primary atypical pneumonia	D. Viruses
___	5. Measles	E. Helminths
___	6. Typhus	F. Rickettsiae
___	7. Common cold	
___	8. Rocky Mountain spotted fever	
___	9. Tapeworm infection	
___	10. Ringworm	

XV. List 6 factors that must occur in order for human infectious disease to occur.

1.

2.

3.

4.

5.

6.

XVI. List 3 common portals of entry.

1.

2.

3.

XVII. List 5 symptoms of localized infections.

1.

2.

3.

4.

5.

XVII. List 6 symptoms of generalized infections.

1.

2.

3.

4.

5.

6.

XIX.   List 2 types of acquired infections.

  1.

  2.

XX.   Indicate which diseases are (A) community acquired and which are (B) hospital acquired.

____   1.   Urinary tract infections   A.   Community acquired

____   2.   Food-borne illness   B.   Hospital acquired

____   3.   Hepatitis B

____   4.   Nosocomial infection

____   5.   Superinfection

____   6.   Syphilis

____   7.   Gonorrhea

____   8.   Iatrogenic infection

____   9.   Tuberculosis

____ 10.   Hepatitis A

____ 11.   Septicemia

____ 12.   AIDS

XXI.   List 3 barriers to providing immunizations to everyone.

  1.

  2.

  3.

XXII.   List 8 ways in which the transmission of infectious agents can be interrupted.

  1.   5.

  2.   6.

  3.   7.

  4.   8.

XXIII.   Fill in the blank.
         Nosocomial infections are much more serious than those acquired in the community because:

XXIV.   List 3 ways by which the resistance cycle can be broken.

  1.

  2.

  3.

XXV. List 4 reasons why resistant bacterial strains develop.

1.

2.

3.

4.

XXVI. List 3 common sites for nosocomial infections in hospitalized patients.

1.

2.

3.

XXVII. List 4 examples of clean technique (medical asepsis) which help prevent infection in hospitalized patients.

1.   3.

2.   4.

XXVIII. List 8 types of isolation techniques.

1.   5.

2.   6.

3.   7.

4.   8.

XXIX. List 3 reasons why patients are being discharged early from the hospital with home health care ordered.

1.

2.

3.

XXX. For each disease or condition listed on the left, indicate all of the protective measure(s) on the right are appropriate.

_____ 1. Mumps   A. Strict isolation

_____ 2. Scabies   B. Contact isolation

_____ 3. Conjunctivitis   C. Respiratory isolation

_____ 4. Cholera (and poor hygiene) D. Enteric precautions

_____ 5. Impetigo   E. Drainage/secretion precautions

_____ 6. Measles

_____ 7. Hepatitis A (and poor hygiene)

_____ 8. Varicella (chickenpox)

_____ 9. Infected decubitus ulcer

_____ 10. Rubella

XXXI. Choose the most appropriate answer.

1. Which layers of the skin protect the body from penetrating and thermal injury that could permit the invasion of microorganisms?
   A. dermis and subcutaneous layer
   B. subcutaneous and muscle layers
   C. epidermis and subcutaneous layers
   D. epidermis and dermis

2. Which membrane in the respiratory tract traps foreign material, keeping it away from the smaller airways?
   A. mucous membrane
   B. serous membrane
   C. synovial membrane
   D. cutaneous membrane

3. One important protective function of the liver is that it:
   A. detoxifies drugs, alcohol, and environmental poisons
   B. manufactures bile
   C. stores red blood cells
   D. produces acidic secretions that protect against growth of bacteria and fungi

4. The protective function of the vagina is that it:
   A. produces alkaline secretions
   B. produces acidic secretions
   C. protects the body from chemical injury
   D. detoxifies poisons

5. Which types of leukocytes are especially involved with fighting infection?
   A. erythrocytes and neutrophils
   B. neutrophils and monocytes
   C. monocytes and thrombocytes
   D. eosinophils and neutrophils

6. Physical agents that cause inflammation include:
   A. insect venom, other chemicals
   B. bacteria, viruses
   C. excessive sunlight, x-rays
   D. x-rays, bacteria

7. The literal meaning of inflammation is:
   A. red flame
   B. great fire
   C. inner infection
   D. fire within

8. The increase in blood flow to an inflamed area is partially responsible for:
   A. warmth and redness
   B. swelling and pain
   C. warmth and pain
   D. swelling and redness

9. The increase in blood flow to an inflamed area is due to:
   A. increased permeability
   B. chemical mediators
   C. hemodynamic changes
   D. hormonal factors

10. The process by which the increased blood flow brings leukocytes to line the small blood vessel walls near the inflamed site is called:
    A. phagocytosis
    B. leukocytosis
    C. pavementing
    D. vasodilation

11. The hemodynamic changes and vascular permeability in inflammation occur with the help of:
    A. hormonal factors
    B. chemical mediators
    C. erythrocytes
    D. thrombocytes

12. Vasoactive amines (histamine, serotonin), acidic lipids (prostaglandins), and lysosomal enzymes are examples of:
    A. hormonal factors
    B. chemical mediators
    C. erythrocytes
    D. thrombocytes

13. The action of cortisol on the inflammation process is to:
    A. slow the release of histamine, stabilize lysosomal membranes, and prevent the chemotaxis of leukocytes
    B. slow the release of histamine, depress lysosomal membrane activity, and prevent the chemotaxis of leukocytes
    C. increase the release of histamine, stabilize lysosomal membranes, and prevent the chemotaxis of leukocytes
    D. increase the release of histamines, depress lysosomal membrane activity, and stimulate the chemotaxis of leukocytes

14. Cells that are produced to clean up inflammatory debris are called:
    A. fibroblast cells
    B. platelet cells
    C. neutrophil cells
    D. macrophage cells

15. When a wound has become infected, has been cleaned and debrided, and is sutured closed after infection is no longer present, this is called:
    A. phagocytosis
    B. chemical mediation
    C. hemodynamics
    D. delayed primary closure

16. One-celled microorganisms capable of multiplying rapidly within a susceptible host are called:
    A. fungi
    B. protozoa
    C. bacteria
    D. mycoplasmas

17. Many childhood illnesses, such as measles and chickenpox, and some forms of hepatitis are caused by:
    A. viruses
    B. bacteria
    C. protozoa
    D. fungi

18. The best way to fight viral illness is:
    A. antibiotics
    B. prevention
    C. drug therapy
    D. vitamin therapy

19. It is seldom possible to kill viruses because:
    A. replication of the virus occurs within the host cell
    B. the cell wall can be destroyed with drugs
    C. the cell wall requires oxygen for functions
    D. the host cell is separate from the virus

20. Vegetable-like organisms that exist by feeding on organic matter are called:
    A. bacteria
    B. viruses
    C. protozoa
    D. fungi

21. Ringworm (tinea corporis) and athlete's foot (tinea pedis) are examples of disease caused by:
    A. bacteria
    B. viruses
    C. fungi
    D. protozoa

22. One-celled organisms that produce diseases such as malaria and amoebic dysentery are called:
    A. fungi
    B. protozoa
    C. viruses
    D. helminths

23. Microorganisms between the size of bacteria and viruses that are transmitted to humans through the bites of fleas and ticks are called:
    A. rickettsiae
    B. protozoa
    C. helminths
    D. mycoplasmas

24. Parasites that are found in soil and water and are generally transmitted from hand to mouth are called:
    A. ricksettiae
    B. protozoa
    C. helminths
    D. mycoplasmas

25. Gram-negative, multishaped organisms without cell walls known as pleuropneumonia-like organisms are called:
    A. helminths
    B. protozoa
    C. mycoplasmas
    D. viruses

26. Microorganisms present in sufficient number and virulence to damage human tissue are called:
    A. reservoirs
    B. causative agents
    C. portals of exit
    D. portals of entrance

27. When a reservoir of microorganisms occurs in the tissues of a human, the human is called a:
    A. host
    B. portal of exit
    C. mode of transfer
    D. portal of entry

28. The route by which the infectious agent leaves one host and travels to another is called:
    A. portal of entry
    B. mode of transfer
    C. host
    D. portal of exit

29. Common portals of exit for organisms spread by droplet contamination through sneezing or coughing are:
    A. the gastrointestinal tract
    B. wounds
    C. the urinary tract
    D. the nose and mouth

30. A common portal of exit is the:
    A. gastrointestinal tract
    B. urinary tract
    C. kidney tract
    D. cardiovascular tract

Introductory Nursing Care of Adults

31. The means by which a microorganism is transported to a host is called:
    A. portal of entry
    B. mode of transfer
    C. portal of exit
    D. reservoir

32. Areas through which infectious agents can enter the body are referred to as:
    A. portals of exit
    B. vector transmissions
    C. portals of entry
    D. common vehicle transmissions

33. Two groups of patients who are most susceptible to hospital-acquired infections include those with:
    A. pneumonia and patients requiring insulin
    B. myocardial infarction and tachycardia
    C. AIDS and cancer patients receiving chemotherapy
    D. emphysema and bronchitis

34. The development of a urinary tract infection when a Foley catheter was inserted using improper technique is an example of:
    A. sexually transmitted infection
    B. superinfection
    C. iatrogenic infection
    D. fungal infection

35. The overgrowth of a second microorganism that can cause illness following antibiotic therapy for one microorganism is called:
    A. thrombophlebitis
    B. superinfection
    C. sexually transmitted infection
    D. septicemia

36. Limiting the spread of microorganisms as much as possible is called:
    A. surgical asepsis
    B. medical asepsis
    C. isolation
    D. contamination

37. The most basic and effective method of preventing cross-contamination is:
    A. hand washing
    B. antibiotics
    C. isolation
    D. use of gown and gloves

38. The primary cause of nosocomial infections is:
    A. soiled hands
    B. faulty equipment
    C. airborne droplets
    D. open wounds

39. The rubbing together of hands during hand washing should last for at least:
    A. 5 seconds
    B. 10 seconds
    C. 15 seconds
    D. 30 seconds

40. Clean technique is to medical asepsis as sterile technique is to:
    A. clean asepsis
    B. medical technique
    C. surgical asepsis
    D. surgical technique

41. The elimination of microorganisms from any object that comes in contact with the patient is called:
    A. medical asepsis
    B. clean technique
    C. isolation technique
    D. surgical asepsis

42. When patients are kept in a private room with the door closed; gown, gloves and mask required; and restricted visitors, this type of isolation is called:
    A. contact isolation
    B. enteric precautions
    C. respiratory isolation
    D. strict isolation

43. A ventilation system that prevents contaminated air from being vented outside the room is part of:
    A. respiratory isolation
    B. tuberculosis isolation
    C. strict isolation
    D. contact isolation

44. How much fluid is required by patients with infection?
    A. 1 liter per day
    B. 2 liters per day
    C. 5 liters per day
    D. 10 liters per day

XXXII. Match the definition on the left with the most appropriate term on the right.

___ 1. Measures often employed for more virulent infections that are spread easily, such as diphtheria or chickenpox

___ 2. Measures employed for patients with active pulmonary tuberculosis

___ 3. Measures previously called "reverse" isolation; designed to protect patients who have decreased immunity to infection

___ 4. Measures necessary for patients with infected wounds

___ 5. Measures employed when infection can be spread by coming into direct contact with infected surfaces

___ 6. Measures necessary when there is danger of microorganisms being spread by droplets

___ 7. Measures employed for patients with infections that reside primarily in the gastrointestinal tract

___ 8. Measures based on the assumption that everyone with whom they come in contact carries the human immunodeficiency virus

A. Respiratory isolation

B. Universal blood and body fluid precautions

C. Tuberculosis isolation

D. Enteric precautions

E. Strict isolation

F. Care of severely compromised patients

G. Contact isolation

H. Drainage and secretion precautions

CHAPTER 1

Immunity

OBJECTIVES

1. Describe the two major types of immunity: natural and acquired.
2. Identify blood cells involved in immunity.
3. Identify organs involved in immunity.
4. Identify nonspecific defense mechanisms.
5. Describe the nonspecific defense mechanisms.
6. Differentiate between humoral and cell-mediated immunity.
7. Describe the three types of disorders of the immune system.
8. Give examples of each type of immune system disorder.
9. Develop a nursing care plan for the patient with an immune system disorder.

LEARNING ACTIVITIES

I.   Match the definition on the left with the most appropriate term on the right.

____   1. A condition in which the immune system is unable to defend the body against a foreign invasion of antigens

____   2. An immediate response to specific antigens involving B lymphocytes and the production of antibodies

____   3. A delayed response to injury or infection involving T cells and the production of substances that enhance the immune response and influence the destruction of antigens

____   4. Temporary immunity acquired after receiving antibodies or lymphocytes produced by another individual

____   5. A condition in which the body is unable to distinguish self from nonself causing the immune system to react and destroy its own tissues

____   6. Immunity acquired after birth as a result of the body's natural immune responses to antigens

____   7. Immunity that is present at birth

____   8. Immunity developed after direct contact with an antigen through illness or vaccination

A. Acquired immunity

B. Cell-mediated immunity

C. Passive acquired immunity

D. Natural immunity

E. Immunodeficiency

F. Humoral Immunity

G. Autoimmunity

H. Active acquired immunity

II. Match the definition on the left with the most appropriate term on the right.

____ 1. The clean-up cells of the body that engulf and destroy microorganisms and cellular debris through a process known as *phagocytosis*

____ 2. A substance produced in viral infections that inhibits the replication of viruses

____ 3. White blood cells that play a key role in immune responses toward infectious organisms and other antigens

____ 4. Any substance that invades the body and is capable of stimulating a response from the immune system

____ 5. A series of proteins that enhance the inflammatory process and immune response

____ 6. A condition in which a normally inoffensive substance stimulates an atypical immune response

____ 7. A protein that is created in response to a specific antigen

____ 8. A substance released in inflammation that causes body temperature to increase

____ 9. An antigen that causes a hypersensitive reaction

A. Leukocytes

B. Allergen

C. Antibody (immunoglobulin)

D. Phagocytes

E. Complement

F. Antigen

G. Allergy

H. Pyrogen

I. Interferon

III. Fill in the blanks.

1. The body's resistance to invading organisms and its ability to fight off invaders once they have gained access to the body is called _____.

2. The system that provides adequate protection from most infections and diseases in a healthy individual is the

_____ _____.

IV. List 5 factors that can compromise the immune system.

1.

2.

3.

4.

5.

V. List 5 examples of antigens.

1.   4.

2.   5.

3.

VI. Fill in the blanks.

1. When healthy, the body protects what it recognizes as self and attempts to destroy that which is

_____.

2. Antibodies are also known as _____.

VII. List 3 examples of situations in which tissue that is normally recognized as self may be seen as nonself by the immune system.

1.

2.

3.

VIII. Match the examples of diseases or conditions on the left with the type of vaccination or method of vaccination preparation on the right. Answers may be used more than once.

___ 1. Pertussis

___ 2. Tetanus toxoid

___ 3. Measles

___ 4. Exposure to hepatitis

___ 5. Poliomyelitis

___ 6. Rabies

___ 7. Snakebite

___ 8. Diphtheria

A. Destroying bacterial toxins that act as antigens

B. Using dead organisms that can no longer cause disease

C. Using immune globulin or antiserum that contains antibodies for a specific agent

D. Altering the structure of live organisms so that they are unable to cause disease yet maintain their antigenic properties to prevent many diseases

IX. Match the definition on the left with the most appropriate term on the right.

___ 1. Participate in the surveillance of abnormal cell growth, allergic reactions, autoimmune diseases, and rejection of foreign tissue; 20–35% of WBCs

___ 2. Participate in inflammatory and allergic responses by releasing substances such as histamine, heparin, and serotonin; 0.2–0.5% of WBCs

___ 3. Ingest large foreign particles, cell fragments, necrotic tissue, or other debris in the circulation; powerful phagocytes that operate as "seek and destroy" scavengers; 2–6% of WBCs

___ 4. Migrate to areas of inflammation or bacterial invasion, where they ingest and kill invading organisms; 40–75% of WBCs

___ 5. Migrate to infected or inflamed areas, where they engulf and destroy antigens; also important in allergic reactions and autoimmune diseases; 2–5% of WBCs

A. Basophils

B. Neutrophils

C. Monocytes

D. Eosinophils

E. Lymphocytes

X.   List 5 body organs that are involved in immunity.

1.

2.

3.

4.

5.

XI.   List 3 functions of chemical mediators when injury to tissues occurs.

1.

2.

3.

XII. List 4 signs and symptoms of inflammation that are caused by chemically mediated responses.

1.

2.

3.

4.

XIII. Fill in the blanks.

1. When the body's self-defenses against foreign invasion fail to function normally, this state is called

   _____.

2. The primary clinical clue to immunodeficiency, whatever the cause, is the tendency to develop

   _____.

3. Two age groups that are at risk for infection are: _____.

XIV. List 8 causes of acquired immunodeficiencies.

1.   5.

2.   6.

3.   7.

4.   8.

XV. List 5 classifications of medications that often place patients at risk for infection.

1.

2.

3.

4.

5.

XVI. List 2 invasive procedures that bypass the patient's first line of defense and increase risk of infection.

1.

2.

XVII. List 5 factors that set the hospitalized patient up for infection.

1.

2.

3.

4.

5.

XVIII. State the usual medical treatment of congenital immunodeficiencies.

XIX. List the primary nursing responsibility in cases of immunodeficiency.

XX. Fill in the blanks.

1. A life-threatening allergic reaction that can quickly deteriorate into shock, coma, and death is called

_____.

2. The main side effect of antihistamines is _____.

3. The classification of drugs that should not be given to patients with asthma because severe bronchospasm may result is _____.

4. The 2 classifications of drugs that are used in the medical treatment of asthma are _____

_____.

5. One classification of drugs that is used in the medical treatment of allergies is _____.

6. The single most important measure for personnel and visitors in preventing infection in the immunodeficient patient is _____.

XXI. List 4 ways by which HIV is spread.

1.   3.

2.   4.

XXII. List 3 types of laboratory work that may document immunodeficiency.

1.

2.

3.

XXIII. Match the intervention on the left with its purpose on the right. Answers may be used more than once.

____ 1. Bone marrow transplant

____ 2. Bactrim

____ 3. AZT

____ 4. Septra

____ 5. Chemotherapy

____ 6. Interleukin-2

____ 7. Pantamidine isethionate (Pentam 300)

____ 8. WBC transfusion

____ 9. Interferon

A. Boost immune system

B. Treat Kaposi's sarcoma

C. Prevent viral replication

D. Treat *P. carinii* pneumonia

XXIV. List 8 goals of nursing care for the patient with AIDS.

1.

2.

3.

4.

5.

6.

7.

8.

XXV. Match the organ on the left with the most appropriate function on the right. Answers may be used more than once.

____ 1. Lymph nodes

____ 2. Liver

____ 3. Bone marrow

____ 4. Spleen

____ 5. Thymus

A. Participate(s) in formation and maturation of immune system cells

B. Act(s) as filter to remove dead cells, debris, and foreign molecules from the blood

C. Filter(s) lymph drained from a region of tissues

D. Filter(s) blood, plays a part in production of specific immunoglobulins

XXVI. Match the example of antigen on the left with the most appropriate classification on the right. Answers may be used more than once.

___ 1. Food

___ 2. Fungi

___ 3. Parasites

___ 4. Organ transplant cells

___ 5. Penicillin

___ 6. Bacteria

___ 7. Insect venoms

___ 8. Pollens

___ 9. Viruses

___ 10. Blood transfusion cells

A. Environmental substances

B. Drugs

C. Microorganisms

D. Transplanted cells

XXVII.   List 9 common allergens.

1.   6.

2.   7.

3.   8.

4.   9.

5.

XXVIII.   List 5 effects of histamine on the body when it is released during anaphylaxis.

1.

2.

3.

4.

5.

XXIX.   List 8 signs and symptoms of anaphylaxis.

1.   5.

2.   6.

3.   7.

4.   8.

XXX. List 6 causes of anaphylaxis.

1.   4.

2.   5.

3.   6.

XXXI.   List 3 nursing goals for a patient with anaphylaxis.

   1.

   2.

   3.

XXXII.   List 3 factors that may initiate autoimmunity.

   1.

   2.

   3.

XXXIII.   List 3 ways in which autoimmune diseases may cause injury.

   1.

   2.

   3.

XXXIV.   List 13 nursing diagnoses for the patient with an autoimmune disorder.

1.	8.
2.	9.
3.	10.
4.	11.
5.	12.
6.	13.
7.	

XXXV.   List 4 goals of nursing care for patients with autoimmune disorders.

   1.

   2.

   3.

   4.

XXXVI.   List 6 goals for nursing intervention of patients with systemic lupus erythematosus.

   1.

   2.

   3.

   4.

   5.

   6.

XXXVII. List the 3 stages of phagocytosis outlined in Figure 10–1. (Figure from Black, J.M., & Matassarin-Jacobs, E. [1993]. *Luckmann and Sorensen's medical-surgical nursing: A psychophysiologic approach* [4th ed., p. 533]. Philadelphia: W. B. Saunders.)

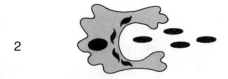

1

Macrophage

Microorganisms

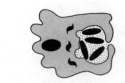

2

3

1.

2.

3.

XXXVIII. List local manifestations of allergic reactions as shown in the figure below.

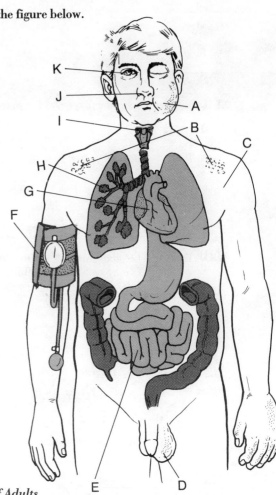

A.

B.

C.

D.

E.

F.

G.

H.

I.

J.

K.

Introductory Nursing Care of Adults

XXXIX. Match the type of white blood cells on the left with its function on the right . Answers may be used more than once.

___ 1. Basophils

___ 2. Lymphocytes

___ 3. Neutrophils

___ 4. Monocytes

___ 5. Eosinophils

A. Immunity; produce antibodies

B. Phagocytosis

C. Release histamine and heparin

D. Allergy; counteract histamine in allergic reactions

XL. List 5 risk factors for transmission of HIV.

1.

2.

3.

4.

5.

XLI. List 12 symptoms of HIV infection and AIDS.

1.

2.

3.

4.

5.

6.

7.

8.

9.

10.

11.

12.

XLII. List 10 nursing diagnoses for persons with AIDS.

1.

2.

3.

4.

5.

6.

7.

8.

9.

10.

XLIII. Match the allergic reactions on the left with the most appropriate stimuli on the right. Answers may be used more than once.

___ 1. Gastrointestinal allergies

___ 2. Atopic dermatitis (eczema)

___ 3. Asthma

___ 4. Urticaria (hives)

___ 5. Allergic contact dermatitis

___ 6. Allergic rhinitis

___ 7. Anaphylaxis

A. Pollens, dust, molds, animal dander

B. Antibiotics (penicillin), blood transfusions, insect venom

C. Soaps, cosmetics, chemicals, fabrics

D. Food, drugs

E. Pollens, dust, molds, cigarette smoke, air pollutants, animal dander

F. Plants (poison ivy); metals (nickel); chemicals, cosmetics; latex gloves

XLIV. Match the disorders of the left with the most appropriate tissue affected on the right. Answers may be used more than once.

___ 1. Idiopathic lymphopenia

___ 2. Pemphigus vulgaris

___ 3. Crohn's disease

___ 4. Systemic lupus erythematosus

___ 5. Cardiomyopathy

___ 6. Autoimmune thrombocytopenic purpura

___ 7. Autoimmune thyroiditis

___ 8. Psoriasis

___ 9. Insulin-dependent diabetes mellitus

___ 10. Idiopathic neutropenia

___ 11. Scleroderma

___ 12. Ulcerative colitis

___ 13. Multiple sclerosis

___ 14. Rheumatoid arthritis

___ 15. Rheumatic fever

___ 16. Addison's disease

___ 17. Goodpasture's syndrome

___ 18. Graves' disease

___ 19. Myasthenia gravis

___ 20. Autoimmune hemolytic anemia

A. Heart

B. Skin

C. Colon

D. Multiple tissues

E. Brain and spinal cord

F. Pancreas

G. Lung, Kidney

H. Thyroid

I. Joints

J. Adrenal gland

K. Red blood cells

L. Lymphocytes

M. Platelets

N. Ileum

O. Neutrophils

P. Neuromuscular junctions

XLV. Choose the most appropriate answer.

1. The body's defense network against infection is the:
   A. cardiovascular system
   B. respiratory system
   C. immune system
   D. circulatory system

2. Proteins that are created in response to antigens are called:
   A. antibodies
   B. mutagens
   C. enzymes
   D. allergens

3. The type of immunity that is present at birth and that is not dependent on a specific immune response or previous contact with an infectious agent is called:
   A. acquired immunity
   B. active immunity
   C. phagocytic immunity
   D. natural immunity

4. The type of immunity newborns acquire from their mothers through the placenta or through ingestion of breast milk (especially colostrum) is called:
   A. passive phagocytosis
   B. active acquired immunity
   C. active natural immunity
   D. passive acquired immunity

5. The blood cells that play a key role in immune responses toward infectious organisms and antigens are:
   A. leukocytes
   B. erythrocytes
   C. thrombocytes
   D. osteocytes

6. Neutrophils, eosinophils, and basophils are examples of:
   A. granulocytes
   B. nongranulocytes
   C. erythrocytes
   D. thrombocytes

7. Phagocytes that are important in allergic reactions and autoimmune diseases are called:
   A. neutrophils
   B. eosinophils
   C. basophils
   D. monocytes

8. Cells that participate in inflammatory and allergic responses by releasing substances such as histamine, heparin, and serotonin are called:
   A. eosinophils
   B. neutrophils
   C. basophils
   D. monocytes

9. Monocytes and lymphocytes are types of:
   A. granular leukocytes
   B. erythrocytes
   C. nongranular leukocytes
   D. thrombocytes

10. Which organ attacks antigens and debris in the interstitial fluid and filters the lymph?
    A. thymus
    B. bone marrow
    C. spleen
    D. lymph node

11. The body's first line of defense is:
    A. skin and inflammation
    B. phagocytosis and kidney
    C. blood vessels and kidney
    D. skin and mucous membranes

12. The cilia in the respiratory tract, the motility of the gastrointestinal tract, and the sloughing of dead skin cells are examples of:
    A. inflammation and peristalsis barriers
    B. physical and chemical barriers
    C. phagocytosis and immune barriers
    D. interferon and complement barriers

13. A series of proteins that enhance the inflammatory process and the immune response by stimulating chemotaxis, phagocytosis, and the activity of antibodies is called:
    A. pyrogen
    B. interferon
    C. complement
    D. histamine

14. Humoral immunity is:
    A. immediate
    B. delayed
    C. cell-mediated
    D. altered

15. A delayed response to injury or infection is called:
    A. humoral immunity
    B. interferon immunity
    C. cell-mediated immunity
    D. pyrogen immunity

16. The human immunodeficiency virus (HIV) is a highly infectious virus that is transmitted through:
    A. sexual contact and respiratory droplets
    B. sexual contact and contact with contaminated blood or blood products
    C. contact with blood or blood products and skin contact
    D. sharing eating utensils and contact with bed linens

17. The most common opportunistic infection seen in AIDS is:
    A. hepatitis B
    B. *Pneumocystis carinii*
    C. *Haemophilus influenzae*
    D. streptococcal pneumonia

18. The most frequent malignancy seen in AIDS is:
    A. Kaposi's sarcoma
    B. *Pneumocystis carinii*
    C. candidiasis
    D. hepatitis B

19. Antiviral medications are given to AIDS patients to:
    A. prevent viral replication and destroy infected cells
    B. destroy viral cells that are infected
    C. prevent viral replication to protect cells that are not yet infected
    D. destroy bacteria and prevent infection

20. The most widely used antiviral drug used for AIDS patients is:
    A. streptomycin
    B. azidothymidine (AZT)
    C. penicillin
    D. erythromycin

21. What percentage of the U.S. population suffers from allergies of some sort?

    A. 20–25%
    B. under 5%
    C. 40–45%
    D. 50–75%

22. Someone who is prone to allergies may be referred to as:

    A. infectious
    B. immunocompromised
    C. atopic
    D. symptomatic

23. Antigens that cause hypersensitive reactions are called:

    A. antibodies
    B. complement
    C. allergens
    D. interferon

24. Allergy testing is performed by injecting small amounts of allergen:

    A. intradermally
    B. intramuscularly
    C. intravenously
    D. interstitially

25. In anaphylaxis, what causes bronchospasm, vasodilation, and increased vascular permeability?

    A. interferon
    B. pyrogen
    C. phagocytosis
    D. histamine

26. Drugs used in the treatment of anaphylaxis include diphenhydramine, corticosteroids, and:

    A. morphine and atropine
    B. ibuprofen and propranolol
    C. epinephrine and propranolol
    D. epinephrine and aminophylline

27. The body's ability to determine self from nonself is called:

    A. tolerance
    B. phagocytosis
    C. immunity
    D. inflammation

28. Autoimmunity can involve any tissue or organ system. In multiple sclerosis, what is affected?

    A. heart and kidney tissue
    B. white matter of brain and spinal cord
    C. lung tissue and liver cells
    D. spleen tissue and thymus gland

29. Common problems of SLE are:

    A. headache and chills
    B. palpitations and restlessness
    C. fatigue and joint stiffness
    D. bleeding and hypotension

30. When an organ is irreversibly damaged and unable to function yet is necessary to sustain life, what is recommended?

    A. surgical repair
    B. transplant
    C. plasmapheresis
    D. phagocytosis

31. Because transplanted tissue is at risk for destruction by the immune response, donor tissue needs to be:

    A. closely matched to that of the recipient
    B. taken from a close family member
    C. kept in frozen storage before use
    D. matched with blood type

32. Two central nervous system autoimmune disorders are:

    A. ulcerative colitis and Crohn's disease
    B. rheumatoid arthritis and SLE
    C. hyperthyroidism and Addison's disease
    D. multiple sclerosis and myasthenia gravis

CHAPTER

11

Fluid and Electrolytes

OBJECTIVES

1. Describe extracellular, intracellular, and transcellular fluid compartments.
2. Describe the composition of extracellular and intracellular body fluid.
3. Discuss the mechanisms of fluid transport and fluid balance.
4. Identify the causes, signs and symptoms, and treatment of fluid imbalance.
5. Describe the major functions of the major electrolytes: sodium, potassium, calcium, and magnesium.
6. Identify the causes, signs and symptoms, and treatment of electrolyte imbalances.
7. Discuss the nursing management of persons with fluid and electrolyte imbalances.
8. Describe the major considerations in relation to fluid and electrolyte balance in the elderly.
9. List the four types of acid-base imbalances.
10. Identify the major causes of each acid-base imbalance.

LEARNING ACTIVITIES

I. Match the definition on the left with the most appropriate term on the right.

_C_ 1. A tendency of biologic systems to maintain stability of the internal environment while continously adjusting to changes necessary for survival

_F_ 2. Movement of water across a membrane from a less concentrated solution to a more concentrated solution

_B_ 3. The random movement of particles in all directions through a solution

_A_ 4. Transfer of water and solutes through a membrane from a region of high pressure to a region of low pressure

_D_ 5. Measurement of the ratio of water to solutes in a solution

_B_ 6. Movement of solutes across membranes using greater energy of force

A. Filtration

B. Active transport

C. Homeostasis

D. Osmolality

E. Diffusion

F. Osmosis

II. Match the definition on the left with the most appropriate term on the right.

_B_ 1. Membranes that separate fluid compartments of the body that permit movement of water and certain solutes from one compartment to another

_A_ 2. A substance that develops an electrical charge when dissolved in water

_A_ 3. An increase in extracellular fluid

_I_ 4. A solution containing a low number of hydrogen ions

_D_ 5. Fluid outside the cell

_C_ 6. The homeostasis of the hydrogen ion (H+) concentration in the body fluids

_E_ 7. Fluid within the cell

_J_ 8. A solution containing a high number of hydrogen ions

_G_ 9. A decrease in extracellular fluid

_PH_ 10. The symbol used to indicate hydrogen ion balance.

A.   Fluid volume excess

B.   Selectively permeable membranes

C.   Acid-base balance

D.   Extracellular fluid

E.   Intracellular fluid

F.   pH

G.   Fluid volume deficit

H.   Alkaline or base

I.   Acid

J.   Electrolyte

III. List 3 factors that affect the percentage of body weight that is water.

1. _Edema_

2.

3.

IV. Match the body water status on the left with the most appropriate condition on the right

_D_ 1. Body water decreases

_C_ 2. Contain less water than other cells

_A_ 3. Body water percentage less than males

_B_ 4. Lower percentage of body water

A.   Females

B.   Obese persons

C.   Advancing age

D.   Increased fat cells

V. List 6 examples of electrolytes.

1. _Sodium_
2. _Potassium_
3. _Calcium_
4. _Chloride_
5. _bicarbonate_
6. _magnesium_

VI. Indicate whether the substances on the left are electrolytes or nonelectrolytes.

B 1. Bilirubin

A 2. Urea

A 3. Magnesium

A 4. Phosphate

B 5. Creatinine

A 6. Bicarbonate

A 7. Potassium

B 8. Protein

A 9. Chloride

A 10. Calcium

A. Electrolytes

B. Nonelectrolytes

VII. Fill in the blanks.

1. The purpose of selective permeability is to _____
_____

2. The process that controls water movement and distribution in body fluid compartments by regulating the concentration of fluid in each compartment is called _____

3. The osmolality of the intracellular fluid is maintained primarily by _____

4. The osmolality of the extracellular fluid is maintained primarily by _____

5. The two body systems that accomplish regulation of fluid balances in the body are _____ and _____

6. The main monitor of fluid balance in the body is the _____

7. The nephrons conduct the work of the kidney through the processes of reabsorption, secretion, and _____

8. The primary activity of the kidney nephron is _____

9. The filtered plasma, or filtrate, moves through the tubules and changes until it becomes _____

10. The process that is important for adjusting the volume and composition of the filtrate and for preventing excessive fluid loss through the kidneys is called _____

11. The phase during which the filtrate is transformed into urine is called _____

12. Two hormones that have a major effect on fluid balance are _____ and _____

13. The hormone that increases the reabsorption of sodium and decreases the reabsorption of potassium is _____

14. When there are increased potassium levels and decreased sodium levels in the blood, the adrenal gland releases the hormone known as _____

15. The hormone that causes the kidney tubules to reabsorb more water is called _____

Introductory Nursing Care of Adults

VIII. List 4 ways by which water is transported between intracellular and extracellular fluid compartments.

1.

2.

3.

4.

IX. List 2 ways by which fluids are gained in a healthy person.

1.

2.

X. List 4 parts of the body through which fluids are lost.

1.   3.

2.   4.

XI. List 4 factors that cause an increase in water loss through the skin and lungs.

1.
                                                   3.
2.
                                                   4.

XII. Match the definition on the left with the most appropriate term on the right.

___ 1. The filtering portion of the nephron   A. Nephron

___ 2. The functioning unit of the kidney; more than   B. Tubule
         a million per kidney
                                                       C. Glomerulus
___ 3. Responsible for reabsorption

XIII. An increase in plasma osmolality (less fluid in the plasma) stimulates the release of antidiuretic hormone (ADH) into the blood stream to replenish needed fluid in the body. List 5 other factors which stimulate the release of ADH related to situations in which there may be less fluid volume.

1.

2.

3.

4.

5.

XIV. List 4 examples that can cause fluid volume deficit or hypovolemia.

1.

2.

3.

4.

XV. List 4 conditions that may cause hypervolemia.

1.   3.

2.   4.

XVI. List 4 functions of sodium in the body.

1.   3.

2.   4.

XVII. List 2 causes of hypokalemia.

1.   2.

XVIII. List 2 functions of chloride.

1.   2.

XIX. List 2 causes of hypochloremia.

1.   2.

XX. List 3 functions of calcium

1.   3.

2.

XXI. List 3 causes of hypocalcemia.

1.   3.

2.

XXII. List 6 functions of magnesium.

1.   4.

2.   5.

3.   6.

XXIII. Match the definition on the left with the most appropriate term on the right.

____ 1. The movement of water across a membrane   A. Filtration
         from a less concentrated solution to a more
         concentrated solution   B. Osmosis

____ 2. Movement of solutes across membranes using   C. Diffusion
         greater force
                                                         D. Active transport
____ 3. The transfer of water and solutes through a
         membrane from an area of high pressure to an
         area of low pressure

____ 4. The random movement of particles in all
         directions through a solution

Introductory Nursing Care of Adults

XXIV. List 10 disease or trauma states that have great potential for altering fluid balance.

1.	6.
2.	7.
3.	8.
4.	9.
5.	10.

XXV. List 5 measurements and observations to be made in collecting data for assessment of patients with fluid and electrolyte imbalances.

1.	4.
2.	5.
3.	

XXVI. List 3 locations where skin turgor is best measured.

1.

2.

3.

XXVII. List 4 parts of the body against which skin is pressed to test for edema.

1.	3.
2.	4.

XXVIII. In addition to poor skin turgor, list 10 general signs and symptoms of fluid volume deficit (or dehydration).

1.	6.
2.	7.
3.	8.
4.	9.
5.	10.

XXIX. List 2 nursing interventions for persons with fluid volume deficit who are receiving intravenous fluid replacement therapy.

1.

2.

XXX. List 5 common signs of dehydration in the elderly.

   1.   4.

   2.   5.

   3.

XXXI. List 1 major cause of severe fluid volume excess which occurs in hospitalized patients.

   1.

XXXII. List 9 signs and symptoms of fluid volume excess.

   1.   6.

   2.   7.

   3.   8.

   4.   9.

   5.

XXXIII. List 7 signs and symptoms of hyponatremia.

   1.   5.

   2.   6.

   3.   7.

   4.

XXXIV. List 7 signs and symptoms of hypernatremia.

   1.   5.

   2.   6.

   3.   7.

   4.

XXXV. List 4 observations that need to be made in assessment of patients with hypernatremia.

   1.

   2.

   3.

   4.

XXXVI. List 7 signs and symptoms of patients with hypokalemia.

   1.   5.

   2.   6.

   3.   7.

   4.

XXXVII. List 4 observations that need to be made in assessment of patients with hypokalemia.

1. diuretic

2.

3.

4.

XXXVIII. List 9 signs and symptoms of hyperkalemia.

1. renal damage   6.

2. limiting the ability of kidney   7.

3. Nerve stimulus conduction   8.

4. muscle active   9.

5. CVA

XXXIX.   Match the numerical values on the left with the pH categories on the right.

B   1. pH between 7.35 and 7.45   A. alkaline

C   2. pH less than 7.35   B. neutral

A   3. pH greater than 7.45   C. acidic

XL.   List 3 mechanisms that maintain normal acid-base balance.

1.

2.

3.

XLI.   List the 4 major types of acid-base imbalances.

1.   3.

2.   4.

XLII.   List 8 causes of acute respiratory acidosis.

1.   5.

2.   6.

3.   7.

4.   8.

XLIII. List 6 common clinical signs and symptoms of respiratory acidosis.

1.   4.

2.   5.

3.   6.

XLIV. List 10 causes of respiratory alkalosis.

1.   6.

2.   7.

3.   8.

4.   9.

5.   10.

XLV. List 10 clinical signs and symptoms of respiratory alkalosis.

1.   6.

2.   7.

3.   8.

4.   9.

5.   10.

XLVI. List 6 causes of metabolic acidosis.

1.   4.

2.   5.

3.   6.

XLVII. List 4 causes of loss of hydrogen ions.

1.   3.

2.   4.

XLVIII. List 2 causes of retention of bicarbonate ions.

1.

2.

IL. List 10 common signs and symptoms of metabolic alkalosis.

1.   6.

2.   7.

3.   8.

4.   9.

5.   10.

L.   Indicate which solution, A or B, in Figure 11–1, has the greater osmolality. (Figure from Black, J.M., & Matassarin-Jacobs, E. [1993]. *Luckmann and Sorensen's medical-surgical nursing: A psychophysiologic approach* [4th ed., p.262]. Philadelphia: W. B. Saunders.)

A chang in osmolality of intracellular fluid affects the osmol of intracellular fluid and viceversa

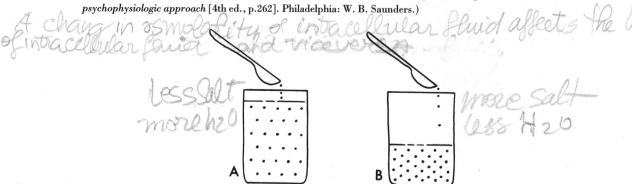

less salt more h2o   *more salt less H2O*

A   B

LI.   Label the parts of the urinary system (A–I) in Figure 11–2. (Figure from Guyton, A. C. [1991]. *Textbook of medical physiology* [8th ed., p. 287]. Philadelphia: W. B. Saunders.)

A. *Renal vein*

B. *Renal artery*

C. *Pelvic*

D. *Cortex*

E. *medulla*

F. *left kidney*

G. *ureters*

H. *urinary bladder*

I. *Right kidney*

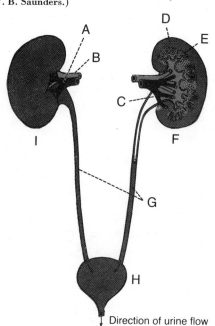

Direction of urine flow

LII. In regulation of body fluid volume, match the conditions on the left with all appropriate effects on the right.

A   1. Hypervolemia   A. Stimulates ADH

D   2. Hypovolemia   B. Inhibits ADH

                                           C. Stimulates aldosterone

                                           D. Inhibits aldosterone

Introductory Nursing Care of Adults

LIII. Match the assessments on the left with the most appropriate conditions on the right. (More than one condition may be appropriate for an assessment.)

___ 1. Bounding pulse	A. Electrolyte imbalances
___ 2. Weak, irregular, and rapid pulse	B. Increased metabolism, with fluid loss
___ 3. Increased pulse	C. Metabolic acidosis
___ 4. Decreased pulse	D. Sodium excess
___ 5. Changes in respiratory function	E. Severe potassium excess
___ 6. Deep, fast respirations	F. Magnesium excess
___ 7. Slow, shallow respirations with intermittent periods of apnea	G. Metabolic alkalosis
	H. Magnesium deficit
___ 8. Fall in systolic blood pressure > 10 mm Hg from lying to standing or from lying to sitting position	I. Fluid volume excess
	J. Fluid volume deficit
___ 9. Fever	K. Increased respiratory rate, with loss of water vapor from lungs
	L. Sodium deficit

LIV. Fill in the arrows in Table 11-11: Mechanisms of Respiratory and Metabolic Acidosis and Alkalosis.

MECHANISMS OF RESPIRATORY AND METABOLIC ACIDOSIS AND ALKALOSIS

CONDITION	CAUSE	pH	H^+	HCO_3^-	$Paco_2$
Respiratory acidosis	Hypoventilation				
Respiratory alkalosis	Hyperventilation				
Metabolic acidosis	Diabetic ketoacidosis Lactic acidosis Diarrhea Renal insufficiency				
Metabolic alkalosis	Vomiting HCO_3 retention Volume depletion K^+ depletion				

LV. Choose the most appropriate answer.

1. Fluid within a cell is called:
   A. extracellular
   B. interstitial
   C. intravascular
   D. intracellular

2. Fluids found in the blood vessels in the form of plasma or serum are called:
   A. intravascular
   B. intracellular
   C. interstitial
   D. intervolemic

3. Fluids surrounding the cells, including lymph fluid, are called:
   A. intravascular
   B. interstitial
   C. intracellular
   D. intervolemic

4. Electrolytes that develop a positive charge when dissolved in water are called:
   A. anions
   B. molecules
   C. cations
   D. elements

5. Sodium, potassium, calcium, and magnesium are examples of:
   A. anions
   B. cations
   C. filtrates
   D. enzymes

6. Chloride, bicarbonate, and phosphate are examples of:
   A. cations
   B. anions
   C. filtrates
   D. enzymes

7. The concentration of electrolytes in a solution or body fluid compartment is measured in:
   A. milligrams (mg)
   B. grams (g)
   C. milliliters (ml)
   D. milliequivalents (mEq)

8. What stimulates osmoreceptors in the hypothalamus to give the sensation of thirst?
   A. increased plasma osmolality
   B. decreased plasma osmolality
   C. less concentrated urine
   D. decreased urine volume

9. Water loss via the skin and lungs increases in a:
   A. hot, moist environment
   B. hot, dry environment
   C. cool, dry environment
   D. cool, moist environment

10. A decrease in extracellular fluid is called:
    A. fluid volume excess
    B. osmosis
    C. edema
    D. fluid volume deficit

11. A measurement of the ratio of the water to the solutes is called:
    A. osmosis
    B. diffusion
    C. osmolality
    D. filtration

12. What percentage of the plasma is filtered by the glomerulus?
    A. 5%
    B. 20%
    C. 50%
    D. 80%

13. Because the retention of sodium causes water retention, aldosterone acts as a:
    A. weight regulator
    B. blood regulator
    C. cardiac regulator
    D. volume regulator

14. One way the body tries to compensate for fluid volume deficits is to:
    A. increase heart rate
    B. decrease heart rate
    C. increase blood pressure
    D. decrease blood pressure

15. An increase in extracellular fluid is called:
    A. fluid volume deficit
    B. fluid volume excess
    C. osmosis
    D. filtration

16. The body tries to compensate for fluid volume excess by:
    A. increasing the filtration and excretion of sodium and water by the kidneys and increasing the production of ADH
    B. decreasing the filtration and excretion of sodium and water by the kidneys and decreasing the production of ADH
    C. increasing the filtration and excretion of sodium and water by the kidneys and decreasing the production of ADH
    D. decreasing the filtration and excretion of sodium and water by the kidneys and increasing the production of ADH

17. A lower than normal concentration of sodium in the blood stream is known as:
    A. hypernatremia
    B. hyponatremia
    C. hyperkalemia
    D. hypokalemia

18. When there is a loss of sodium or an excess loss of body water, what occurs?
    A. hypokalemia
    B. hyperkalemia
    C. hyponatremia
    D. hypernatremia

19. When there is a deficiency in sodium ions in the extracellular fluid, the body attempts to compensate by:
    A. decreasing the amount of water excreted from the kidneys
    B. increasing the amount of water excreted from the kidneys
    C. decreasing the amount of water in blood vessels
    D. increasing the amount of water in the extracellular fluid

20. What results from an increased intake of sodium or a decrease in body water?
    A. hyperkalemia
    B. hypokalemia
    C. hypernatremia
    D. hyponatremia

21. When the kidneys excrete too much potassium, what results?
    A. hyperkalemia
    B. hypokalemia
    C. hypercalcemia
    D. hypocalcemia

22. An extracellular anion that is usually bound with

other ions, especially sodium or potassium, is:
    A. chloride
    B. magnesium
    C. calcium
    D. iron

23. Low serum chloride, or hypochloremia, usually occurs with the loss of:
    A. phosphate
    B. bicarbonate
    C. iron
    D. sodium

24. Ninety-nine percent of the body's calcium is concentrated in the:
    A. blood and muscles
    B. liver and brain
    C. bones and teeth
    D. kidneys and adrenal gland

25. If more calcium is needed in the bones, it is taken from the blood as well as reabsorbed through the:
    A. lungs
    B. kidneys
    C. heart
    D. liver

26. Next to potassium, the most abundant cation in the intracellular fluid is:
    A. calcium
    B. sodium
    C. chloride
    D. magnesium

27. Hypomagnesemia is frequently associated with hypocalcemia and:
    A. hypokalemia
    B. hyponatremia
    C. hypochloremia
    D. hypotension

28. An increased pulse rate can signal:
    A. loss of sodium ions
    B. excess of magnesium ions
    C. excess of sodium ions
    D. loss of chloride ions

29. One liter of fluid retention equals a weight gain of:
    A. 1 pound
    B. 2.2 pounds
    C. 5.4 pounds
    D. 10 pounds

30. How much fluid can a patient accumulate before pitting edema is present?
    A. 1 pound
    B. 5 pounds
    C. 10 pounds
    D. 20 pounds

31. Puffy eyeballs and fuller cheeks suggest:
    A. fluid volume excess
    B. fluid volume deficit
    C. potassium excess
    D. potassium deficit

32. Older people generally have a slower return to normal following a pinch of the skin to check for turgor, so assessment of the elderly should also include:
    A. pitting peripheral edema
    B. range of motion
    C. shortness of breath
    D. mucous membrane moisture

33. If a depression remains in the tissue after pressure is applied with a fingertip, the edema is described as:
    A. excessive
    B. pitting
    C. depressed
    D. minimal

34. A deep and persistent pit that is approximately 1 inch is described as:
    A. 1+
    B. 2+
    C. 3+
    D. 4+

35. When the edema is so severe that pitting is not possible and the tissue feels hard, the edema is described as:
    A. 10+
    B. 5+
    C. tenacious
    D. brawny

36. When the tongue is red and swollen, this suggests:
    A. potassium excess
    B. calcium excess
    C. sodium excess
    D. magnesium excess

37. A dry mouth may be the result of:
    A. fluid volume excess
    B. fluid volume deficit
    C. hypochloremia
    D. hyperchloremia

38. Distention of the jugular neck vein can indicate:
    A. fluid volume excess
    B. fluid volume deficit
    C. hypocalcemia
    D. hypercalcemia

39. When the hands are placed in a dependent position, and the veins take longer than 3 to 5 seconds to fill, the patient may have:
    A. hypokalemia
    B. hyperkalemia
    C. fluid volume deficit

D. fluid volume excess

40. A measure of hydrogen ions in the urine is called:
    A. urinalysis
    B. urine specific gravity
    C. urine pH
    D. urine glucose

41. The normal range for urine pH is:
    A. 2.0 to 7.0
    B. 2.0 to 12.0
    C. 4.6 to 8.0
    D. 7.0 to 12.0

42. A urine specimen that is not tested within 4 hours of collection may become:
    A. alkaline
    B. acidic
    C. more concentrated
    D. less concentrated

43. A measure of the kidney's ability to conserve water or concentrate urine is called:
    A. pH
    B. urine potassium
    C. creatinine clearance
    D. specific gravity

44. In most instances, normal urine specific gravity is between:
    A. 1.001 and 1.035
    B. 2.001 and 4.035
    C. 4.001 and 6.035
    D. 5.0 and 7.0

45. A good indicator of fluid balance is:
    A. urine sodium
    B. urine creatinine clearance
    C. urine specific gravity
    D. urine potassium

46. A more precise measurement of the kidney's ability to concentrate urine than the specific gravity is:
    A. urine sodium
    B. urine pH
    C. urine osmolality
    D. urine potassium

47. A measure of the number of dissolved particles in a solution is:
    A. pH
    B. creatinine clearance
    C. urine potassium
    D. osmolality

48. A 24-hour urine specimen is required for:
    A. creatinine clearance
    B. pH
    C. specific gravity
    D. osmolality

49. The normal hematocrit for adult males is:
    A. 12%
    B. 30%
    C. 44%
    D. 60%

50. Blood urea nitrogen (BUN) provides a measure of:
    A. blood volume
    B. renal function
    C. cardiac function
    D. liver function

51. When a patient has an elevated BUN, the hematocrit should be monitored because a high BUN can cause:
    A. breakdown of red blood cells
    B. fluid volume excess
    C. hemorrhage
    D. fluid volume deficit

52. A measure of blood concentration is:
    A. hematocrit
    B. hemoglobin
    C. serum osmolality
    D. serum electrolytes

53. An example of severe fluid volume deficit is:
    A. diarrhea
    B. vomiting
    C. acute hemorrhage
    D. edema

54. In patients with fluid volume deficit, assessment of vital signs is important to detect:
    A. postural hypotension, increased temperature, and increased pulse
    B. postural hypotension, decreased temperature, and decreased pulse
    C. postural hypertension, increased temperature, and increased pulse
    D. postural hypertension, decreased temperature, and decreased pulse

55. What amounts of fluid per day are needed by the average person for adequate hydration?
    A. 500–700 ml/day
    B. 800–1000 ml/day
    C. 1500–2000 ml/day
    D. 3500–5000 ml/day

56. When breathing problems occur in patients with fluid volume excess, patients should:
    A. lie flat in bed
    B. have head of bed elevated 30 degrees
    C. ambulate frequently
    D. be in side-lying position

57. If pitting edema is present in patients with fluid volume excess, patients should:
    A. be turned every 2 hours
    B. cough every 2 hours
    C. ambulate every 2 hours
    D. have blood pressure checked every 2 hours

58. To prevent hyponatremia in patients with feeding tubes, what should be used for irrigation?
    A. sterile water
    B. normal glucose
    C. normal saline
    D. sterile dextrose

59. The heart rate of patients on digitalis should be closely watched, because hypokalemia can cause:
    A. congestive heart failure
    B. pericarditis
    C. digitalis toxicity
    D. diuresis

60. In order to prevent gastrointestinal irritation, oral potassium supplements should be given with:
    A. meals
    B. a full glass of water or fruit juice
    C. a full glass of milk
    D. a teaspoon of water

61. What must be checked before starting an intravenous infusion of potassium?
    A. blood pressure
    B. temperature
    C. weight
    D. urine output

62. Serum potassium levels greater than 5.0 mEq/L can cause:
    A. cardiac arrest
    B. fever
    C. increased urine output
    D. pneumonia

63. The homeostasis of the hydrogen ion concentration in the body fluids is:
    A. acid-base balance
    B. active transport
    C. adaptation
    D. osmosis

64. The respiratory system regulates the pH by:
    A. removing oxygen from the blood
    B. removing carbon dioxide from the blood
    C. removing sodium from the blood
    D. removing chloride from the blood

65. When the respiratory system falls to eliminate the appropriate amount of carbon dioxide to maintain the normal acid-base balance, what occurs?
    A. respiratory alkalosis
    B. respiratory acidosis
    C. metabolic acidosis
    D. metabolic alkalosis

66. As the body attempts to eliminate the excessive carbon dioxide in the lungs, the:
    A. respiratory rate increases, and respirations are shallow
    B. respiratory rate increases, and respirations are deep
    C. respiratory rate decreases, and respirations are shallow
    D. respiratory rate decreases, and respirations are deep

67. The most common cause of respiratory alkalosis is:
    A. hypoventilation
    B. hyperventilation
    C. drowning
    D. obesity

68. A solution containing a higher number of hydrogen ions is:
    A. alkaline
    B. acidic
    C. hypernatremic
    D. hyperkalemic

69. Hyperventilation is characterized by:
    A. slow, deep respirations
    B. slow, shallow respirations
    C. rapid, deep respirations
    D. rapid, shallow respiration

70. When patients with respiratory alkalosis are hyperventilating, they should be encouraged to breathe:
    A. rapidly into a paper bag
    B. shallow breaths
    C. panting breaths
    D. slowly into a paper bag

71. When the body retains too many hydrogen ions or loses too many bicarbonate ions, what occurs?
    A. respiratory acidosis
    B. respiratory alkalosis
    C. metabolic acidosis
    D. metabolic alkalosis

72. With too many acids and too few bases present in metabolic acidosis, the:
    A. blood $PaCo^2$ increases
    B. blood pH remains the same
    C. blood pH rises
    D. blood pH drops

73. With acidosis, the skin is:
    A. warm and diaphoretic
    B. warm and puffy
    C. cool and clammy
    D. cool and edematous

74. Acidosis is usually treated with intravenous infusion of:
    A. potassium chloride
    B. normal saline
    C. calcium salts
    D. sodium bicarbonate

75. An increase in bicarbonate levels or a loss of hydrogen ions results in:
    A. metabolic acidosis
    B. metabolic alkalosis
    C. respiratory alkalosis
    D. respiratory acidosis

12

Nutrition

OBJECTIVES

1. Discuss the role of the alimentary system in the digestion of food.
2. Discuss the digestion and absorption of food.
3. List the functions of each of the six classes of essential nutrients.
4. List the functions of proteins, carbohydrates, and fats.
5. List the food sources of proteins, carbohydrates, and fats.
6. List the food sources of dietary fiber.
7. List the possible health benefits of dietary fiber.
8. List the food sources of each of the vitamins and minerals.
9. Discuss the changes in nutrient needs as the individual ages.
10. Distinguish between anorexia nervosa and bulimia.
11. Discuss the different types of nutritional support.
12. Identify guidelines for the nutritional assessment.

LEARNING ACTIVITIES

I. Match the definition on the left (1-16) with the most appropriate term on the right.

M 1. Lipid-wrapped proteins carried into the blood stream; includes high-density and low-density lipoproteins, which carry cholesterol

G 2. Small amounts of metals (calcium, sodium and potassium) and nonmetals (chloride, phosphate) that are essential to the body; can build up

C 3. Neutral fats found in plant and animal food sources

J 4. Combination of incomplete proteins that provide all nine essential amino acids when consumed together

P 5. Compounds that come chiefly from animal sources and are usually solid at room temperature; also coconut and palm oils

O 6. Large organic compounds made of various combinations of amino acids, found in meat, milk, fish, and eggs

A. Saturated fatty acids
B. Incomplete protein
C. Triglycerides
D. Calorie
E. Vitamins
F. Lipids
G. Minerals
H. Basal metabolic rate
I. Amino acids
J. Complementary protein
K. Complete protein
L. Insoluble fiber
M. Lipoproteins
N. Resting metabolic rate
O. Proteins
P. Unsaturated fatty acids

I. *Continued*

_____ 7. Organic compounds supplied by food that the body requires for normal growth and development

_____ 8. A group of 22 substances that can be bonded in different ways to make a variety of proteins. The body can manufacture sufficient amounts of these provided the nine essential amino acids are derived from the diet

_____ 9. Indigestible roughage found in plant cells; aids in stool formation and elimination

_____ 10. Compounds that come from plants or fish and are generally liquid at room temperature; can be monounsaturated (olive, peanut, canola, and avocado oils) or polyunsaturated (corn, safflower, and sesame oils)

_____ 11. Measurement of energy expenditure taken in the morning after awakening and approximately 10 to 12 hours after the last meal

_____ 12. Plant protein lacking one or more essential amino acids

_____ 13. Fats in solid or liquid form; store energy, carry fat-soluble vitamins, maintain healthy skin and hair; supply essential fatty acids and promote a feeling of fullness (satiety)

_____ 14. Standard unit for measuring energy; the amount of heat needed to raise the temperature of 1 ml of water at a standard temperature by 1 degree centigrade

_____ 15. Measurement of energy expenditure taken at any time of the day and 3 to 4 hours after the last meal

_____ 16. Protein containing all nine essential amino acids; usually of animal origin (e.g., meat, eggs)

A. Saturated fatty acids

B. Incomplete protein

C. Triglycerides

D. Calorie

E. Vitamins

F. Lipids

G. Minerals

H. Basal metabolic rate

I. Amino acids

J. Complementary protein

K. Complete protein

L. Insoluble fiber

M. Lipoproteins

N. Resting metabolic rate

O. Proteins

P. Unsaturated fatty acids

II. List 3 functions of the gastrointestinal system.

1.

2.

3.

III. List 5 ways that hormones help regulate the process of digestion.

1.

2.

3.

4.

5.

IV. List the 3 areas of the gastrointestinal system in which the digestion of food occurs.

1.

2.

3.

V. List the 6 nutrients.

1.   4.

2.   5.

3.   6.

VI. List 3 factors that affect the digestion of food.

1.

2.

3.

VII. List 5 factors that can cause the metabolic rate to vary.

1.   4.

2.   5.

3.

VIII. List 5 hormones that affect the basal metabolic rate.

1.   4.

2.   5.

3.

IX. List 6 physiologic factors that affect basal metabolic rate.

1.   4.

2.   5.

3.   6.

X.   List 2 reasons why the BMR of a sleeping person is lower than that of an awake, alert person.

1.

2.

XI.   List 3 major food sources of monosaccharides.

1.

2.

3.

XII.   List 5 hormones that are involved in the regulation of blood glucose levels.

1.   4.

2.   5.

3.

XIII.   List 3 effects of ketosis on the body.

1.

2.

3.

XIV.   List the number of calories per gram provided by fats, carbohydrates, and protein.

1.   Fats _____

2.   Carbohydrates _____

3.   Protein _____

XV.   List 5 functions of lipids.

1.

2.

3.

4.

5.

XVI.   List 3 examples of saturated fats.

1.

2.

3.

XVII. Match characteristics on the left with the corresponding type of fats on the right.

____ 1. Olive, corn and peanut oils

____ 2. Come chiefly from animal sources

____ 3. Consist of 3 fatty acids attached to a glycerol molecule

____ 4. Liquid at room temperature

____ 5. Butter, milk fat, fat from meat

____ 6. Neutral fats

____ 7. Come from plants and fish

____ 8. Made of as many hydrogen atoms as they can carry

____ 9. Coconut and palm oils

A. Triglycerides

B. Unsaturated fats

C. Saturated fats

XVIII. List 6 sources of complete proteins in foods.

1.   4.

2.   5.

3.   6.

XIX. Explain why it is important to eat a diet that contains all of the essential amino acids, plus enough additional amino acids to allow for synthesis of the nonessential amino acids.

XX. Explain why protein must be eaten in the diet each day.

XXI. List 7 signs of protein deficiency.

1.   5.

2.   6.

3.   7.

4.

XXII. List 8 vitamins of the B complex group.

1.   5.

2.   6.

3.   7.

4.   8.

XXIII. List 5 functions of water in the body.

1.   4.

2.   5.

3.

XXIV. List 4 ways in which water is lost from the body.

1.   3.

2.   4.

XXV. Explain why it is essential that all living things replenish water <u>daily</u> to maintain health and efficiency.

XXVI. List 5 areas to cover in a nutritional assessment.

1.   4.

2.   5.

3.

XXVII. List 6 signs of malnourishment.

1.   4.

2.   5.

3.   6.

XXVIII. List 5 areas to include when taking a dietary history.

1.   4.

2.   5.

3.

XXIX. List 7 diseases with which obesity is associated.

1.   5.

2.   6.

3.   7.

4.

XXX. List 5 causes that contribute to problems with being underweight.

1.   4.

2.   5.

3.

XXXI. List 6 symptoms of bulimia.

1.   4.

2.   5.

3.   6.

XXXII. List 6 conditions that interfere with taking in liquids orally which may require enteral tube feedings.

1.   4.

2.   5.

3.   6.

XXXIII. List 8 complications of enteral tube feedings.

1.   5.

2.   6.

3.   7.

4.   8.

XXXIV. List 3 causes of complications of enteral tube feedings.

1.
                                           3.
2.

XXXV. List 7 frequently occurring complications of patients who are being fed parenterally.

1.   5.

2.   6.

3.   7.

4.

XXXVI. List the 5 major food groups that make up the food guide pyramid. What are the recommended amounts of each group?

1.

2.

3.

4.

5.

XXXVII. Label the feeding tubes in Figure 12–4. (Figure from Mahan, L. K., & Arlin, M. [1992]. *Krause's food, nutrition & diet therapy* [8th ed., p. 509]. Philadelphia: W. B. Saunders.)

A.

B.

C.

D.

E.

F.

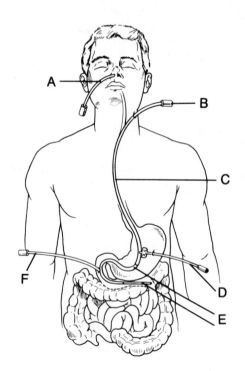

XXXVIII. Choose the most appropriate answer.

1. The gastrointestinal system is also known as the:
   A. endocrine system
   B. alimentary system
   C. urinary system
   D. excretory system

2. The digestion of food is made possible by:
   A. diffusion
   B. osmosis
   C. homeostasis
   D. hydrolysis

3. Digestion begins in the mouth where starches are digested by an enzyme called:
   A. chyme
   B. pepsin
   C. ptyalin
   D. insulin

4. What process moves the food through the esophagus into the stomach?
   A. osmosis
   B. hydrolysis
   C. peristalsis
   D. active transport

5. Gastric juices include:
   A. hydrochloric acid, enzymes, mucus, and gastrin
   B. hydrochloric acid, enzymes, mucus, and bile
   C. hydrochloric acid, enzymes, bile, and insulin
   D. ptyalin, enzymes, mucus and bile

6. The stomach is normally emptied in:
   A. 30–60 minutes
   B. 1–4 hours
   C. 5–8 hours
   D. 10–12 hours

7. The function of the cardiac sphincter is to:
   A. prevent the backflow of the food mass from the duodenum into the stomach
   B. prevent the backflow of the food mass from the stomach into the pharynx
   C. prevent the backflow of blood from the left ventricle into the left atrium
   D. prevent the backflow of the food mass from the large intestine into the small intestine

8. The primary organ of absorption is the:
   A. mouth
   B. stomach
   C. small intestine
   D. large intestine

9. The folds of the small intestine are covered with finger-like projections called:
   A. cilia
   B. flagella
   C. villi
   D. valves

10. Absorption is accomplished by the processes of:
    A. osmosis and hydrolysis
    B. diffusion and hydrolysis
    C. osmosis and active transport
    D. diffusion and active transport

11. The movement of particles from an area of higher concentration to an area of lower concentration is called:
    A. hydrolysis
    B. active transport
    C. filtration
    D. diffusion

12. The movement of particles across a membrane that requires the input of energy is called:
    A. diffusion
    B. active transport
    C. osmosis
    D. filtration

13. What is one type of carbohydrate that cannot be digested and is excreted unchanged in the feces?
    A. fiber
    B. glucose
    C. glycogen
    D. monosaccharide

14. Fats are broken down in the stomach into:
    A. fatty acids and glycerol
    B. glucose and glycerol
    C. fatty acids and glucose
    D. glycogen and glycerol

15. The emotions of fear, anger, and worry can cause the hypothalamus to stimulate the autonomic nervous system, which:
    A. stimulates peristalsis, depresses the gastric secretions, and slows the movement of food through the intestines.
    B. stimulates peristalsis, increases gastric secretions, and speeds the movement of food through the intestines.
    C. inhibits peristalsis, depresses the gastric secretions, and slows the movement of food through the intestines.
    D. inhibits peristalsis, stimulates the gastric secretions, and speeds the movement of food through the intestines.

16. Very little bacterial action occurs in the stomach due to the presence of:
    A. bile
    B. chyme
    C. hydrochloric acid
    D. pepsin

17. Bacterial action is most intense in the:
    A. small intestine
    B. large intestine
    C. stomach
    D. liver

18. Which foods are the most easily digested?
    A. raw foods
    B. cooked foods
    C. fried foods
    D. foods with additives

19. The metabolic rate is affected significantly by the amount of heat lost to the atmosphere from the skin through the process of:
    A. radiation
    B. convection
    C. diffusion
    D. evaporation

20. The BMR of a sleeping person is how much lower than that of an awake, alert person?:
    A. 5%
    B. 10%
    C. 50%
    D. 75%

21. The standard unit for measuring energy is the:
    A. calorie
    B. milliliter
    C. milligram
    D. kilogram

22. A calorie is the amount of heat energy required to raise the temperature of 1 ml of water at a standard initial temperature by:
    A. 1 degree C.
    B. 10 degrees C
    C. 25 degrees C.
    D. 50 degrees C.

23. The measurement used most often in nutritional guidelines is:
    A. calorie
    B. kilocalorie
    C. milliliter
    D. kilogram

24. Carbohydrates are organic compounds that consist of:
    A. nitrogen, carbon, and hydrogen
    B. carbon, hydrogen, and oxygen
    C. oxygen, nitrogen, and carbon
    D. carbon, hydrogen, and calcium

25. The simplest form of carbohydrates is:
    A. disaccharides
    B. oligosaccharides
    C. polysaccharides
    D. monosaccharides

26. Glucose, fructose, and galactose are examples of:
    A. disaccharides
    B. oligosaccharides
    C. polysaccharides
    D. monosaccharides

27. Sucrose is found in:
    A. fruits
    B. vegetables
    C. maple syrup
    D. margarine

28. Which carbohydrates are usually insoluble (indigestible)?
    A. monosaccharides
    B. polysaccharides
    C. oligosaccharides
    D. disaccharides

29. When excess carbohydrates are taken in by the body, they are converted to:
    A. glycogen
    B. glucose
    C. sucrose
    D. fructose

30. When glycogen is needed by the body, it is converted to glucose by a process called:
    A. glycogenesis
    B. glucogenesis
    C. osmosis
    D. diffusion

31. What acts like a sponge to absorb many times its weight in water and helps provide a full feeling long after eating?
    A. soluble fiber
    B. monosaccharides
    C. insoluble fiber
    D. glycerols

32. Diets without at least 50 to 100 grams of carbohydrates per day are likely to lead to:
   A. ketosis
   B. alkalosis
   C. hyperglycemia
   D. hypernatremia

33. Butter, margarine, and salad dressing are all:
   A. more than half carbohydrate
   B. more than half fat
   C. more than half protein
   D. more than half polysaccharides

34. Lipids are made of:
   A. nitrogen, hydrogen and oxygen
   B. carbon, hydrogen, and oxygen
   C. hydrogen, carbon, and nitrogen
   D. carbon, oxygen, and nitrogen

35. Which nutrient can be stored in the body compactly with little or no water?
   A. carbohydrate
   B. fat
   C. protein
   D. glucose

36. Neutral fats, or the most common fats found in foods of both plant and animal origin, are called:
   A. corticosteroids
   B. insoluble fibers
   C. soluble fibers
   D. triglycerides

37. Adipose cells can store up to 95% of their volume as:
   A. glucose
   B. glycogen
   C. amino acids
   D. triglycerides

38. Most human adipose cells are in the form of white fat, which accumulates in:
   A. subcutaneous tissue
   B. epidermis
   C. dermis
   D. muscles

39. Lipids are a major source of energy for:
   A. subcutaneous tissue
   B. epidermis tissue
   C. muscle tissue
   D. mucous membrane

40. Where are most lipids carried to be converted to energy or used in the synthesis of new triglycerides?
   A. gall bladder
   B. liver
   C. heart
   D. kidney

41. After absorption, lipids are carried in the blood stream in packages called:
   A. saturated fats
   B. lipoproteins
   C. adipose
   D. unsaturated fats

42. Most nutritionists recommend that the daily fat intake should be what percentage of the daily caloric intake?
   A. 50% or less
   B. 30% or less
   C. 15% or less
   D. 10% or less

43. To minimize the risk of heart disease, people should eat more:
   A. saturated fats
   B. polysaturated fats
   C. glycerol fats
   D. unsaturated fats

44. The main source of saturated fats in the American diet comes from:
   A. vegetable oils
   B. cottonseed oil
   C. animal products
   D. safflower oil

45. The basic material of life is considered to be:
   A. fat
   B. carbohydrate
   C. protein
   D. glucose

46. The basic structure of protein is:
   A. amino acids
   B. glucose
   C. monosaccharides
   D. fatty acids

47. When various incomplete proteins are consumed at the same time, the body can use them together to obtain a balance of the essential amino acids; incomplete proteins consumed together are called:
   A. uncomplementary proteins
   B. complementary proteins
   C. animal proteins
   D. enzyme proteins

48. The nine amino acids that must be obtained from the diet are called:
    A. dietary amino acids
    B. essential amino acids
    C. incomplete amino acids
    D. complementary amino acids

49. Which of the following foods has the highest protein content?
    A. cereals
    B. beans
    C. poultry
    D. lentils

50. Vitamins A, D, E, and K are:
    A. fat soluble
    B. water soluble
    C. insoluble
    D. complementary

51. In addition to fat-soluble vitamins, which group of nutrients needs bile and pancreatic juices for absorption?
    A. carbohydrates
    B. proteins
    C. amino acids
    D. lipids

52. Extra amounts of fat-soluble vitamins are stored in the:
    A. liver
    B. gall bladder
    C. fat cells
    D. epidermis

53. The intake of water is controlled by:
    A. exercise
    B. thirst
    C. metabolism
    D. stress

54. How much water should adults drink daily?
    A. 500 ml
    B. 1000 ml
    C. 2500 ml
    D. 5000 ml

55. The diet for the elderly should include:
    A. protein and carbohydrates
    B. carbohydrates and lipids
    C. all the food groups
    D. protein and lipids

56. Older adults with chronic diseases have an increased risk for:
    A. protein deficiency and negative nitrogen balance
    B. vitamin deficiency and positive nitrogen balance
    C. mineral deficiency and negative nitrogen balance
    D. carbohydrate deficiency and positive nitrogen balance

57. Guidelines for the amounts of nutrients that healthy people should consume daily are called:
    A. basic four food groups
    B. recommended daily allowances
    C. food pyramids
    D. minimum food requirements

58. Overweight individuals are considered obese if their weight is what percent above the ideal body weight?
    A. 5% or more above
    B. 10% or more above
    C. 20% or more above
    D. 30% or more above

59. Enteral tubes may enter the body through the nose, esophagus, stomach, or:
    A. ileum
    B. jejunum
    C. duodenum
    D. large intestine

60. A method of administering nutrients only if the gastrointestinal tract cannot be used is called:
    A. enteral tube feedings
    B. nasogastric tube feedings
    C. duodenal tube feedings
    D. parenteral nutrition

61. Central parenteral nutrition or TPN feedings usually are used for patients who are debilitated and malnourished with a weight loss of what percent of body weight?
    A. 10% or more
    B. 20% or more
    C. 50% or more
    D. 75% or more

62. Total parenteral nutrition can supply up to:
    A. 100 kcal per day
    B. 1000 kcal per day
    C. 2000 kcal per day
    D. 4000 kcal per day

63. What type of solution is administered through a Hickman or Broviac-type catheter?
    A. hypotonic
    B. hypertonic
    C. isotonic
    D. glucose and sterile water

64. It is important that transitional feedings be done:
    A. gradually
    B. abruptly
    C. orally
    D. parenterally

65. If patients who have been without food for an extended period of time are given food too quickly, they may develop:
    A. hypernatremia
    B. hypercalcemia
    C. hypophosphatemia
    D. hyperphosphatemia

First Aid and Emergency Care

OBJECTIVES

1. List the principles of emergency and first aid care.
2. List the steps of the initial assessment and interventions for the person requiring emergency care.
3. Describe the components of the nursing assessment of the person requiring emergency care.
4. Outline the steps of the nursing process for emergency or first aid treatment of victims of cardiopulmonary arrest, choking, shock, hemorrhage, traumatic injury, burns, heat or cold exposure, poisoning, bites, and stings.
5. Explain the legal implications of administering first aid in emergency situations.

LEARNING ACTIVITIES

I. Match the definition on the left (1-15) with the most appropriate term on the right.

____ 1. Tearing away of tissue

____ 2. Presence of air in the pleural cavity that causes the lung on the affected side to collapse

____ 3. Loss of a large amount of blood

____ 4. An injury to muscle tissue or the tendons that attach them to bones, or both

____ 5. A severe, potentially fatal, allergic reaction characterized by hypotension and bronchial constriction

____ 6. Presence of blood in the pleural cavity causing the lung on the affected side to collapse

____ 7. Elevation of body core temperature above 99°F

____ 8. Inadequate circulation caused by falling blood pressure

____ 9. Nosebleed

____ 10. Decrease in body core temperature below 95°F

____ 11. An injury to a ligament

A. Shock

B. Hypothermia

C. Cardiopulmonary arrest

D. Hemothorax

E. Epistaxis

F. Sprain

G. Evisceration

H. Avulsion

I. Hemorrhage

J. Hyperthermia

K. Strain

L. Poison

M. Respiratory arrest

N. Pneumothorax

O. Anaphylactic shock

I. *Continued*

    12. Any substance that, in small quantities, is capable of causing illness or harm following ingestion, inhalation, injection, or contact with the skin

    13. Absence of breathing

    14. Protrusion of internal organs through a wound

    15. Absence of heartbeat and breathing

A. Shock

B. Hypothermia

C. Cardiopulmonary arrest

D. Hemothorax

E. Epistaxis

F. Sprain

G. Evisceration

H. Avulsion

I. Hemorrhage

J. Hyperthermia

K. Strain

L. Poison

M. Respiratory arrest

N. Pneumothorax

O. Anaphylactic shock

II. List 3 measures that nurses can teach people to reduce the risk of choking.

1.

2.

3.

III. List 4 measures to be taken to prevent carbon monoxide poisoning.

1.

2.

3.

4.

IV. List 6 teaching points to include when working with patients who are allergic to insect bites concerning treatment and prevention of insect bites.

1.

2.

3.

4.

5.

6.

V. Choose the most appropriate answer.

1. General guidelines for first aid treatment of emergency patients include:
   A. Cover with wool blanket to prevent chilling
   B. Remove penetrating objects
   C. Splint injured parts in the position they are found
   D. Give orange juice with sugar if unconscious

2. Data in emergency situations should include the:
   A. chief complaint, nursing care plan, and allergies to drugs
   B. treatment given, complete physical assessment, and relevant medical history
   C. treatment given, nursing diagnosis, and current medications
   D. chief complaint, treatment given, and relevant medical history

3. The first assessment priorities must be:
   A. observation of uncontrolled bleeding or shock
   B. systematic head-to-toe assessment
   C. airway, breathing, and circulation
   D. palpation of carotid and peripheral pulses

4. The systematic assessment begins with inspection of the:
   A. head
   B. chest
   C. abdomen
   D. lungs

5. When the heart stops beating, a person is in:
   A. pulmonary arrest
   B. anaphylactic shock
   C. cardiac arrest
   D. cardiopulmonary arrest

6. When respirations cease, the person is in:
   A. cardiac arrest
   B. anaphylactic shock
   C. cardiopulmonary arrest
   D. respiratory arrest

7. In most cases, the brain begins to die after 4 minutes without oxygen due to:
   A. heart tissue's susceptibility to hypoxia
   B. nerve tissue's susceptibility to hypoxia
   C. lung tissue's susceptibility to hypoxia
   D. blood vessel tissue's susceptibility to hypoxia

8. Prompt recognition and treatment of cardiopulmonary arrest is so important due to the need to maintain the oxygen supply to the:
   A. heart
   B. brain
   C. lungs
   D. blood vessels

9. The goal of CPR is to maintain:
   A. the heartbeat until respirations are restored
   B. respirations until the heartbeat is restored
   C. circulation until the heartbeat and respirations are restored
   D. oxygenation until the heartbeat and respirations are restored

10. When cardiopulmonary arrest is suspected, the first step is to:
    A. tap the victim urgently and ask "Are you okay?"
    B. place the victim supine on a firm, flat surface
    C. put your ear near the victim's nose and mouth to listen for breathing
    D. give two full breaths

11. Check for cardiac arrest in the adult by palpating the:
    A. brachial artery on the arm nearest you
    B. brachial artery on the arm away from you
    C. carotid artery on the side of the neck nearest you
    D. carotid artery on the side of the neck away from you

12. Airway obstruction caused by a foreign body that enters the airway is:
    A. cardiac arrest
    B. respiratory arrest
    C. choking
    D. cardiopulmonary arrest

13. Grabbing the throat with one or both hands is the universal sign for:
    A. heart attack
    B. choking
    C. danger
    D. loss of consciousness

14. If the choking victim is conscious, the rescuer performs:
    A. the Heimlich maneuver
    B. CPR
    C. 15 chest compressions
    D. assessment of breathing

15. If a choking victim loses consciousness, the rescuer does a finger sweep, attempts to ventilate, straddles the victim's thighs, and gives:
    A. 5 chest compressions
    B. 15 chest compressions
    C. 5 abdominal thrusts
    D. 10 abdominal thrusts

16. Evidence of effective treatment of choking includes:
    A. expulsion of obstructing object, restoration of heartbeat, normal skin color, and decreased anxiety
    B. expulsion of obstructing object, spontaneous respirations, normal skin color, and decreased anxiety
    C. spontaneous respirations, spontaneous heartbeat, normal skin color, and decreased anxiety
    D. spontaneous respirations, expulsion of obstructing object, decreased heart beat, and decreased anxiety

17. Conditions that may lead to shock include:
    A. blood loss, electrocution, drowning
    B. severe allergic reactions, myocardial infarction, lung failure
    C. overwhelming infection, kidney failure, myocardial infarction
    D. blood loss, severe allergic reactions, overwhelming infection

18. In shock, the pulse becomes:
    A. rapid and weak, thready, imperceptible
    B. rapid and weak, bounding, perceptible
    C. slow and weak, thready, imperceptible
    D. slow and weak, bounding, imperceptible

19. In shock, blood pressure:
    A. increases
    B. stays the same
    C. expands
    D. decreases

20. In shock, the urine output:
    A. is unchanged
    B. is tinged with blood
    C. decreases
    D. increases

21. For the patient in shock, the first priority is to maintain blood flow to the:
    A. heart
    B. brain
    C. lungs
    D. kidneys

22. The legs of the patient in shock may be elevated when:
    A. the shock is caused by congestive heart failure
    B. the shock is caused by postoperative abdominal hemorrhage
    C. the shock is caused by bleeding of the head or neck
    D. intracranial pressure is increased

23. The patient in shock should be protected from:
    A. cold and given fluids
    B. heat and left uncovered
    C. cold but not overheated
    D. heat and covered up

24. In patients in shock, blood is shunted to vital internal organs as a protective response to:
    A. falling temperature
    B. rising temperature
    C. falling blood pressure
    D. rising blood pressure

25. Excessively warming the patient in shock causes blood vessels in the skin to:
    A. dilate, bringing blood supply to the vital organs
    B. dilate, bringing blood supply away from vital organs
    C. constrict, bringing blood supply away from vital organs
    D. constrict, bringing blood supply to the vital organs

26. The loss of a large amount of blood is:
    A. hemostasis
    B. homeostasis
    C. hematocrit
    D. hemorrhage

27. In an adult, what amount of blood loss may result in hypovolemic shock?
    A. 30 ml or more
    B. 1 pint or more
    C. 1 liter or more
    D. 10 liters or more

28. With external bleeding, when fracture is not suspected, the injured part is:
    A. elevated and immobilized
    B. elevated and massaged
    C. lowered and immobilized
    D. lowered and massaged

29. If direct wound pressure and elevation fail to control bleeding, pressure is applied to the:
    A. coronary heart vessels
    B. cerebral blood vessels
    C. main artery that supplies the area
    D. main vein that supplies the area

30. A break in a bone is called a:
    A. hemorrhage
    B. sprain
    C. strain
    D. fracture

31. A fracture that does not break the skin is:
    A. compound
    B. open
    C. simple (closed)
    D. complete

32. A fracture in which the ends of the broken bone protrude through the skin is:
    A. compound
    B. simple
    C. closed
    D. incomplete

33. A fracture in which the broken ends are separated is:
    A. compound
    B. simple
    C. complete
    D. incomplete

34. A fracture in which the bone ends are not separated is:
    A. complete
    B. incomplete
    C. compound
    D. simple

35. The primary symptom of fracture is:
    A. nausea
    B. itching
    C. pain
    D. hemorrhage

36. Goals of emergency nursing intervention for a patient with fractures are:
    A. avoidance of additional trauma and pain
    B. increased cardiac output and reduced fear
    C. improved cerebral blood flow and reduced fear
    D. restored patient airway and normal respirations

37. The key to emergency management of fractures is:
    A. application of cold
    B. elevation of injury
    C. immobilization
    D. application of heat

38. Injuries to muscles and/or the tendons that attach them to bones are called:
    A. dislocations
    B. strains
    C. sprains
    D. fractures

39. Emergency treatment for sprains and strains include:
    A. direct wound pressure and elevation
    B. immobilization and elevation
    C. application of heat
    D. maintenance of blood flow to brain

40. Nursing diagnoses that might apply to the patient with a head injury during the emergency phase of treatment include:
    A. decreased cardiac output related to hypovolemia, and fear related to possible impending death
    B. altered cerebral tissue perfusion related to hypovolemia, and anxiety related to panic
    C. ineffective breathing pattern related to neurologic trauma, and high risk for injury related to increasing intracranial pressure
    D. ineffective breathing pattern related to neurologic trauma, and high risk for injury related to decreasing intracranial pressure

41. The goals of emergency nursing care of the patient with a head injury are:
    A. avoidance of additional trauma and pain
    B. adequate ventilation and absence of further injury
    C. increased cardiac output and reduced fear
    D. improved cerebral blood flow and reduced fear

42. The victim of a head or neck injury must be kept flat with:
    A. head elevated at 45° angle
    B. head elevated at 90° angle
    C. cold packs applied to the head and neck
    D. proper alignment of the head and neck

43. Criteria for evaluating the achievement of nursing goals for the emergency care of the head injury patient include:
    A. immobilization of injured parts without evidence of additional injury or pain
    B. improved pulse quality, cessation of bleeding, and reduced anxiety
    C. normal respiratory rate and depth, normal pulse rate, and stable neurologic status with secure spinal immobilization
    D. increased pulse strength, increased blood pressure, and reduced fear

44. After a diving injury, while removing the victim from the water, efforts are made to:
    A. immobilize the extremities
    B. immobilize the neck and back
    C. turn the victim in a prone position
    D. turn the victim in a supine position

45. The priority nursing goal for the patient with a neck or spinal injury is to:
    A. provide adequate ventilation
    B. increase cardiac output
    C. reduce fear
    D. avoid additional injury

Introductory Nursing Care of Adults

46. Successful nursing intervention for the patient with a neck or spinal injury is based on:
    A. continuous monitoring for signs of increased intracranial pressure and oxygenation
    B. continuous immobilization of the back and spine, and transport for medical care
    C. prevention of aspiration and maintenance of circulation
    D. prevention of skin breakdown and shock

47. Nursing diagnoses for the patient with an eye injury include:
    A. impaired self-image related to change in physical capacity, and high risk for depression related to dependence
    B. impaired coping related to change in vision, and high risk for impaired tissue integrity related to irritation
    C. high risk for impaired skin integrity related to immobility, and self-care deficits related to impaired eyesight
    D. high risk for injury related to foreign body in eye, and impaired tissue integrity related to chemical trauma

48. When chemicals come in contact with the eye, the nurse should:
    A. flush with tap water to irrigate the eye for 30 minutes
    B. flush with sterile normal saline or water to irrigate the eye for 30 minutes
    C. cover with a sterile cloth and page physician immediately
    D. place patient in shower under cold water until pain is relieved

49. If bleeding is under control, the priority nursing diagnosis for a traumatic injury to the auricle is:
    A. impaired body image related to injury
    B. anemia related to blood loss
    C. impaired tissue integrity related to mechanical obstruction
    D. decreased cardiac output related to blood loss

50. The most critical chest injuries include:
    A. tension pneumothorax, ulcer, and bowel obstruction
    B. pericarditis, lung contusion, and flail chest
    C. open pneumothorax, flail chest, and cardiac tamponade
    D. lung concussion, closed pneumothorax, and pericarditis

51. Any injury at or below the nipple may cause both:
    A. chest and head injuries
    B. chest and neck injuries
    C. chest and shoulder injuries
    D. chest and abdominal injuries

52. Signs and symptoms of chest injuries that impair respirations are:
    A. dyspnea, tachycardia, decreased blood pressure, and unequal pupils
    B. dyspnea, tachycardia, restlessness, and cyanosis
    C. shallow respirations, bradycardia, lethargy and edema
    D. tachypnea, bradycardia, confusion, and cyanosis

53. Open chest wounds that penetrate the pleural cavity allowing air to enter are referred to as:
    A. pneumothorax
    B. cardiac tamponade
    C. flail chest
    D. hemothorax

54. The pneumothorax wound should be covered with which type of dressing:
    A. saline
    B. occlusive
    C. vented
    D. porous

55. The term used when several adjacent ribs are broken in more than one place is:
    A. pneumothorax
    B. cardiac tamponade
    C. flail chest
    D. hemothorax

56. The abnormal chest wall movement in flail chest would be described as what sort of motion?
    A. sawing
    B. paradoxical
    C. pulsating
    D. rhythmic

57. The abnormal chest wall action in flail chest causes:
    A. altered tissue perfusion
    B. increased cardiac output
    C. increased pulse strength
    D. impaired gas exchange

58. The accumulation of blood in the pleural cavity that causes the lung to collapse is:
    A. pneumothorax
    B. cardiac tamponade
    C. flail chest
    D. hemothorax

59. The protrusion of internal organs through a wound is called:
    A. avulsion
    B. hemorrhage
    C. evisceration
    D. decubitus

60. The main criterion for evaluating emergency nursing care of the patient with an eviscerated abdominal wound is:
    A. protection of the wound
    B. control of bleeding
    C. restoration of a strong pulse
    D. reduction in fear

61. First aid for minor superficial burns is to:
    A. apply butter to the burn
    B. apply petroleum jelly to the burn
    C. cover with cloth
    D. immerse the injured body part in cool water for 2–5 minutes

62. When a large body surface area is burned, or any area is severely burned, the nurse should:
    A. apply mediations to the burn
    B. cover the burn with a clean, dry dressing or cloth
    C. cover the burn with a cool, wet dressing or cloth
    D. apply ice to the burn

63. Evaluation of emergency care of the burn victim is based on finding:
    A. immobility as well as circulatory and respiratory status maintained
    B. absence of symptoms of shock, burned areas covered, coping supported
    C. absence of symptoms of respiratory distress, skin surfaces free of burning materials, pain reduction
    D. absence of symptoms of ileus, monitoring for signs of gastrointestinal bleeding, monitoring of circulation

64. A condition in which body temperature rises above 99°F is:
    A. hypothermia
    B. hyperthermia
    C. hypoglycemia
    D. hyperkalemia

65. Heat exhaustion is treated by:
    A. pushing fluids with caffeine
    B. warming and ambulating the victim
    C. cooling and hydrating the victim
    D. placing victim in ice

66. A patient with heat exhaustion would be considered stable when the patient exhibits:
    A. urine output of at least 10 ml/hr; pulse rate of 100 or more
    B. ability to take a regular diet without nausea
    C. below normal body temperature; bradycardia
    D. lowered body temperature; intake and retention of fluids

67. A body core temperature of 106°F or greater is:
    A. hyperthermia
    B. hypothermia
    C. heatstroke
    D. heat exhaustion

68. The skin is red, hot, and dry, and perspiration is absent in:
    A. heatstroke
    B. heat exhaustion
    C. hyperthermia
    D. hypothermia

69. Nursing diagnoses for the patient with heatstroke include:
    A. sexuality patterns, altered, related to impotence
    B. thermoregulation, ineffective, related to disease process
    C. post-trauma response related to illness
    D. hyperthermia related to heat, dehydration, and inappropriate clothing

70. Mild tissue damage caused by cold is called:
    A. frostbite
    B. frostnip
    C. hypothermia
    D. hyperthermia

71. When the body is exposed to extreme cold, blood vessels in the skin and extremities:
    A. dilate
    B. enlarge
    C. constrict
    D. swell

72. The priority nursing diagnosis for the victim of frostbite is:
    A. sensory/perceptual alterations related to decreased circulation
    B. high risk for impaired skin integrity related to vascular changes caused by extreme cold exposure
    C. high risk for infection related to tissue damage
    D. disuse syndrome related to vascular changes

73. The immediate treatment of mild cold injury is:
    A. rapid rewarming
    B. massaging to increase circulation
    C. covering with dressing
    D. immersing in tepid water

74. A decrease in the body core temperature below 95°F is:
    A. frostnip
    B. frostbite
    C. cold exhaustion
    D. hypothermia

75. Nursing diagnoses for the elderly patient with hypo-thermia include:
    A. impaired tissue perfusion related to lack of oxygen
    B. increased cardiac output related to dysrhyth-mias associated with rewarming
    C. thought process, altered, related to rewarming
    D. severe hypothermia related to exposure to cold

76. Any substance that, in small quantities, is capable of causing illness or harm following ingestion is:
    A. antitoxin
    B. emetic
    C. poison
    D. antiemetic

77. Carbon monoxide poisoning occurs because carbon monoxide:
    A. is blown off too rapidly during exhalation
    B. binds to hemoglobin and occupies sites needed to transport oxygen to the cells
    C. binds to white blood cells and causes infection
    D. is retained and prevents oxygen from being inhaled in adequate amounts

78. The primary nursing diagnosis for the victim of carbon monoxide poisoning is:
    A. impaired gas exchange related to carbon mon-oxide poisoning
    B. ineffective breathing pattern related to thick secretions
    C. high risk for aspiration related to difficulty swallowing
    D. anxiety related to ineffective breathing pat-tern

79. The primary nursing diagnosis for the victim of drug or chemical poisoning is:
    A. altered thought process related to lack of oxy-gen to the brain
    B. high risk for infection related to break in skin
    C. high risk for injury related to poison
    D. high risk for suffocation related to chemical injury of oral airway

80. Nursing diagnoses for the patient who has been bitten include:
    A. decreased cardiac output related to dysrhyth-mias
    B. high risk for infection related to bite, and high risk for injury related to exposure to allergens or toxins
    C. fear related to effects of epinephrine
    D. high risk for suffocation related to swelling of airway

81. Goals of nursing care for the emergency treatment of bite victims include:
    A. disinfection and isolation of area
    B. control of toxic effects of epinephrine re-lease
    C. wound cleanliness, and absence of allergic re-action or toxic effects
    D. prevention of further injury

82. Local effects of venom on blood and blood vessels include:
    A. skin breakdown, petechiae, and clubbing of nails
    B. coolness of extremities, shiny skin, and blood clots
    C. discoloration, pain, and edema
    D. brittle nails, hair loss, and cellulitis

83. After a bite, epinephrine may be given to prevent:
    A. hypotension
    B. aspiration
    C. blood clots
    D. anaphylaxis

84. A victim of a bite would be considered improved when:
    A. wound has only clear or white drainage, pulse is 100 or less, and respiratory rate is in-creased
    B. patient is sleepy but able to be aroused, wound has only slight drainage, and only slight toxic effect are noted
    C. patient is alert, respiratory rate is 30 or more, and blood pressure is normal
    D. wound is free of debris, patient is alert with-out dyspnea, and specific toxic effects are absent

85. Injuries to ligaments are called:
    A. strains
    B. fractures
    C. sprains
    D. dislocations

Surgical Care

OBJECTIVES

1. State the purpose of each type of surgery: diagnostic, exploratory, curative, palliative, and cosmetic.
2. List data to be included in the nursing assessment of the preoperative patient.
3. Identify the nursing diagnoses, goals, and interventions during the preoperative phase of the surgical experience.
4. Outline a preoperative teaching plan.
5. List the responsibilities of each member of the surgical team.
6. Explain the nursing implications of each type of anesthesia.
7. Explain how the nurse can help prevent postoperative complications.
8. List data to be included in the nursing assessment of the postoperative patient.
9. Identify nursing diagnoses, goals, and interventions for the postoperative patient.
10. Explain patient needs to be considered in discharge planning.

LEARNING ACTIVITIES

I.   Match the definition on the left with the most appropriate term on the right.

____ 1. Relieves symptoms or improves function without correcting the basic problem

____ 2. Bloody

____ 3. Protrusion of body organs through an open wound

____ 4. Containing serum

____ 5. Separation of previously joined edges: reopening of a surgical wound

____ 6. Made up of blood and serum

A. Sanguineous

B. Serous

C. Serosanguineous

D. Dehiscence

E. Evisceration

F. Palliative

II.   Match the definition on the left with the most appropriate term on the right.

____ 1. A device that uses a photoelectric sensor to measure the oxygen saturation of the blood

____ 2. A physician who specializes in the administration of anesthetics and monitors the patient while under anesthesia

____ 3. An agent that abolishes the pain

____ 4. Reduction in body temperature

____ 5. A registered nurse who specializes in the administration of anesthetics and monitors the condition of patients receiving anesthetics

A. Anesthesiologist

B. Hypothermia

C. Anesthetic

D. Nurse anesthetist

E. Oximeter

III.   Match the definition or example on the left with the most appropriate term on the right.

____ 1. Repair of congenitally damaged structures

____ 2. Surgery to flatten the abdomen or change the size of the breasts

____ 3. Ablation, or removal of tissue

____ 4. Biopsy of skin lesion or lump in breast tissue

____ 5. Surgery to change the shape of facial features or remove wrinkles

____ 6. Repair of damaged tissue

____ 7. Opening a body cavity to diagnose and find out the extent of a disease process

____ 8. Surgery to relieve symptoms or improve function without correcting the basic problem

____ 9. Cleft lip repair

____ 10. Use of specialized scopes inserted into the body through small incisions

A. Cosmetic surgery

B. Palliative surgery

C. Curative surgery

D. Exploratory surgery

E. Diagnostic surgery

IV.   List 3 reasons why older persons are often at greater risk for surgical complications.

1.

2.

3.

V.   Match the surgical complications on the left with the related conditions on the right. Answers may be used more than once.)

1. Increased risk of pulmonary complications as a result of anesthesia or hypotension

____ A. Liver disease

____ B. Chronic respiratory disease

2. Excessive bleeding

____ C. Bleeding disorders

3. Impaired wound healing

____ D. Diabetes mellitus

4. Cardiac complications related to anesthesia and stress of surgery

____ E. Heart disease

5. Heal more slowly

6. Drug toxicity due to inability to metabolize drugs effectively

7. Greater risk for infection

VI.   List 2 reasons why smoking increases the risk of pulmonary complications.

1.

2.

VII.   List 3 goals of nursing care for the patient during the preoperative phase.

1.

2.

3.

VIII.   List 4 diagnostic test that are done preoperatively.

1.   3.

2.   4.

IX.   List 5 factors related to the patient's past medical history that need to be recorded before surgery.

1.   4.

2.   5.

3.

X.   List data to be collected as part of the physical examination of a surgical patient. Fill in the blanks.

1. Skin: Inspect for _____ , _____ , and _____ .

2. Skin: Palpate to assess _____ , _____ ,

_____ , and _____ .

Introductory Nursing Care of Adults
Copyright © 1995 by W.B. Saunders Company. All rights reserved.

3. Thorax: Observe respiratory _____ , _____ , and

   _____ .

4. Thorax: Auscultate lungs to assess _____ .

5. Thorax: Assess apical heart beat for _____ and _____ .

6. Abdomen: Inspect for _____ and _____ .

7. Abdomen: Auscultate for _____ .

8. Extremities: Inspect for _____ , _____ ,

   _____ , and _____ .

9. Extremities: Assess _____ ; listen for _____ ; note

   _____ or _____ .

10. Prosthesis: Note presence of any prosthetic devices, such as _____ , _____ ,

    _____ , _____ , and _____ .

XI.   List 2 nursing diagnoses for the preoperative patient, and 2 nursing goals of preoperative
       care.

   Nursing diagnoses:

   1.

   2

   Nursing goals:

   1.

   2.

XII.   List 3 factors to tell the family as a part of preoperative teaching.

   1.

   2.

   3.

XIII.   List the 4 components of a consent form for surgery.

   1.   3.

   2.   4.

XIV.   What preparation of the digestive tract is done for patients having surgery on the abdomen
        or the digestive tract itself?

XV.   List 3 purposes of bowel cleansing.

1.

2.

3.

XVI.   Explain why adult patients are given nothing by mouth from midnight before the scheduled surgery.

XVII.   List 3 classifications of drugs that are given preoperatively.

1.

2.

3.

XVIII.   List 2 factors the patient should be told following administration of preoperative medications.

1.

2.

XIX.   List 3 nursing interventions following administration of the preoperative medication.

1.

2.

3.

XX.   List 6 parts of the preoperative checklist which must be completed before surgery.

1.

2.

3.

4.

5.

6.

XXI.   List 2 criteria for achievement of nursing goals for the preoperative patient.

1.

2.

XXII.   Match the definition on the left with the most appropriate term on the right.

_____   1. Person who administers anesthesia and monitors the patient's status throughout the procedure

_____   2. Person who assesses the patient, plans intraoperative nursing care, and maintains patient safety; person in charge of the operating room

_____   3. Physician who specializes in anesthesia

_____   4. Person who handles instruments within the sterile field during surgery

_____   5. Person who operates the heart bypass machine during open heart surgery

_____   6. Registered nurse with special training in anesthesia

_____   7. Person who actually performs the surgical procedure

A. Scrub nurse or scrub tech

B. Surgeon

C. Circulating registered nurse

D. Nurse anesthetist

E. Nurse anesthetist or anesthesiologist

F. Perfusionist

G. Anesthesiologist

XXIII.   List 3 ways by which local anesthetics may be administered.

1.

2.

3.

XXIV.   List 3 complications of local anesthesia.

1.

2.

3.

XXV.   List 4 methods by which general anesthetic agents can be given.

1.   3.

2.   4.

XXVI.   List 2 reasons for inserting an endotracheal tube into the patient's trachea during surgery.

1.

2.

XXVII. List 5 nursing diagnoses and 5 nursing goals for patients in the intraoperative phase.

Nursing Diagnoses

1.
2.
3.
4.
5.

Nursing Goals

1.
2.
3.
4.
5.

XXVIII. List 3 factors that may cause complications of surgery.

1.
2.
3.

XXIX. List 2 reasons why shock is likely to occur in the immediate postoperative period.

1.
2.

XXX. List 3 causes of postoperative low blood volume (hypovolemia).

1.
2.
3.

XXXI. List 4 reasons why hypoxia may occur in the immediate postoperative period.

1.
2.
3.
4.

XXXII. Match the conditions which may cause postoperative hypoxia on the left with the effect on the right.

____ 1. Spasm of larynx or bronchi

____ 2. General anesthesia

____ 3. Anesthesia

____ 4. Patient is unconscious

A. Depress cough and swallowing reflex

B. Narrows airway and obstructs air flow

C. Tongue falls back and blocks airway

D. Depress respirations

XXXIII. List 3 classifications of drugs that depress respiratory function and cause pulmonary
secretions to be drier and thicker.

1.

2.

3.

XXXIV. List 3 complications of postoperative wound healing.

1.

2.

3.

XXXV. Match each description on the left with the appropriate wound complication on the right.

____ 1. Most likely to occur between the 5th and 12th
postoperative days

____ 2. Protrusion of body organs through the open
wound

____ 3. Reopening of the surgical wound

____ 4. Likely to happen when there is excessive strain
on the suture line

A. Dehiscence

B. Evisceration

XXXVI. List 4 common gastrointestinal problems that follow surgery.

1.

2.

3.

4.

XXXVII. List 5 factors that cause postoperative gastrointestinal problems.

1.

2.

3.

4.

5.

XXXVIII. List 4 factors that may cause peristalsis to be impaired after surgery.

1.

2.

3.

4.

XXXIX. List 3 causes of urinary retention following surgery.

1.

2.

3.

XL. List 5 nursing diagnoses for the patient in the immediate postoperative phase when the patient is recovering from anesthesia, as well as 5 nursing goals for this phase.

1.   1.

2.   2.

3.   3.

4.   4.

5.   5.

XLI. List 4 signs and symptoms of impending shock.

1.

2.

3.

4.

XLII. List 3 measures to reduce the risk of shock.

1.

2.

3.

XLIII. List 3 nursing measures to reduce the risk of hypoxia during the immediate postoperative period.

1.

2.

3.

XLIV. List 5 criteria for evaluating the outcomes of nursing goals in the immediate postoperative phase.

1.

2.

3.

4.

5.

XLV.   List 5 conditions that determine when the patient can be moved from the recovery room to the nursing unit.

1.   4.

2.   5.

3.

XLVI.   List 4 safety precautions that should be taken when the patient is transferred to his or her own bed on the nursing unit.

1.   3.

2.   4.

XLVII.   List 5 critical elements of the assessment of the postoperative patient.

1.   4.

2.   5.

3.

XLVIII. List 11 nursing diagnoses of the postoperative period.

1.

2.

3.

4.

5.

6.

7.

8.

9.

10.

11.

IL.   List 12 goals of nursing care after recovery from anesthesia.

1.   7.

2.   8.

3.   9.

4.   10.

5.   11.

6.   12.

L. List 4 nursing measures for pain management in the early postoperative phase.

1.

2.

3.

4.

LI. List 5 classic signs and symptoms of wound infection.

1.

2.

3.

4.

5.

LII. List 2 principles of prevention of wound infection.

1.

2.

LIII. List 4 nursing measures to prevent the introduction of infectious organisms to a wound.

1.

2.

3.

4.

LIV. List 2 measures to support the patient's healing and resistance to infection.

1.

2.

LV. List 6 signs and symptoms of pneumonia for which the nurse should observe postoperatively.

1.   4.

2.   5.

3.   6.

LVI. List 3 types of surgeries in which coughing is contraindicated.

1.

2.

3.

LVII.   List 3 measures to prevent thrombophlebitis and related pulmonary emboli.

1.

2.

3.

LVIII.   List 4 signs and symptoms that would alert the nurse to possible pulmonary emboli.

1.   3.

2.   4.

LIX.   List 5 measures which may be ordered in the *early* postoperative period to promote the passage of flatus.

1.   4.

2.   5.

3.

LX.   List 4 characteristics of paralytic ileus.

1.   3.

2.   4.

LXI.   List 11 criteria for evaluating the outcomes of nursing goals for the surgical patient listed below.

1. Pain:

2. Impaired tissue integrity:

3. High risk for infection:

4. Impaired gas exchange:

5. Urinary retention:

6. Colonic constipation:

7. High risk for fluid volume deficit:

8. Altered nutrition: less than body requirements:

9. Impaired physical mobility:

10. Body image disturbance:

11. Knowledge deficit:

LXII. Using Figure 14–10, label each method of wound closure (A–E). (Figure from Ignatavicius, D. D., & Bayne, M. V. [1991]. *Medical-surgical nursing: A nursing process approach.* Philadelphia: W. B. Saunders.)

A.

B.

C.

D.

E.

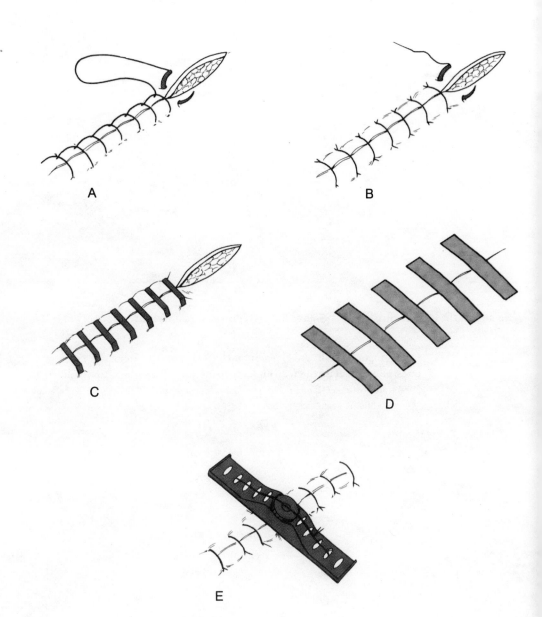

LXIII. Using Figure 14–9, label each (A and B) complication of wound healing. (Figure from Ignatavicius, D. D., & Bayne, M. V. [1991]. *Medical-surgical nursing: A nursing process approach.* Philadelphia: W. B. Saunders.)

A.

B.

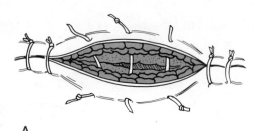

LXIV. Using Figure 14–8, label each part (A–H) of the drawing representing inhalation anesthesia given through an endotracheal tube. (Figure from Ignatavicius, D. D., & Bayne, M. V. [1991]. *Medical-surgical nursing: A nursing process approach.* Philadelphia: W. B. Saunders.)

A.

B.

C.

D.

E.

F.

G.

H.

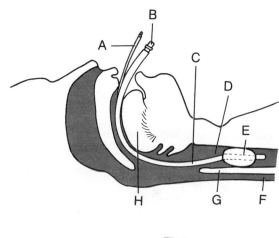

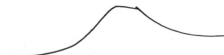

LXV. Match each preoperative medication on the left with every appropriate classification and action on the right.

___ 1. glycopyrrolate (Robinul)

___ 2. chloral hydrate (Noctec)

___ 3. promethazine hydrochloride (Phenergan)

___ 4. pentobarbital sodium (Nembutal)

___ 5. diazepam (Valium)

___ 6. hydroxyzine hydrochloride (Vistaril, Atarax)

___ 7. atropine sulfate

___ 8. meperidine hydrochloride (Demerol)

___ 9. secobarbital sodium (Seconal Sodium)

___ 10. morphine sulfate (MS Contin, Duramorph)

A. narcotic analgesic

B. anticholinergic

C. sedative or hypnotic

D. antiemetic

E. skeletal muscle relaxant

F. antimotion sickness

LXVI. The patient who has had surgery is at risk for a number of complications. List 8 surgical complications which may occur in the postoperative period.

1.

2.

3.

4.

5.

6.

7.

8.

LXVII. Choose the most appropriate answer.

1. The surgical patient who is malnourished is at risk for:
   A. excessive bleeding and hemorrhage
   B. drug toxicity and ineffective metabolism
   C. cardiac complications and dyspnea
   D. poor wound healing and infection

2. Obese surgical patients are likely to have postoperative:
   A. infection and increased temperature
   B. excessive bleeding and hemorrhage
   C. headache and bradycardia
   D. respiratory and wound complications

3. Excess body fluid in the surgical patient can overload the:
   A. brain
   B. heart
   C. muscles
   D. lungs

4. Electrolyte imbalances may predispose the surgical patient to:
   A. cardiac arrhythmias
   B. lung complications
   C. liver malfunctions
   D. bone tissue loss

5. Before surgery, a patient must sign a legal document called a(n):
   A. bill of rights
   B. consent form
   C. advanced directive
   D. living will

6. If the patient is a minor, who signs the surgical consent form?
   A. physician
   B. registered nurse
   C. parent or guardian
   D. close relative

7. Shaving the skin in preparation for surgery is often delayed until shortly before surgery in order to:
   A. improve wound healing
   B. control bleeding
   C. allow less time for organisms to multiply
   D. prevent postoperative edema

8. The use of local anesthetics that block the conduction of nerve impulses in a specific area is called:
   A. general anesthesia
   B. sedative anesthesia
   C. anticonvulsant anesthesia
   D. regional anesthesia

9. The injection of an anesthetic agent into and under the skin around the area of treatment is called:
   A. local infiltration
   B. topical administration
   C. nerve block technique
   D. intravenous infusion

10. One complication of spinal anesthesia is:
    A. tachycardia
    B. hemorrhage
    C. headache
    D. shock

11. Postspinal headache can be relieved by:
    A. elevating the head of the bed
    B. lying flat
    C. early ambulation
    D. coughing and deep breathing

12. A "blood patch" may help treat:
    A. hemorrhage
    B. postspinal headache
    C. shock
    D. tachycardia

13. Signs and symptoms of local anesthesia toxicity include:
    A. initially, CNS depression, then CNS and cardiovascular stimulation
    B. initially, CNS stimulation, then cardiovascular stimulation
    C. initially, CNS depression, then cardiovascular depression
    D. initially, CNS stimulation, then CNS and cardiovascular depression

14. Inhalation anesthetic agents and the endotracheal tube can causes irritation of the:
    A. lungs and the brain
    B. skin and the heart
    C. kidney and the liver
    D. respiratory tract and the larynx

15. A life-threatening complication of inhalation anesthesia characterized by increasing body temperature and metabolic rate, tachycardia, hypotension, cyanosis, and muscle rigidity is called:
    A. anaphylactic shock
    B. malignant hyperthermia
    C. hypotensive shock
    D. hyperglycemia

16. Inadequate oxygenation of body tissues is called:
    A. hypotension
    B. hypovolemia
    C. hypoxia
    D. hypoglycemia

17. An infection of the lungs due to immobility is called:
    A. hypovolemic pleurisy
    B. hypertensive bronchitis
    C. hypostatic pneumonia
    D. hyperglycemic asthma

18. When peristalsis is slow, gas builds up, causing:
    A. cramping pain and distention
    B. diarrhea and tachycardia
    C. fever and infection
    D. nausea and vomiting

19. "Gas pains" typically occur:
    A. during surgery
    B. immediately after surgery
    C. 6 hours after surgery
    D. second or third day after surgery

20. With urinary retention, the kidneys:
    A. produce no urine and the patient is unable to empty the bladder
    B. produce urine and the patient is able to empty the bladder
    C. produce no urine and the patient is able to empty the bladder
    D. produce urine but the patient is unable to empty the bladder

21. The inflammation of veins with the formation of blood clots is:
    A. hemorrhage
    B. shock
    C. thrombophlebitis
    D. pericarditis

22. Clots that cling to the walls of blood vessels are called:
    A. emboli
    B. platelets
    C. thrombi
    D. anticoagulants

23. If pain is felt when the foot is dorsiflexed to assess for pain in the calf, this finding is called:
    A. negative Homans's sign
    B. positive Chvostek's sign
    C. negative Chvostek's sign
    D. positive Homans's sign

24. If intravenous fluids are given too rapidly postoperatively, they can overload the circulatory system, causing:
    A. lung failure
    B. heart failure
    C. brain failure
    D. kidney failure

25. What is used to monitor the oxygenation of the blood?
    A. sphygmomanometer
    B. ECG
    C. oximeter
    D. stethoscope

26. When regional block anesthesia is used during surgery, the nurse must remember that after surgery:
    A. sensation in the area is impaired
    B. circulation in the area is impaired
    C. infection is likely to occur
    D. fever may make the patient drowsy

27. Once the immediate postoperative phase has passed, what risks lessen?
    A. fever and infection
    B. pneumonia and atelectasis
    C. shock and hypoxia
    D. thrombophlebitis and decubitus ulcer

28. Two common narcotic analgesics that are given postoperatively are:
    A. Tylenol and aspirin
    B. meperidine and morphine
    C. codeine and tincture of opium
    D. alprazolam and diazepam

29. Clean sutured incisions heal by:
    A. first intention
    B. second intention
    C. third intention
    D. fourth intention

30. After the first 24 hours following surgery, what should be reported to the physician, if observed?
    A. respirations of 20
    B. temperature of 98.8°F
    C. blood pressure of 110/70
    D. continued or excessive bleeding

31. A soft tube that permits passive movement of fluids from the wound is called a:
    A. active drain
    B. Hemovac
    C. Penrose drain
    D. Jackson-Pratt

32. In the immediate postoperative phase, wound drainage is often bright red; as the amount of blood in the drainage decreases, the fluid becomes:
    A. straw colored, then clear and pink
    B. clear, then pink and straw colored
    C. pink, then clear and straw colored
    D. pink, then straw colored and clear

33. What may precede wound dehiscence?
    A. a sudden decrease in wound drainage
    B. a sudden increase in wound drainage
    C. a sudden increase in temperature
    D. a sudden decrease in appetite

34. If evisceration occurs, the usual practice is to cover the wound with:
    A. dry sterile dressings
    B. saline-soaked gauze with a dry dressing over it
    C. antibiotic ointment and dry dressings
    D. steroid ointments and dry dressings

35. Signs and symptoms of wound infection usually do not develop until the:
    A. first hour after surgery
    B. sixth hour after surgery
    C. first day after surgery
    D. third to fifth day after surgery

36. What specimen should be taken before antibiotics are begun?
   A. urine sample
   B. blood test
   C. stool culture
   D. wound culture

37. While awaiting results of the culture and sensitivity test, the physician often orders a:
   A. narcotic analgesic
   B. bronchodilator
   C. broad-spectrum antibiotic
   D. cholinergic blocker

38. To prevent pneumonia, the patient must be assisted to turn initially every:
   A. 5 minutes
   B. 15 minutes
   C. 2 hours
   D. 6 hours

39. A device used to promote lung expansion is the:
   A. Penrose drain
   B. sphygmomanometer
   C. inhaler
   D. incentive spirometer

40. If patients develop pneumonia, they are treated with rest, oxygen, and:
   A. antibiotics
   B. narcotics
   C. anticholinergics
   D. vasopressors

41. Emboli may be treated with:
   A. Dilantin and anticonvulsants
   B. morphine and analgesics
   C. heparin and thrombolytic agents
   D. Lasix and diuretics

42. In the early postoperative phase, the nurse must monitor signs of:
   A. diuresis or kidney failure
   B. urinary retention or kidney failure
   C. urinary retention or deep breathing
   D. deep breathing and coughing

43. Urinary function is monitored postoperatively by monitoring:
   A. intake and output and bladder distention
   B. vital signs and kidney pain
   C. cramping and abdominal pain
   D. peripheral edema and chest distention

44. If the patient is unable to void, what is necessary?
   A. vital signs
   B. daily weights
   C. catheterization
   D. clear liquid diet

45. Some agencies have policies that limit the amount of urine that can be drained from a full bladder at one time; these limits are usually:
   A. 5–10 ml
   B. 50–100 ml
   C. 400–500 ml
   D. 750–1000 ml

46. Most patients pass flatus:
   A. 15 minutes after surgery
   B. 1 hour after surgery
   C. 48 hours after surgery
   D. 1 week after surgery

47. The best way to prevent gastrointestinal discomfort postoperatively is:
   A. administration of antacids
   B. early, frequent ambulation
   C. administration of laxatives
   D. early, frequent meals

48. Which surgical drain works by creating negative pressure when the receptacle is compressed?
   A. Penrose
   B. urinary
   C. Hemovac
   D. passive

49. A clean wound with minimal tissue destruction and minimal tissue reaction begins to heal as the edges are:
   A. left open
   B. joined by sutures or staples
   C. allowed to heal from the inside out
   D. closed surgically

50. A "hairline" or fine scar is seen in healing with:
   A. first intention
   B. second intention
   C. third intention
   D. fourth intention

51. One way to prevent shock as a surgical complication is to:
   A. keep airway in place until patient is alert
   B. splint incision during activity
   C. keep IV fluid rate on schedule
   D. change position at least every 3 hours

LXVIII. Match the treatment on the left with the complication for which it is used on the right. (Some answers may be used more than once.)

___ 1. Administer oxygen

___ 2. Catheterization as ordered

___ 3. Give intravenous fluids as ordered. Encourage oral intake when allowed.

___ 4. Ambulate frequently when permitted. Laxatives or enemas, or both, as ordered.

___ 5. Vasopressors (drugs to raise blood pressure) as ordered

___ 6. Suction as necessary

___ 7. Cover the open wound with a sterile dressing. If organs protrude, saturate the dressing with normal saline. Notify physician. Keep patient still and quiet.

___ 8. Antiemetic drugs as ordered

___ 9. Encourage deep breathing and coughing

___ 10. Bedrest. Anticoagulant therapy as ordered.

___ 11. Rectal tube, heat to abdomen, bisacodyl suppositories as ordered. Position on right side. Nasogastric intubation with suction as ordered.

___ 12. Fluid or blood replacement

___ 13. Rest. Oxygen and antibiotics as ordered.

___ 14. Additional surgery to control bleeding

A. Fluid and electrolyte imbalances

B. Altered elimination

C. Impaired wound healing

D. Shock

E. Digestive disturbances

F. Hypoxia

G. Thrombophlebitis

H. Inadequate oxygenation; pneumonia

15

Intravenous Therapy

OBJECTIVES

1. Identify the indications for intravenous fluid therapy.
2. Describe the types of fluids used for intravenous fluid therapy.
3. Describe the types of venous access devices used for intravenous therapy.
4. Given the prescribed hourly flow rate, calculate the correct drop rate for an intravenous fluid.
5. Explain the causes, signs and symptoms, and nursing implications of the complications of intravenous fluid or drug therapy.
6. Explain the nursing responsibilities when a patient is receiving intravenous therapy.

LEARNING ACTIVITIES

I.   Match the definition on the left with the most appropriate term on the right.

____ 1. A liquid containing one or more dissolved substances

____ 2. A term used to describe a solution that has a higher concentration of electrolytes than normal body fluids

____ 3. Stationary blood clot

____ 4. An obstruction of a blood vessel created by a trapped blood clot or other substance

____ 5. A term used to describe a solution that has the same concentration of electrolytes as normal body fluids

____ 6. An unattached blood clot or other substance in the circulatory system

____ 7. A collection of infused fluid in tissues surrounding a cannula inserted for intravenous therapy

____ 8. A term used to describe a solution that has a lower concentration of electrolytes than normal body fluids

____ 9. A tube that can be inserted into a body cavity or duct; needle or catheter employed for intravenous therapy

____ 10. A measure of the concentration of electrolytes in a fluid.

____ 11. Escape of fluid or blood from a blood vessel into body tissue

____ 12. Inflammation of blood vessel

A.   Embolism

B.   Hypotonic

C.   Cannula

D.   Phlebitis

E.   Solution

F.   Embolus

G.   Hypertonic

H.   Extravasation

I.   Isotonic

J.   Infiltration

K.   Tonicity

L.   Thrombus

II. Match the definition or description on the left with the most appropriate term on the right.

____ 1. Used for in-and-out therapy; therapy of short duration; for infants; adults with poor veins; occasionally for peripheral IV therapy

____ 2. Hickman-Broviac catheters inserted by physicians

____ 3. Small, plastic tubes that fit over or inside needles

____ 4. Needles and catheters

____ 5. Inserted in antecubital space, advanced into axillary subclavian vein or superior vena cava

A. Catheters

B. Winged infusion needle

C. Tunneled catheters

D. Cannulas

E. Peripherally inserted central catheters

III. Match the definition or description on the left with the most appropriate term on the right.

____ 1. Main infusion rate set by nurses, saves time, prevents accidental delivery of large amounts of fluid

____ 2. Implanted under skin, allows immediate access to vein without repeated venipunctures

____ 3. Short cannula with attached injection port; usually flushed with dilute heparin or saline solution

____ 4. Given through injection port in tubing of continuous infusion

A. Piggyback infusion

B. Infusion port

C. Heparin lock (saline lock)

D. Infusion pump

IV. Match the description on the left with the corresponding IV complication on the right.

____ 1. Piece of catheter breaks off in vein

____ 2. Skin torn or irritated by tape or insertion of cannula

____ 3. Attached blood clot

____ 4. Obstruction caused by trapped embolus

____ 5. Collection of infused fluid in tissue surrounding the cannula

____ 6. Unattached blood clot

____ 7. Inflammation of the vein

A. Thrombus

B. Embolism

C. Infiltration; extravasation

D. Catheter embolus

E. Embolus

F. Trauma

G. Phlebitis

. Match the signs and symptoms on the left with the complications on the right.

___ 1. Decreased blood pressure

___ 2. Site red and warm, with purulent drainage

___ 3. Shortness of breath, shock, hypotension

___ 4. Rising blood pressure, bounding pulse, edema

___ 5. Redness, warmth, tenderness near insertion site

___ 6. Pain, burning sensation, pale and puffy site, may feel hard and cool

A. Infection

B. Phlebitis

C. Air embolism

D. Infiltration

E. Blood loss

F. Fluid volume excess

I. Fill in the blanks.

1. Irrigation of an occluded IV cannula is not recommended because _____

_____.

2. If air accidentally enters a central line, the patient should be positioned so that he or she is _____

_____.

VII. Choose the most appropriate answer.

1. Tonicity of IV fluid is important because it affects:
   A. blood excretion
   B. blood volume
   C. blood weight
   D. blood vessels

2. The most commonly used IV solutions include:
   A. water with dextrose and sodium chloride solutions
   B. water with packed cells, blood, and glucose
   C. saline with albumin
   D. saline with dextrose

3. Normal saline is:
   A. 0.25% sodium chloride
   B. 0.5% sodium chloride
   C. 0.9% sodium chloride
   D. 1.5% sodium chloride

4. An IV solution of 0.45% sodium chloride is:
   A. hypertonic
   B. isotonic
   C. hypotonic
   D. equivalent

5. An IV solution of 0.45% sodium chloride is given if the patient's body fluids are:
   A. dilute
   B. isotonic
   C. alkaline
   D. concentrated

6. Advantages of PIC (peripherally inserted central catheters) over peripheral cannulas include:
   A. they can be left in place longer, create some arm restriction, replacement once a week
   B. dressing changes every week, can infuse medications more safely, smaller cannula
   C. can infuse medications more quickly, smaller dressing, smaller cannula
   D. they can be left in place longer, create less arm restriction, less traumatic to vein

7. Advantages of PIC (peripherally inserted central catheters) over other central catheters include:
   A. smaller needle, cost savings, no risk of infection
   B. easier insertion, less expensive, reduced risk of infection
   C. remaining in place longer, fewer dressing changes, no risk of dislodgement
   D. easier insertion, cost savings, reduced risk of pneumothorax or air embolism

8. The IV cannula and tubing are usually changed every:
   A. hour, up to a maximum of 2 hours
   B. 4 hours, up to a maximum of 8 hours
   C. 48 hours, up to a maximum of 72 hours
   D. 120 hours, up to a maximum of 168 hours

9. Factors affecting IV infusion rates include:
   A. Needle diameter, venting of fluid container, and respiratory status
   B. Height of container, volume of fluid in container, needle diameter
   C. Position of extremity, glomerular filtration rate, and venous valves
   D. Height of the bed, position of all extremities, and venous return

10. In order to calculate the IV infusion rate, the nurse must know:
    A. ordered fluid volume per hour and number of drops equal to 1 ml in tubing set
    B. how to set the ml per minute on the IV infusion pump
    C. ordered fluid volume minus urine output
    D. ordered fluid volume and the prior 24 hour IV intake

11. Symptoms of an air embolus include:
    A. pulmonary edema, frothy, pink sputum, feeling of doom
    B. chest pain, diminished respirations, lethargy
    C. shortness of breath, hypotension, possibly shock and cardiac arrest
    D. nausea, vomiting and diarrhea, hepatomegaly, pink sputum

12. Edema, coolness, and pain at the IV insertion site is an indication of:
    A. thrombophlebitis
    B. infection
    C. air embolus
    D. infiltration

13. Redness, swelling, and warmth characterize:
    A. inflammation and infection
    B. infiltration and air embolus
    C. blood loss and hemorrhage
    D. catheter embolus and fluid volume loss

14. Signs of fluid volume excess include:
    A. dry mouth, confusion, nausea
    B. increasing blood pressure, bounding pulse, dyspnea
    C. inflammation, redness, purulent drainage
    D. increased urine output, shock, weakness

15. If signs of fluid volume excess occur, the nurse:
    A. slows the infusion rate, turns the patient to the right side, and gives pain medication
    B. slows the infusion rate, elevates the head of the bed, and notifies the physician or charge nurse
    C. elevates the head of the bed, checks the vital signs, and calls the charge nurse
    D. stops the infusion, lowers the head of the bed and notifies the physician or charge nurse

16. Irrigation of an occluded cannula is not recommended because it may:
    A. damage a venous valve
    B. introduce an air embolus
    C. force clots into the bloodstream
    D. cause the patient pain

17. If air accidentally enters a central line, the patient is
    A. turned on the left side with head lowered
    B. turned on the left side with the head of bed raised at 30° angle
    C. turned on the right side with the head of bed raised at 30° angle
    D. turned on the right side with the head of the bed lowered

18. The patient with an air embolus is placed in a special position to:
    A. trap air in the left atrium so it can be gradually absorbed
    B. trap air in the right ventricle so it is not transferred to the lungs
    C. trap air in the left ventricle so it is not transferred to the lungs
    D. trap air in the right atrium so it can be gradually absorbed

19. When a central catheter is inserted or removed, the patient is instructed to:
    A. take a deep breath and hold it for 30 seconds
    B. take a deep breath and bear down
    C. breathe normally
    D. hold breath for 30 seconds

When a central catheter is inserted or removed, it is important to:
A. help prevent air from entering the lungs
B. help prevent air from entering the blood stream
C. help air enter the blood stream
D. help air enter the lungs

The criteria for evaluating the nursing care of a patient with an IV include the absence of:
A. palpitations, pain and redness at the infusion site
B. blood return, swelling and pain at the infusion site
C. edema, pallor, redness, and drainage at the infusion site
D. movement, erythema, and firmness at the infusion site

As you are making your morning rounds at 7:00 a.m., you note that Ms. Cadena's IV has 900 ml and is running at 75 ml/hour. When you check the IV on your 10:00 a.m. rounds, you note that she now has only 100 ml remaining. What signs and symptoms do you need to be alert for with this patient?
A. bounding pulse
B. nausea and vomiting
C. dehydration
D. productive cough

Which nursing intervention may prevent fluid volume excess from occurring?
A. Encourage the patient to ambulate
B. Encourage the patient to cough
C. Time tape the IV bag and monitor closely
D. Keep an accurate Intake and Output record

While observing your patient, you note that he is complaining of crushing chest pain, difficulty breathing, and has a rapid thready pulse. You suspect he is experiencing an air embolism. What interventions are appropriate?
A. Turn the patient to the left side, raise the head of the bed, and notify the charge nurse or physician.
B. Turn the patient to the left side, lower the head of the bed, and notify the charge nurse or physician.
C. Place the patient on his back, lower the head of the bed, and notify the charge nurse.
D. Ambulate the patient for 15 minutes and notify the charge nurse.

Which of the following are indications for initiating IV therapy?
A. maintenance of intake and output
B. maintenance of fluid and electrolyte balance
C. decreasing body temperature
D. increasing rate and rhythm of respirations

26. The patient is not systemically edematous. However, the hand in which the IV catheter was inserted is puffy and cool. This is a sign of:
A. phlebitis
B. infection
C. infiltration
D. air embolus

27. When the IV line has infiltrated, nursing interventions include:
A. discontinue IV, apply ice, and place area lower than the heart
B. slow down the IV rate, apply ice, and elevate affected arm
C. discontinue IV and have it restarted in a different vein; elevate affected arm
D. slow down the IV rate, apply warm compresses, and place the area lower than the heart

28. You check your patient's IV site and find that his vein is cordlike. The IV is running well, but the site is red and the patient tells you the site is "sore when touched." These are signs of:
A. infiltration
B. catheter embolus
C. air embolus
D. phlebitis

29. What does "a tubing has a drop factor of 15" mean?
A. The tubing will deliver 15 ml of fluid for every drop.
B. The tubing will deliver 1 ml of fluid for every 15 drops.
C. The tubing will deliver 1 ml of fluid in 15 minutes.
D. The tubing will deliver 15 ml of fluid in 1 minute.

30. The nurse checked the patient's IV 1 hour ago and it was running at the correct rate of 50 ml/hour. Now the nurse finds that the IV is running at 100 ml/hour. What may be the cause of this increased rate?
A. the tubing has a kink in it
B. the clamp has been tightened
C. the fluid container is too high
D. the filter is blocked

31. How much air does it take to cause an air embolism in an adult?
A. as little as 10 cc
B. 20 to 30 cc
C. 50 to 100 cc
D. 150 to 200 cc

Introductory Nursing Care of Adults

16

Pain Management

OBJECTIVES

1. Define pain.
2. Explain the physiologic basis for pain.
3. Identify situations in which patients are likely to experience pain.
4. Explain the relationships between past pain experiences, anticipation, culture, anxiety, activity, and a patient's response to pain.
5. Identify differences in duration and patient response with acute and chronic pain.
6. Explain the special needs of the elderly patient who has pain.
7. List the data to be collected in assessing pain.
8. Describe interventions used in the management of pain.
9. Describe nursing care of patients receiving opioid and nonopioid analgesics for pain.
10. List the factors that should be considered when pain is not relieved with analgesic medications.

LEARNING ACTIVITIES

I.   Match the definition on the left (1-10) with the most appropriate term on the right.

___ 1. Process of pain transmission; usually related to pain sensation resulting from stimulation of pain receptors and transmission of stimuli to pain fibers, spinal cord, and brain

___ 2. Unpleasant sensory and emotional experience associated with actual or potential tissue damage existing whenever the person says it does; a unique, private experience involving the holistic person in a time dimension of past, present, and future and influenced by internal and external environment

___ 3. Drug that acts on the nervous system to relieve or reduce the suffering or intensity of pain

___ 4. A physiologic result of repeated doses of an opioid where the same dose is no longer effective in achieving the same analgesic effect; a larger dose of opioids is required to achieve the same analgesic effect

A.   Pain

B.   Addiction

C.   Acute pain

D.   Pain tolerance

E.   Nociception

F.   Physical dependence

G.   Tolerance

H.   Chronic pain

I.   Pain threshold

J.   Anaglesic

I. *Continued*

_____ 5. Behavioral pattern of compulsive drug use characterized by craving for an opioid and obtaining and using the drug for effects other than pain relief

_____ 6. Physiologic adaptation of the body to an opioid so a person exhibits withdrawal symptoms when the opioid is stopped abruptly after repeated administration

_____ 7. Amount of pain a person is willing to endure before taking action to relieve pain

_____ 8. Pain that lasts longer than 6 months

_____ 9. Level of intensity that causes the sensation of feeling of pain

_____ 10. Pain that lasts less than 6 months, has an identifiable cause, and goes away as healing occurs

A. Pain

B. Addiction

C. Acute pain

D. Pain tolerance

E. Nociception

F. Physical dependence

G. Tolerance

H. Chronic pain

I. Pain threshold

J. Anaglesic

II. Indicate for each factor on the left whether it will (A) increase or (B) decrease endorphins.

_____ 1. TENS

_____ 2. Laughter

_____ 3. Prolonged use of alcohol

_____ 4. Acupuncture

_____ 5. Brief stress

_____ 6. Brief pain

_____ 7. Prolonged stress

_____ 8. Exercise

_____ 9. Placebos

_____ 10. Prolonged pain

A. Increase

B. Decrease

III. Indicate for each statement on the left whether it (A) opens the gate or (B) closes the gate according to gate-control theory.

____ 1. Distraction

____ 2. Tissue damage

____ 3. Massage

____ 4. Heat application

____ 5. Position change

____ 6. Fear of pain

____ 7. Guided imagery

____ 8. Monotonous environment

____ 9. Cold application

____ 10. Preparatory information

A. Opens the gate

B. Closes the gate

IV. Match the description on the left with the most appropriate factor affecting pain response on the right.

____ 1. A patient who has received nitrous oxide during surgery and who says he does not have pain post-op

____ 2. An older person who is stoic and does not want to bother the nurse

____ 3. Pain associated with childbirth is usually short-lived, whereas cancer pain may be chronic

____ 4. Anger, fatigue, insomnia, depression

____ 5. A patient who prays and believes that divine intervention will help him to endure pain

A. Situational factors

B. Pain threshold

C. Religious beliefs

D. Age

E. Anesthetic

V. For each characteristic on the left, indicate whether it refers to (A) acute or (B) chronic pain.

____ 1. No report of pain unless questioned

____ 2. Pain from migraine headaches and neuralgia

____ 3. Increased heart rate, blood pressure, respiratory rate

____ 4. Limited, short duration

____ 5. Normal heart rate, blood pressure, respiratory rate

____ 6. Less responsive to analgesics

____ 7. Additional drugs seldom needed to manage pain

____ 8. Lasts 6 months or longer

____ 9. Tempory pain

____ 10. Phantom limb pain

A. Acute pain

B. Chronic pain

VI. Fill in the blanks below, indicating how these barriers to pain assessment for the older adult affect their responses to pain.

1. Visual, verbal, hearing and motor impairments _____

   _____.

2. Cognitive impairment may make patients _____.

3. Pain itself may cause _____.

VII. List 2 advantages of using a pain scale, such as the VAS scale.

1.

2.

VIII. A 42-year-old male with multiple fractures in the right arm used the numeric scale from 1 to 10 for rating pain. The patient complained of throbbing in his right arm and a backache. He rated the intensity of both pains at 7 on the scale at 8:00 p.m. The nurse applied heat to the lower back as ordered, massaged his back, and administered 10 mg of morphine intramuscularly. At 9:00 p.m., the patient rated intensity of both pains at 2 and stated that the pain was slowly going away.

Were the interventions effective in relieving the pain? What evidence do you have that the pain was or was not relieved?

IX. Indicate for each factor on the left whether it acts as an (A) aggravating factor or (B) alleviating factor for pain.

___ 1. Elevation and rest of affected limb   A. Aggravating factor

___ 2. Application of cold   B. Alleviating factor

___ 3. Certain times of day or night

___ 4. Application of menthol

___ 5. Physical activities that reduce pain in specific areas

___ 6. Application of heat

___ 7. Certain temperatures

X. List 6 nursing diagnoses related to pain.

1.

2.

3.

4.

5.

6.

XI. Indicate for each nonpharmacologic intervention on the left whether it is an (A) physical or (B) psychological intervention.

___ 1. Music

___ 2. Progressive muscle relaxation

___ 3. Massage

___ 4. Cold

___ 5. Educational instruction

___ 6. Simple imagery

___ 7. TENS

___ 8. Jaw relaxation

___ 9. Heat

A. Physical

B. Psychological

XII. Match the characteristic on the left with the most appropriate term on the right.

___ 1. Physiologic changes that occur from repeated doses of opioids where a larger dose is required to achieve the same effect

___ 2. Compulsive obtaining and use of drug for psychic effects

___ 3. Withdrawal symptoms may occur if the opioid is stopped abruptly (e.g., irritability, chills, sweating, nausea)

___ 4. Psychological dependence characterized by continued craving for opioid for other than pain relief

___ 5. The need for higher doses to achieve pain relief

A. Addiction

B. Tolerance

C. Physical dependency

XIII. List 4 nursing measures for patients who have constipation as a result of taking opioid analgesics.

1.

2.

3.

4.

XIV. List 7 factors which influence response to pain.

1.

2.

3.

4.

5.

6.

7.

XV. List 6 factors which lower the pain threshold.

1.

2.

3.

4.

5.

6.

XVI. Choose the most appropriate answer.

1. An unpleasant sensory and emotional experience associated with actual or potential tissue damage is:
   A. pain
   B. opioid
   C. analgesic
   D. discomfort

2. Pathways that carry messages to the brain, where the messages are interpreted, are:
   A. internal
   B. external
   C. afferent
   D. efferent

3. Stimulation of which of the following causes diminished pain perception?
   A. small-diameter fibers
   B. large-diameter fibers
   C. arteries
   D. veins

4. Tissue damage and fear of pain cause stimulation of:
   A. small-diameter fibers
   B. large-diameter fibers
   C. arteries
   D. veins

5. Factors influencing the response to pain include pain threshold, pain tolerance, age, physical activity, and the type of surgery. These factors are examples of:
   A. psychosocial factors
   B. emotional factors
   C. sociological factors
   D. physical factors

6. The point at which a stimulus causes the sensation or feeling of pain is the pain:
   A. duration
   B. peak
   C. threshold
   D. tolerance

7. Anger, fatigue, anxiety, and depression cause which effect on the pain threshold?
   A. raise it
   B. lower it
   C. stimulate it
   D. arouse it

8. When the pain threshold is lowered, the person experiences pain:
   A. less easily
   B. more easily
   C. as excruciating
   D. as mild

9. Which age group tends not to report their pain or tends to report their pain as much less severe than it really is?
   A. older patients
   B. middle-age patients
   C. adolescent patients
   D. children

10. Which type of surgery is reported to be the most painful for patients?
    A. skull region
    B. thoracic region
    C. upper abdominal region
    D. lower abdominal region

11. Dilated pupils, perspiration, and pallor are results of which nervous system response to pain?
    A. voluntary
    B. somatic
    C. parasympathetic
    D. sympathetic

12. A temporary pain that serves as a warning of tissue damage and subsides when healing takes place is:
    A. chronic pain
    B. permanent pain
    C. acute pain
    D. pain of unknown cause

13. Pain associated with cancer, arthritis, and peripheral vascular diseases is:
    A. temporary pain
    B. chronic pain
    C. acute pain
    D. joint pain

14. A pain that cannot be explained or that persists after healing has taken place is:
    A. acute benign pain
    B. acute metastatic pain
    C. chronic benign pain
    D. chronic metastatic pain

15. The first step in pain management is:
    A. assessment
    B. planning
    C. intervention
    D. evaluation

16. When possible, the information about pain should be obtained from the:
    A. nurse
    B. patient
    C. doctor
    D. patient's family

17. Factors that make the pain worse are called:
    A. benign factors
    B. stoic factors
    C. psychological factors
    D. aggravating factors

18. The application of heat, cold, and massage and TENS are examples of :
    A. physical comfort measures
    B. cutaneous stimulation
    C. environmental control
    D. psychological comfort measures

19. The application of cold results in:
    A. vasoconstriction
    B. vasodilation
    C. inflammation
    D. blood clots

20. The longest time a cold application can be used without tissue injury would be:
    A. 3 minutes
    B. 15 minutes
    C. 30 minutes
    D. 60 minutes

21. Rubbing, kneading, manipulation, or application of pressure and friction to the body is called:
    A. heat
    B. cold
    C. environmental control
    D. massage

22. Which of the following is the most expensive and least available?
    A. cold
    B. heat
    C. massage
    D. TENS

23. Focusing on stimuli other than pain is called:
    A. massage
    B. stimulation
    C. distraction
    D. acupuncture

24. Relaxation is most effective for:
    A. delusional pain
    B. mild to moderate pain
    C. moderate to severe pain
    D. severe pain

25. Using a person's imagination to help control pain is called:
    A. environmental control
    B. stimulation
    C. imagery
    D. massage

26. When pain is unpredictable, analgesics are more effective when given:
    A. once a day
    B. twice a day
    C. around the clock
    D. PRN

27. The initial treatment choice for mild pain is:
    A. opioid analgesics
    B. nonopioid analgesics
    C. narcotics
    D. anesthetics

28. Aspirin, acetaminophen, and NSAIDs are examples of:
    A. opioid analgesics
    B. nonopioid analgesics
    C. narcotics
    D. anesthetics

29. Ketorolac (Toradol) is generally used for the short-term management of:
    A. cancer pain
    B. congestive heart failure
    C. urinary tract infection
    D. postoperative pain

30. Drugs that do not improve analgesia beyond a certain dosage are said to have a:
    A. peak effect
    B. duration effect
    C. ceiling effect
    D. onset effect

31. A deficiency of platelets in the blood is called:
    A. anemia
    B. thrombocytopenia
    C. hypoglycemia
    D. hyperkalemia

32. Nonopioids should be used cautiously in patients with congestive heart failure or hypertension because of the side effect of:
    A. decreased circulation
    B. depressed respirations
    C. tachycardia
    D. fluid retention

33. Nonopioids tend to block pain transmission:
    A. at the central nervous system
    B. during cell wall synthesis
    C. at the myocardium
    D. peripherally

34. Nalbuphine (Nubain), butorphanol (Stadol), and pentazocine (Talwin) are examples of:
    A. nonopioid analgesics
    B. anticholinergics
    C. opioid agonist-antagonists
    D. opioid agonists

35. A patient receiving 10 mg morphine IM for pain will be given what dose PO to receive an equianalgesic dose?
    A. 10 mg PO
    B. 30 mg PO
    C. 60 mg PO
    D. 80 mg PO

36. If the patient is nauseated or has difficulty swallowing, which route is useful for administering opioids?
    A. oral
    B. rectal
    C. topical
    D. intradermal

37. To evaluate the patient for constipation, the nurse must assess the patient for:
    A. black, tarry stools; anorexia
    B. decreased blood pressure, itching, and respiratory
    C. abdominal distention, cramping, and abdominal pain
    D. intake and output, blood pressure, and pulse

38. Which effect of opioids is not potentiated by the use of promethazine (Phenergan)?
    A. sedation
    B. respiratory depression
    C. hypotension
    D. analgesic

39. Meperidine is not the analgesic of choice for older adults because the risk for toxicity is high; toxic effects include:
    A. analgesia
    B. sedation
    C. seizures
    D. relaxation

40. A patient who has had back surgery complains of muscle spasms. Which drug may be most effective in relieving his pain?
    A. muscle relaxant
    B. opioid
    C. NSAID
    D. aspirin

41. What is the most common problem that nurses encounter?
    A. pain
    B. heart attack
    C. stroke
    D. headache

42. Some parts of the body are more sensitive to pain than other parts, due to:
    A. varied pain thresholds
    B. uneven patterns of addiction
    C. uneven distribution of nociceptors
    D. varied pain tolerance

43. What are the body's natural opioid-like substances that lock into opioid receptors in the brain and spinal cord?
    A. serotonin
    B. endorphins
    C. adrenaline
    D. thyroxines

44. The action of endorphins is to block the transmission of:
    A. painful impulses to the brain
    B. pleasure impulses to the brain
    C. opioid receptors in the brain
    D. anxiety impulses to the brain

Patient Care Settings

OBJECTIVES

1. Describe the principles of rehabilitation.
2. List the four levels of disability.
3. Discuss legislation passed to protect the rights of the disabled.
4. Identify the goals of rehabilitation.
5. Name the members of the rehabilitation team.
6. Compare the differences and similarities between home health nursing and community health nursing.
7. Describe the three levels of prevention.
8. Name the five criteria for Medicare home health nursing reimbursement.
9. Discuss the criteria for admission to hospice care.
10. List the four levels of modern nursing home care.
11. Discuss the effects of institutionalization on the elderly client.
12. Describe the principles of nursing home care.

LEARNING ACTIVITIES

I. Match the definition on the left (1-9) with the most appropriate term on the right.

___ 1. Quantifiable loss of function, usually for the purpose of indicating a diminished capacity for work

___ 2. Certain nursing procedures, such as dressing changes, Foley catheter insertions, and venipuncture

___ 3. Physical or psychological disturbance in functioning

___ 4. Steps taken to increase health of individual by strengthening body systems and preventing disease or injury

___ 5. Inability to perform one or more normal daily activities because of mental or physical disability

___ 6. Used to determine adequacy of home environment, knowledge level of the patient and family regarding care procedures, side effects of treatment, and family's level of comfort in performing specific procedures

A. Primary prevention
B. Impairment
C. Skilled observation and assessment
D. Rehabilitation
E. Tertiary prevention
F. Handicap
G. Secondary prevention
H. Skilled procedures
I. Disability

Introductory Nursing Care of Adults
Copyright © 1995 by W.B. Saunders Company. All rights reserved.

143

I. *Continued*

    ___ 7. Steps taken to prevent disease recurrence or complications

    ___ 8. Steps taken to find disease early and begin treatment as soon as possible

    ___ 9. Process of restoring individual to best possible health and functioning following physical or mental impairment

A. Primary prevention

B. Impairment

C. Skilled observation and assessment

D. Rehabilitation

E. Tertiary prevention

F. Handicap

G. Secondary prevention

H. Skilled procedures

I. Disability

II. Fill in the blanks.

1. The type of quantifiable loss of function of a person who is classified as disabled allows for _____ _____ or _____.

2. Two goals of rehabilitation are to _____ and to _____.

III. Match the description disability on the left with the level of disability on the right.

    ___ 1. Severe limitations in one or more ADS, unable to work

    ___ 2. Slight limitation in one ore more ADS, usually able to work

    ___ 3. Total disability characterized by near complete dependence on others for assistance with ADL, unable to work

    ___ 4. Moderate limitation in one or more ADL, able to work but workplace may need modifications

A. Level I

B. Level II

C. Level III

D. Level IV

IV. Match the definition on the left with the most appropriate term on the right.

    ___ 1. Persons who assists the patient in regaining swallowing or speaking functions

    ___ 2. Person who assists patient with regaining fine motor skills necessary for dressing, eating, and grooming

    ___ 3. Person who assists with coordinating resources for placement in the home or convalescent facility after discharge

    ___ 4. Person who assists patient in all aspects of mobility

A. Physical therapist

B. Occupational therapist

C. Speech therapist

D. Social worker

. List 6 roles that rehabilitation nurses perform to assist the patient and family in returning to a high level of functioning.

1.

2.

3.

4.

5.

6.

I. List 3 levels of prevention in community health nursing intervention.

1.

2.

3.

II. List 3 examples of primary prevention.

1.

2.

3.

VIII. Match the description on the left with the most appropriate individual in the history of home health nursing on the right.

____ 1. Believed that all people had the right to direct access to services of a nurse

____ 2. Organized the Daughters of Charity in 1617

____ 3. Believed that nurses should live in the area where their patients lived to gain insight into the complexity of health care problems and their causes

____ 4. Organized the first district nursing organization

____ 5. Predecessor to modern public health nursing

____ 6. Opened the first training school for visiting nurses

A. William Rathbone

B. Lillian Wald

C. St. Vincent de Paul

IX. List 4 types of agencies that deliver home health nursing.

1.

2.

3.

4.

X. List 4 functions of local, state, and regional health departments.

1.

2.

3.

4.

XI. The nursing divisions of state, regional, or local health departments are usually asked to deliver nursing services to populations at risk. List 3 services that are delivered by health departments to populations at risk.

1.

2.

3.

XII. List 3 principles of delivery of nursing home care.

1.

2.

3.

XIII. List 2 reasons why the profitability of proprietary agencies has expanded.

1.

2.

XIV. What are the 5 basic criteria that must be met in order to receive Medicare reimbursement?

1.

2.

3.

4.

5.

XV. List 3 primary home health care services that are considered to be "skilled."

1.

2.

3.

XVI. List 3 aspects of skilled nursing.

1.

2.

3.

XVII. Match the definition or description on the left with the most appropriate members of the home health care team

____ 1. Assess for assistive devices; work with patients and their families on therapies to regain strength and mobility

____ 2. Perform common household chores such as cooking, light housekeeping, laundry, shopping, and picking up medications

____ 3. Specialists in the care of all types of wounds

____ 4. Work with families to identify problems in the management of the patient's illness in the home; recommend referrals to community resources

____ 5. Work with patients who have speech or swallowing disorders

____ 6. Provide personal care for the patient in the home, such as bathing, ambulating, transferring, skin care, and oral hygiene

____ 7. Help the patient become more safe and independent in the home setting

A. Home health aides

B. Speech therapists

C. Occupational therapists

D. Physical therapists

E. Social workers

F. Enterostomal therapists

G. Homemakers

XVIII. List 5 of the most common intravenous therapies that can be given in the home.

1.   4.

2.   5.

3.

XIX. List 4 requirements for admission to hospice care.

1.   3.

2.   4.

XX. List 5 basic elements of the hospice philosophy of care.

1.   4.

2.   5.

3.

XXI. List 4 types of problems that the team method in hospice care provides for.

1.

2.

3.

4.

XXII. List 6 factors that have a bearing on who requires nursing home placement.

1.

2.

3.

4.

5.

6.

XXIII. List the 4 levels of nursing home care.

1.   3.

2.   4.

XXIV. List 3 methods to provide support and acceptance for families who are relocating a family member into a nursing home.

1.

2.

3.

XXV. List 5 common effects of institutionalization.

1.

2.

3.

4.

5.

XXVI. List 4 sources of revenue for proprietary agencies.

1.   3.

2.   4.

XXVII. Match the nursing interventions on the left with the appropriate principle on the right.

____ 1. Encourage nursing home residents to feed themselves.

____ 2. Allow nursing home residents to assist in establishing care goals.

____ 3. Give nursing home residents choices in activities.

____ 4. Determine possible causes for incontinence.

____ 5. Set specific goals for each resident that encourage independent functioning.

A. Maintenance of function

B. Promotion of independence

C. Maintenance of autonomy

XXVIII. Match the description on the left with the most appropriate level of prevention on the right.

___ 1. Providing Pap smears at reduced cost

___ 2. Efforts to educate people to wear seat belts

___ 3. Teaching a diabetic proper diet and foot care

___ 4. Providing mammograms at reduced cost

___ 5. Use of physical therapy to prevent contractures in a stroke patient

___ 6. Campaigns in schools to prevent children from smoking

___ 7. Exercise programs to increase strength and cardiovascular fitness

A. Primary

B. Secondary

C. Tertiary

XXIX. Choose the most appropriate answer.

1. The process of restoring an individual to the best possible health and functioning following a physical or mental impairment is called:
   A. independent function
   B. home health care
   C. rehabilitation
   D. chronicity

2. A disturbance in functioning that may be either physical or psychological is called:
   A. rehabilitation
   B. impairment
   C. restoration
   D. independence

3. Physical or mental impairment results in a:
   A. loss of independence
   B. loss of dependence
   C. loss of movement
   D. loss of function

4. A quantifiable loss of function, usually indicating diminished capacity for work, is called:
   A. impairment
   B. alteration to integrity
   C. compensation
   D. disability

5. An inability to perform daily activities is called:
   A. impairment
   B. disability
   C. handicap
   D. paralysis

6. The ultimate goal of rehabilitation is to live:
   A. with assistance
   B. with modification
   C. independently
   D. dependently

7. The first law passed to aid the rehabilitation of World War I servicemen by providing job training for injured veterans was the:
   A. Vocational Rehabilitation Act of 1920
   B. Social Security Act of 1935
   C. Medicare Act of 1965
   D. Rehabilitation Act of 1973

8. The first comprehensive approach to problems experienced by the disabled was the:
   A. Vocational Rehabilitation Act of 1920
   B. Social Security Act of 1935
   C. Medicare Act of 1965
   D. Rehabilitation Act of 1973

9. Which act began affirmative action programs to assist in the employment of the disabled and prohibited discrimination against the disabled in programs receiving federal funds?
   A. Vocational Rehabilitation Act of 1920
   B. Social Security Act of 1935
   C. Medicare Act of 1965
   D. Rehabilitation Act of 1973

10. Which law extended the protection given to the disabled in the public sector to the private sector as well?
    A. Vocational Rehabilitation Act
    B. Social Security Act
    C. Rehabilitation Act
    D. Americans with Disabilities Act

11. Which law mandates that any business endeavor designed to serve the public must ensure that its services are accessible to the disabled?
    A. Social Security Act
    B. Medicare Act
    C. Americans with Disabilities Act
    D. Rehabilitation Act

12. Effective rehabilitation commences:
    A. immediately after an injury
    B. when the patient goes home from the hospital
    C. 1 week after surgery
    D. when the patient has had time to adjust to the injury

13. Caretakers who intervene too soon in the rehabilitation of a disabled person encourage:
    A. independence
    B. dependence
    C. responsibility
    D. freedom

14. When nurses help families of disabled persons adapt routines to the home setting and prioritize routines, the nurse is functioning in the role of:
    A. counselor/mentor
    B. coordinator/tutor
    C. caregiver/teacher
    D. advocate/mediator

15. The synthesis of public health concepts and nursing practice make up:
    A. primary care nursing
    B. nursing administration
    C. community health nursing
    D. team nursing

16. The placement of the focus of attention on improving the health of communities and aggregates is called:
    A. community health
    B. public health
    C. occupational health
    D. home health

17. The use of physical therapy to prevent contractures in a stroke patient is an example of what type of prevention?
    A. total
    B. primary
    C. secondary
    D. tertiary

18. The synthesis of direct nursing care and community health nursing is called:
    A. home health nursing
    B. community health nursing
    C. public health nursing
    D. school nursing

19. Community-based services and access to health care are key issues of:
    A. Social Security Act
    B. Americans with Disabilities Act
    C. Nursing's Agenda for Health Care Reform
    D. Medicare/Medicaid Act

20. Agencies supported by tax dollars and authorized by law to deliver services to a defined area or community are called:
    A. voluntary agencies
    B. proprietary agencies
    C. official agencies
    D. hospital-based agencies

21. The most important source of home health care funding is:
    A. private insurance
    B. Medicare
    C. Medicaid
    D. private pay clients

22. Medicare law defines that care:
    A. must be given by nurses only
    B. is standard for a particular disease
    C. is reimbursable under the law
    D. is quality care

23. By providing clear documentation of functional losses and goals for care, the nurse is meeting the Medicare criterion of:
    A. skilled care
    B. reasonable and necessary care
    C. homebound patient
    D. intermittent care

24. The Medicare criterion, that the patient must be homebound, is referring to the fact that the patient must:
    A. be bedridden
    B. be well enough to go to the doctor's office
    C. require considerable effort to leave home
    D. be able to make small, frequent trips to the store

25. Relaying information to the patient and family at a pace they can handle is an example of:
    A. teaching skills
    B. assessment skills
    C. counselor skills
    D. skilled procedures

26. The criterion for Medicare reimbursement related to intermittent care means that:
    A. the patient is seen daily
    B. the patient is intermittently sick
    C. visits will be made by a variety of health care workers
    D. visits occur periodically and do not usually exceed 28 hours per week

Introductory Nursing Care of Adults

27. A stroke patient who is aphasic will need the services of a(n):
    A. occupational therapist
    B. physical therapist
    C. speech therapist
    D. social worker

28. Patients and their families needing assistance to manage chronic illness in the home will need the services of a:
    A. speech therapist
    B. social worker
    C. occupational therapist
    D. physical therapist

29. Facilities providing basic room, board, and supervision are called:
    A. domiciliary care facilities
    B. sheltered housing
    C. intermediate care
    D. skilled care

30. Facilities that contain modification to provide care for the frail elderly and usually include community dining facilities are called:
    A. domiciliary care facilities
    B. sheltered housing
    C. intermediate care
    D. skilled care

31. Treating patients primarily in light of their diagnosis or dysfunctional behavior patterns is an example of:
    A. indignity
    B. regression
    C. social withdrawal
    D. depersonalization

32. Being left in bed a great part of the day, finding it difficult to walk, and losing skills of conversation are examples of:
    A. social withdrawal
    B. indignity
    C. regression
    D. depersonalization

Falls

OBJECTIVES

1. Define falls.
2. List the incidence of falls.
3. Describe predisposing factors related to falls.
4. Discuss the relationship among restraint use and falls, types of restraints, and regulations for restraint use.
5. Demonstrate knowledge of fall-prevention techniques.
6. Describe nursing interventions to be used when a fall occurs.

LEARNING ACTIVITIES

I.   Match the definition on the left with the most appropriate term on the right.

_____ 1. Anything that restricts movement

_____ 2. Circumstance in which one unintentionally falls to the ground or hits an object such as a chair or stair

_____ 3. Factors related to the internal functioning of an individual, such as the aging process or physical illness

_____ 4. Psychotropic medications given to subdue agitated or confused patients

_____ 5. Law enacted in 1987 to protect patients in nursing homes

_____ 6. Factors in the environment that can cause falls

A.   Chemical restraints

B.   Extrinsic factors

C.   Fall

D.   Omnibus Reconciliation Act (OBRA)

E.   Physical restraint

F.   Intrinsic factors

II. For each factor on the left, indicate whether it is an (A) intrinsic factor or (B) extrinsic factor.

___ 1. Central nervous system diseases causing dizziness and gait disorders

    A. Intrinsic factor

    B. Extrinsic factor

___ 2. Overestimation of abilities

___ 3. Confusion

___ 4. Wet or excessively waxed floors

___ 5. Pets

___ 6. Depression

___ 7. Imposed mobility

___ 8. Physical restraints

___ 9. Unstable and defective equipment

___ 10. Nonfunctioning brake locks on wheelchairs

___ 11. Multiple medications related to increased incidence of chronic illness

___ 12. Trailing electrical wires

III. List 7 factors associated with people at greatest risk for injury from falls.

1.

2.

3.

4.

5.

6.

7.

IV. List 9 damaging psychological effects on older patients caused by restraints.

1.

2.

3.

4.

5.

6.

7.

8.

9.

V.　List 3 alternatives to physical restraints.

1.

2.

3.

VI.　Match each risk factor on the left with the most appropriate intervention on the right.

___　1.　Musculoskeletal disorders

___　2.　Impaired dark adaptation

___　3.　Balance disorders

___　4.　Stroke

___　5.　Reduced visual acuity

___　6.　Postural hypotension

___　7.　Impacted cerumen (ear wax)

___　8.　Peripheral neuropathy

___　9.　Impaired color perception

___ 10.　Foot disorders

___ 11.　Presbycusis

A.　Maintain adequate lighting; reduce glare from shiny floors and allow time to adjust to light levels—e.g., from a dark room to outside. Use night light in bedroom and bathroom.

B.　Trim toenails. Use appropriate footwear.

C.　Speak slowly; use low voice; decrease background noise. Encourage use of hearing aid.

D.　Remove ear wax.

E.　Use bright colors as markers, especially oranges, yellows, and reds.

F.　Be sure individual wears glasses, if appropriate. Keep glasses clean. Encourage regular eye examinations.

G.　Use correctly sized footwear with firm soles.

H.　Encourage balance and gait training and muscle–strengthening exercises.

I.　Encourage dorsiflexion exercises. Use pressure-graded stockings (TEDs). Elevate head of bed. Teach individual to get up from chair or bed slowly. Individual should avoid tipping head backward.

J.　Encourage balance exercises.

K.　Call bell in visual field and within reach of arm that has use. Anticipate needs for toileting, dressing, eating, and bathing. Assist with transfer. Provide passive range of motion exercises to improve functional ability.

VII.　List 4 basic strategies for reducing all types of falls.

1.

2.

3.

4.

VIII. List 3 important factors to document when a fall occurs.

1.

2.

3.

IX. For each fall-prevention technique listed on the left, indicate the category on the right to which it relates.

___ 1. Clutter-free rooms and hallways	A. Patient education
___ 2. Frequent rounds/checks/observations	B. Environment-oriented
___ 3. Keep patient's belongings close to bed	C. Patient-oriented
___ 4. Note diuretics and laxatives given at night	D. Nursing assessment
___ 5. Place TV controls within reach	E. Activities of daily living
___ 6. Note hypnotic or sedative drugs given at night, especially to elderly or postoperative patients	F. Medications
___ 7. Encourage use of bathroom and corridor handrails	
___ 8. Provide rehabilitation training to improve functional ability	
___ 9. Night lights in rooms	
___ 10. Exercise to strengthen muscles and prevent weakness	

X. Choose the most appropriate answer.

1. What is the estimated number of persons aged 65 or older who fall in a given year?
   A. 1 in 3
   B. 1 in 10
   C. 1 in 20
   D. 1 in 100

2. At what age does there appear to be a steady increase in the number of falls?
   A. 40 and older
   B. 65 and older
   C. 75 and older
   D. 85 and older

3. Of the total number of deaths due to falls, what percent of these deaths occur in the elderly?
   A. 10%
   B. 20%
   C. 50%
   D. 72%

4. What percent of deaths due to falls does the U.S. Public Health Service state are preventable?
   A. one fifth
   B. one third
   C. one half
   D. two thirds

5. Factors, such as the aging process and physical illness, that increase the possibility of falling, are called:
   A. extrinsic factors
   B. environmental factors
   C. intrinsic factors
   D. hospital factors

6. Factors increasing the opportunity to fall are called:
   A. extrinsic factors
   B. aging process factors
   C. intrinsic factors
   D. physical illness factors

7. Of all reported falls, what percentage do not result in injury?
   A. 10 to 20 percent
   B. 25 to 35 percent
   C. 40 to 50 percent
   D. 65 to 75 percent

8. What is the most frequent type of injury, occurring in 25 to 30% of all falls?
   A. deep tissue damage
   B. contusions, cuts, or lacerations
   C. concussion
   D. fractures

9. Geriatric chairs and siderails are examples of:
   A. environmental restraints
   B. social restraints
   C. physical restraints
   D. chemical restraints

10. Older patients are more likely than younger patients to be physically restrained because of their greater likelihood of:
    A. mental decline and weight loss
    B. chronic illness and physical decline
    C. heart disease and insomnia
    D. falling and confusion

11. The major complications from using physical restraints includes:
    A. sedation from medications administered and accidental aspiration
    B. falls from wheelchairs and beds (when patients are able to untie restraints or wriggle out of them) and accidental strangulation
    C. fatigue from fighting the restraints and confusion resulting from fatigue
    D. skin breakdown from friction and wound development

12. Which law was enacted to protect patients from unnecessary restraint in nursing homes?
    A. Medicare Act
    B. Public Health Act
    C. Social Security Act
    D. Omnibus Reconciliation Act

13. The Omnibus Reconciliation Act of 1987 (OBRA) states that nursing home residents have the right to be free from any physical restraints imposed or psychoactive drug administered for the purposes of:
    A. discipline or convenience
    B. safety or public health
    C. exercise or physical therapy
    D. strict confinement

14. Physical restraints should be removed and released every:
    A. hour for 10 minutes
    B. 2 hours for 10 minutes
    C. 4 hours for 10 minutes
    D. 8 hours for 10 minutes

15. Psychoactive drugs should never be used for the purposes of:
    A. relief of headaches
    B. insomnia
    C. discipline
    D. hallucinations

16. Commonly prescribed psychoactive drugs for the elderly include:
    A. Benadryl, Demerol, and Phenergan
    B. Atropine, Thorazine, and Lidocaine
    C. Ibuprofen, Soma, and Xanax
    D. Haldol, Mellaril, and Ativan

17. The best way to prevent falls is to educate patients and caregivers about:
    A. the proper use of physical restraints
    B. ways to prevent falls
    C. the proper use of chemical restraints
    D. ways to treat medical conditions

18. After a fall, the patient should be encouraged to:
    A. begin ambulation as soon as possible to prevent nausea and vomiting
    B. stay in bed on complete bedrest for 24 hours to prevent another fall from occurring
    C. begin ambulation as soon as possible to prevent hazards of bedrest and fear of falling again
    D. stay in bed for at least 8 hours to prevent headaches and muscle aches from getting worse

19. In the "roll" method of getting up from a fall, after rolling onto the right side and bending the right knee, the patient should:
    A. crawl to a chair
    B. shuffle to the stairs
    C. get up on all fours
    D. lever upward to the kneeling position by pressing down on the right forearm

20. In the "crawl" method of getting up from a fall, after rolling to a prone position and getting up on all fours, the patient should:
    A. pull to a sitting position on the floor
    B. crawl to a sturdy couch, chair, or bed and place hands on it
    C. stand up
    D. kneel

21. In the "stair shuffle" method of getting up from a fall, after pulling to a sitting position on the floor and shuffling on the buttocks to the stairs, the patient should:

   A. turn around and kneel on the lowest stair
   B. get up on all fours
   C. turn around and place arms on waist-height stair to support body
   D. gradually move up and backward to a stair height suitable for standing

19

9/17/99

Immobility

OBJECTIVES

1. Describe common problems associated with immobility.
2. Discuss the impact of exercise and positioning on preventing complications related to immobility.
3. Identify risk factors of pressure ulcers.
4. Describe the stages of pressure ulcers.
5. Provide methods of preventing and treating pressure ulcers.
6. Discuss the impact of immobility on respiratory status, nutrition, and elimination.

LEARNING ACTIVITIES

I.   Match the definition on the left with the most appropriate term on the right.

D 1. The inability to move; imposed restriction on entire body

A.   Erythema   *red skin*

E 2. Exercise in which each joint is moved in various directions to the farthest possible extreme

B.   Pressure ulcer

C.   Isometric exercise

I 3. Exercise of the patient that is carried out by the therapist or nurse without the assistance of the patient

D.   Immobility

E.   Range of motion exercise

C 4. Muscle contraction without movement used to maintain muscle tone

F.   Active exercise

F 5. Exercise carried out by the patient

G.   Contracture

A 6. Redness of the skin; usually a sign that capillaries have become congested because of impaired blood flow

H.   Shearing forces

I.   Passive exercise

G 7. Shortening of the muscles and tendons

H 8. Two contacting parts slide on each other.

B 9. An open wound caused by pressure on a bony prominence; also called a "pressure sore"

II. List 4 therapeutic reasons for rest and immobility.

1. relief from pain & further injury
2. reduction of the workload of the heart
3. promotion of healing & repair
4. reversal of the effects of gravity.

III. Match the therapeutic reason for rest and immobility on the left with the most appropriate condition on the right.

_B_ 1. reduction of the workload of the heart   A. abdominal hernias and prolapsed organs

_A_ 2. reversal of the effects of gravity *keep on ground*   B. cardiac or renal condition

_C_ 3. relief from pain and further injury of a part   C. fractured bone

IV. List 4 reasons why the elderly are particularly vulnerable to the effects of immobility.

1. changes that occur c immobility occur c aging
2. tend to have one or more chronic illness
3. pain associate c chronic disease
4. loss of mobility, strength & changes in posture & gait

V. Fill in the blanks.

1. The major motions in range-of-motion exercises include flexion, extension, abduction, adduction, and
   ___rotation___.

2. Exercises performed to maintain muscle tone without moving the joint are called
   ___Isometric___.

3. Pressure points on the skin that tend to break down and form bed sores include bony prominences of the elbow, hips, shoulders, and ___Sacrum___. (back tail)

4. The most frequent site of skin breakdown is the ___Sacrum___.

5. Three causes of constipation include inactivity, decreased fluid intake, and ___lack of adequate jo___

VI. List the 7 elements of a pressure sore prevention protocol.

1. turn 2hr
2. keep bed wrinkle free; dry urinate
3. avoid friction bud designed to reduce pressure
4. use special mattress
5. apply sheep skin
6. take measure to enclourpt mobility
7. instruct pt & family about risk factor

VII. Match the characteristics on the left with the most appropriate stage of pressure ulcer on the right. Answers may be used more than once.

C 1. Wound may be infected, and is usually open and draining

B 2. Some skin loss in the epidermis and/or dermis

A 3. Irregular, ill-defined area of pressure reflecting the shape of the object creating the pressure

C 4. Crater-like sore with a distinct outer margin

B 5. Ulcer is surrounded by a broad, indistinct, painful, reddened area that is hot or warmer than normal

A 6. Nonblanchable erythema

B 7. A shallow ulcer develops and appears blistered, cracked, or abraded

D 8. Ulcer is usually infected and may appear black with exudation, foul odor, and purulent drainage

C 9. Full-thickness skin loss involving damage or necrosis of the dermis and subcutaneous tissues

A 10. Little destruction of tissue, and condition is reversible

D 11. Full-thickness skin loss with extensive destruction of the deeper underlying muscle and possible bone tissue

C 12. Patient may have fever, dehydration, anemia, and leukocytosis

B 13. Pain and tenderness may be present, with swelling and hardening of the tissue and associated heat

A. Stage I

B. Stage II

C. Stage III

D. Stage IV

Treatment of a pressure ulcer is prevention.

VIII. List the 3 major principles of wound management that should be followed in the treatment of decubitus ulcers.

1. clean this area
2. promote formation of granulation tissue.
3. Ensure adequate nutrition intake, vitamine

IX. List 4 examples of individuals who are at risk for impaired respiratory capacity related to immobility.

1. Who have been sedate.
2. Who c tight binder or bandages, that would limit chest expansion;
3. Who have abdominal attention of GAS, fluid abscess Lie on position for long time
4. elder adult

X. List 2 nursing interventions for patients at risk for respiratory complications.

1. frequently turn & positiony.
2. Coughing & deep breathing

XI. In Figure 19–1, label the bony prominences (A–Z).

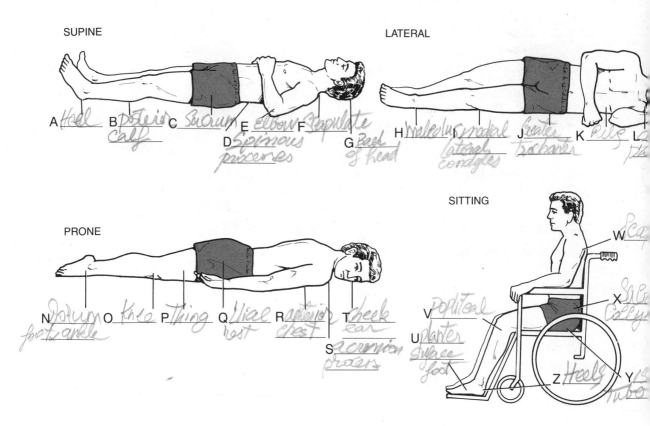

SUPINE

LATERAL

A Heel B posterior calf C Sacrum D Spinous processes E elbow F Scapulate G Back of head

H malerlus lateral condyles I medial J greater trochanter K Rib L

PRONE

SITTING

N dorsum foot ankle O Knee P thing Q Iliac rest R anterior chest S acromion process T cheek ear

V popliteal U plantar surface foot W sca X Sa Co Coccyx Z Heels Y Ischial Tubo

XII. Match the consequences of immobility on the left with the appropriate body system on the right.

B 1. Decreased sensory stimulation (kinesthetic, visual, auditory, tactile); decreased social interaction; changes in affect, cognition, and perception

C 2. General weakening of muscles, causing altered colonic motility, constipation

D 3. arterial oxygen desaturation; increased hypostatic pooling; increased risk of atelectasis and infection

E 4. Thickening of joint capsule; loss of smoothness of cartilage surface; decreased flexibility of connective tissues; changes similar to osteoarthritis—joint contractures, demineralization of bone, bone loss; atrophy and shortening of muscle; decrease in muscle strength; decreased muscle oxidative capacity; decline in aerobic capacity

H 5. Decreased cardiac output and stroke volume; increased peripheral resistance; net loss of total body water and total blood volume

A. Metabolic

B. Sensory

C. Gastrointestinal

D. Pulmonary

E. Musculoskeletal

F. Integumentary

G. Urinary

H. Cardiovascular

A 6. Decreased basal metabolic rate; increased storage of fat or carbohydrate; negative nitrogen and calcium metabolic balance due to decreased absorption of protein and calcium intake; decreased glucose tolerance; metabolic alkalosis

G 7. Increased nitrogen, phosphorus, total sulfur, sodium, potassium, and calcium excretion; renal insufficiency; decreased glomerular filtration rate; loss of ability to concentrate urine; lower creatinine tolerance

E 8. Pressure ulcers

A. Metabolic
B. Sensory
C. Gastrointestinal
D. Pulmonary
E. Musculoskeletal
F. Integumentary
G. Urinary
H. Cardiovascular

III. List 2 reasons why the position of the patient should be changed every 2 hours.

1. PT should turn 2hr prevent und presure skin.
2. maintaining joints in their function position so that they are not abnormally flexed or extended.

IV. Choose the most appropriate answer.

1. The best medicine for immobility is:
A. exercise
B. proper diet
C. skin integrity
D. increased fluid intake

2. Regardless of the acuity of their disease, those who are ill and disabled can:
A. perform aerobic exercise
B. perform anaerobic exercise
C. carry out modified exercise
D. lift heavy weights

3. Extremes to which joints may be moved in various directions refers to:
A. passive exercise
B. active exercise
C. range of motion
D. isometric exercise

4. Little or no motion of the joints results in:
A. tendonitis
B. bursitis
C. skin breakdown
D. contractures

5. In which type of exercise does the nurse ask the patient to contract the muscle and hold it in the position for several seconds, relax the muscle for a few seconds and then contract it again?
A. isotonic
B. isometric
C. passive
D. weight lifting

6. Thirty-five percent of all skin breakdown occurs at the:
A. hip
B. sacrum
C. shoulder
D. elbow

7. A lesion produced by the sloughing of necrotic, inflammatory tissue is called:
A. infection
B. wound
C. laceration
D. ulcer

8. A term used for bed sores is:
A. wound infection
B. cellulitis
C. decubitus ulcer
D. bony pressure

9. An area of redness that is the beginning of a pressure sore is called:
A. erythema
B. inflammation
C. wound
D. hemorrhage

10. Erythema progresses rapidly to an ulcerated stage in persons who are malnourished, obese, aged, or
A. suffering from skin infection
B. suffering from skin inflammation
C. sustaining lacerations
D. suffering from circulatory disease

11. Forces that exert a downward pressure on tissues underlying the skin are called:
    A. positive
    B. shearing
    C. projectile
    D. slanting

12. Pressure sores are expensive to treat, result in longer hospital stays, increase the likelihood of nursing home placement, and:
    A. increase self-esteem
    B. reduce safety needs
    C. reduce infection
    D. increase mortality

13. A useful instrument for identifying those at risk of developing pressure ulcers is the:
    A. pain scale
    B. neurologic scale
    C. Norton scale
    D. Glasgow scale

14. What is NOT recommended for pressure points?
    A. sheepskin
    B. massage
    C. egg crate mattress
    D. trapeze bars

15. Which of the following causes concentrated areas of pressure that puts patients at higher risk for developing pressure ulcers?
    A. sheepskin
    B. egg crate mattresses
    C. trapeze bars
    D. rubber rings and doughnuts

16. An increase in the number of white blood cells in the blood is called:
    A. leukocytosis
    B. thrombocytopenia
    C. agranulocytosis
    D. eosinophilia

17. Leukocytosis, fever, dehydration, and anemia may occur at which stage?
    A. stage I
    B. stage II
    C. stage III
    D. stage IV

18. Wound healing is enhanced when:
    A. the temperature is higher than that of body temperature
    B. the ulcer is completely covered with an impermeable dressing
    C. the ulcer and surrounding tissues can take up oxygen and expel carbon dioxide
    D. the ulcer and surrounding tissues are gently messaged

19. Stage III and IV decubitus ulcers usually require:
    A. culture and sensitivity tests before treatment can begin
    B. a very moist environment at all times
    C. the ulcer to be completely covered with an impermeable dressing
    D. débridement to promote granulation of new healthy tissue

20. The purpose of whirlpool baths for decubitus ulcers is to:
    A. raise the temperature
    B. assist with débridement
    C. decrease granulation
    D. increase leukocytosis

21. When a person remains immobile or does not take deep breaths, which of the following is most likely to occur to the respiratory status?
    A. an accumulation of carbon dioxide, which collects in the alveoli
    B. an accumulation of thick secretions, which pool in the lower respiratory structures
    C. decreased circulation to the lungs
    D. decreased oxygen entering the lungs

22. When thick secretions pool in the lower respiratory structures, these secretions interfere with the:
    A. normal exchange of white blood cells and red blood cells in the capillaries
    B. circulation of blood to the extremities
    C. detoxification process in the liver
    D. normal exchange of oxygen and carbon dioxide in the lungs

23. Patients should be taught that the objective of coughing is to:
    A. rapidly move the secretions upward and cough them out a little at a time
    B. rapidly move the secretions upward and cough them out all at once
    C. gradually move the secretions upward and cough them out all at once
    D. gradually move the secretions upward and cough them out a little at a time

24. When teaching deep breathing to patients, tell them to concentrate on exhaling the air slowly while pursing their lips. While doing this, patients should focus on the:
    A. volume of air being exhaled
    B. volume of air being inhaled
    C. force with which they exhale
    D. force with which they inhale

25. For patients with anorexia, meals should be:
    A. high in sodium
    B. high in fiber
    C. small and frequent
    D. served three times a day

26. When constipated individuals strain to defecate, causing an increase in intra-abdominal pressure, this is called the:
    A. reflux maneuver
    B. vomiting maneuver
    C. Valsalva maneuver
    D. Heimlich maneuver

27. Long-standing constipation can result in:
    A. diarrhea
    B. fecal impaction
    C. nausea
    D. vomiting

28. The urinary system functions best when the person is:
    A. sitting
    B. upright
    C. lying on a side
    D. lying prone

29. The most effective way to prevent urinary incontinence associated with immobility is to set up a:
    A. high-protein diet
    B. cough and deep breathing program
    C. restriction of fluid intake
    D. toileting program

20

Confusion

OBJECTIVES

1. Define delirium and dementia.
2. Identify the causes of acute confusion.
3. Describe the differences between delirium and dementia.
4. Discuss nursing assessment and interventions related to delirium and dementia.

LEARNING ACTIVITIES

I. Match the definition or description on the left with the most appropriate term on the right.

___ 1. An acute organic disorder characterized by disturbances in orientation, short-term memory, and sleep

    A.   Delirium

    B.   Dementia

___ 2. Short-term confusional state

___ 3. Often irreversible confusion

___ 4. Acute confusional state

___ 5. A clinical syndrome characterized by impairment of memory, orientation, and appropriate behavior

___ 6. Chronic confusion

___ 7. A clinical syndrome characterized by impairment of intellectual functions, problem-solving, and judgment

___ 8. Often reversible confusion

___ 9. An acute organic disorder characterized by disturbances in attention, thinking, perception

___ 10. A clinical syndrome or collection of symptoms that is chronic in nature

___ 11. An acute organic disorder usually caused by some underlying illness

II. List 6 areas of disturbance which occur in patients with delirium.

1.

2.

3.

4.

5.

6.

III. Fill in the blanks.

1. Acute confusion that begins abruptly and usually lasts from 1 week to 1 month is _____.

2. Alzheimer's disease, Huntington's disease and Parkinson's disease are conditions associated with

   _____.

3. A type of dementia that affects the neurons in the brain is: _____.

4. A type of dementia that affects the blood vessels in the brain and causes multiple small strokes is:

   _____.

5. The type of affect that is present in dementia is _____.

6. To avoid agitation caused by extraneous stimuli for a patient with delirium, one should keep the lighting in the room soft and diffuse, and the room itself quiet and _____.

IV. Two characteristics of patients with dementia which should be used as a basis for providing care are:

1.

2.

V. Match each clinical feature on the left with the most appropriate condition on the right.

_____ 1. Flat or indifferent affect

_____ 2. Disoriented, with impaired thinking ability

_____ 3. Intermittent fear, perplexity, or bewilderment

_____ 4. Marked contrasts in levels of awareness

_____ 5. Hallucinations vague, fleeting, ill-defined, and in many cases it is difficult to make a clear judgment that they exist

_____ 6. Persecutory delusions are vague, random, contradictory

_____ 7. General intellectual powers preserved during lucid intervals

_____ 8. Lasts a few weeks to 3 months

_____ 9. Not much fluctuation; progressive decline

_____ 10. Hallucinations often disturbing and very clearly defined

A. Delirium

B. Dementia

VI. Choose the most appropriate answer.

1. The first priority for nursing interventions for the patient with delirium is to:
   A. meet basic physiologic needs
   B. take vital signs
   C. force fluids
   D. provide therapeutic touch

2. Because adequate sleep is important for the patient with delirium, which of the following nursing measures would be most appropriate to help the patient fall asleep?
   A. a glass of wine, a shower, and a long walk
   B. pain medication, milk and cookies, and showing a movie
   C. a back rub, a glass of warm milk, soothing conversation
   D. a sedative medication, a large dinner, and physical activity

3. A patient who has been suffering from delirium is now complaining of hallucinations that are frightening to him. In dealing with the patient, the nurse should:
   A. acknowledge the reality of the hallucinations
   B. orient the patient to the proper date and time
   C. orient the patient to the reality of being sick and hospitalized
   D. acknowledge how frightening hallucinations can be

4. When dealing with a delirious patient who is experiencing hallucinations, the best response of the nurse would be:
   A. "What is it that you are seeing on the wall?"
   B. "You are sick in the hospital, and what you are seeing is part of the illness."
   C. "The time is 2:00 P.M. and the date is (_____)."
   D. "Tell me what you are seeing."

5. The use of physical restraints should be avoided with patients with delirium because they tend to:
   A. increase anxiety and increase agitation
   B. decrease anxiety and increase agitation
   C. decrease anxiety and decrease agitation
   D. increase anxiety and decrease agitation

6. The first priority for dementia patients is to meet their:
   A. belonging needs
   B. self-esteem needs
   C. self-actualization needs
   D. basic needs

7. When dementia patients resist activities such as bathing or dressing, the nurse should:
   A. orient the patient to reality
   B. assist the patient in a nonconfrontational manner
   C. state clearly what needs to be done
   D. restrain the patient

8. People with dementia should be offered:
   A. no more than three full meals a day
   B. decreased fluids
   C. a diet high in sugar
   D. finger foods high in protein and carbohydrates

9. When taking care of patients with dementia, it is helpful to remember that they usually:
   A. benefit from reality orientation
   B. forget things quickly
   C. have disturbing hallucinations
   D. are able to learn new things

10. If patients with dementia start to become very restless or agitated, an effective nursing intervention is to:
    A. discuss the cause of their discomfort with them
    B. speak calmly and reassure them constantly
    C. orient them to time and place
    D. divert their attention and gently guide them to a new activity

Incontinence

OBJECTIVES

1. Identify types of urinary and fecal incontinence.
2. Explain the pathophysiology and treatment of specific types of incontinence.
3. Identify common therapeutic measures used for the incontinent patient.
4. List nursing assessment data needed to assist in the evaluation and treatment of incontinence.
5. Specify nursing goals, diagnoses, interventions, and evaluation criteria for the patient with incontinence.

LEARNING ACTIVITIES

I. Match the definition on the left with the most appropriate term on the right.

____ 1. Involuntary loss of urine during physical exertion

____ 2. Uncontrolled passage of stool associated with constipation

____ 3. Fecal incontinence caused by weak perineal muscles, loss of anal reflexes, loss of anal sphincter tone, or rectal prolapse

____ 4. Reflexive uncontrolled bowel movement, usually seen with dementia

____ 5. Inappropriate voiding in the presence of normal bladder and urethral function

____ 6. Incontinence associated with colorectal disease

____ 7. Involuntary loss of urine associated with a full bladder

____ 8. The inability to control the passage of urine

____ 9. Temporary loss of control over voiding

____ 10. The inability to control the passage of feces

____ 11. Involuntary loss of urine, usually shortly after a strong urge to void

____ 12. Condition in which the bladder does not function normally because of some disorder affecting the nerves of the bladder

____ 13. Urinate

____ 14. Expression of urine from the bladder by applying pressure over the lower abdomen

____ 15. Urination

A. Functional incontinence

B. Transient incontinence

C. Void

D. Overflow incontinence (fecal)

E. Micturition

F. Urinary incontinence

G. Urge incontinence

H. Credé's technique

I. Stress incontinence

J. Neurogenic bladder

K. Fecal incontinence

L. Anorectal incontinence

M. Symptomatic incontinence

N. Neurogenic incontinence

O. Overflow incontinence (urine)

II.　Fill in the blanks.

1.　Four factors required for normal controlled voiding include healthy bladder muscles (detrusor muscles), a patent urethra, normal transmission of nerve impulses, and _____.

2.　Five methods of treatment for urge incontinence include antibiotics for infection, removal of impaction, behavioral techniques, anticholinergics, and _____.

3.　Factors that contribute to overflow incontinence include obstruction to urine flow, underactive detrusor muscle, or _____.

4.　Drugs that may cause urinary retention include antihistamines, epinephrine, theophylline, and _____.

5.　A common reason for urethral obstruction in males is _____.

6.　The two groups of patients that usually require intermittent catheterization only once or twice before normal bladder function returns are _____ and _____.

7.　Activities that may lead to stress incontinence include coughing, laughing, sneezing, and _____.

8.　Contributing factors to stress incontinence include pelvic floor muscle relaxation following childbirth, obesity, and _____.

III.　List 6 methods of medical treatment for the patient with overflow incontinence.

1.

2.

3.

4.

5.

6.

IV.　List 6 methods of treatment for a person with stress incontinence.

1.

2.

3.

4.

5.

6.

V.　List 9 classifications of drugs that may contribute to urinary incontinence.

1.　　　　　　　　　　　　　　　6.

2.　　　　　　　　　　　　　　　7.

3.　　　　　　　　　　　　　　　8.

4.　　　　　　　　　　　　　　　9.

5.

Introductory Nursing Care of Adults
Copyright © 1995 by W.B. Saunders Company. All rights reserved.

VI. List 10 nursing diagnoses for the patient with urinary incontinence.

1.

2.

3.

4.

5.

6.

7.

8.

9.

10.

VII. List 3 nursing diagnoses for the patient with fecal incontinence.

1.

2.

3.

VIII. List 3 goals for nursing care of the patient with fecal incontinence.

1.

2.

3.

IX. List 3 criteria for nursing goal achievement for the patient with fecal incontinence.

1.

2.

3.

X. Match the definition or description on the left with the most appropriate diagnostic test or procedure on the right.

____ 1. Used to evaluate the neuromuscular function of the bladder

____ 2. May be ordered to create images of the urinary structures

____ 3. Clean-catch urinalysis, blood urea nitrogen measurement

____ 4. Used to determine whether the patient is emptying the bladder completely

____ 5. Measures voiding duration and the amount and rate of urine voided

____ 6. Uses a scope inserted through the urethra to visualize the urethra and bladder

____ 7. Detects involuntary passage of urine when abdominal pressure increases.

A. Postvoid residual

B. Imaging procedures

C. Cystometry

D. Uroflowmetry

E. Cystoscopy

F. Laboratory tests

G. Provocative stress testing

XI. Match the definition or description on the left with the most appropriate therapeutic measure on the right.

____ 1. Intended to help the patient recognize incontinence and to ask caregivers for help with toileting

____ 2. Voiding schedule based on the patient's usual pattern

____ 3. Includes anticholinergics and smooth muscle relaxants

____ 4. Uses patient education, scheduled voiding, and positive reinforcement

____ 5. Sometimes employed by people with spinal cord injury

____ 6. Uses electronic or mechanical sensors to give feedback about physiologic activity

____ 7. Commonly called Kegel exercises

A. Pelvic muscle exercises

B. Reflex training

C. Bladder training

D. Habit training

E. Drug therapy

F. Biofeedback

G. Prompted voiding

XII. Match the definition or description on the left with the most appropriate urine collection device on the right.

____ 1. External urine collection devices which are useful for males

____ 2. Requires patient dexterity, adequate vision, and ability and motivation to learn

____ 3. Ordered to control urinary incontinence

A. Indwelling catheters

B. External devices

C. Intermittent self-catheterization

XIII. Match the nursing diagnosis on the left with the most appropriate cause on the right.

____ 1. Functional incontinence

____ 2. Reflex incontinence

____ 3. High risk for infection

A. Neurologic impairment

B. Chronic bladder distention or catheterization

C. Physical, cognitive, or environmental barriers

XIV. Match each nursing diagnosis on the left with the most appropriate nursing goal on the right.

____ 1. Reflex incontinence related to neurologic impairment

____ 2. Stress incontinence related to weak pelvic structures, increased intra-abdominal pressure

____ 3. Total incontinence related to neurologic dysfunction

____ 4. Urge incontinence related to decreased bladder capacity or bladder spasms

____ 5. High risk for impaired skin integrity related to the presence of urine on the skin

____ 6. High risk for infection related to chronic bladder distention or catheterization

____ 7. Knowledge deficit of causes of incontinence and corrective measures

____ 8. Functional incontinence related to physical, cognitive, or environmental barriers

____ 9. Social isolation related to fear of embarrassment

____ 10. Situational low self-esteem related to loss of control over voiding

A. Patient understanding of incontinence and its treatment

B. Absence of skin breakdown due to urine

C. Adequate management of irreversible incontinence to prevent spillage

D. Decreased episodes of voiding associated with increased abdominal pressure

E. Continent voiding with appropriate support

F. Absence of urinary tract infection

G. Improved self-esteem

H. Decreased episodes of involuntary voiding due to full bladder

I. Absence of social isolation

J. Ability to hold increased volume of urine

XV. Match each side effect and use on the left to the appropriate drug classification on the right.

____ 1. Postural hypotension, tachycardia, headache, dizziness, nasal congestion

____ 2. Used for urge incontinence; causes delayed desire to void

____ 3. Used for atonic bladder; causes bladder contraction

____ 4. Cardiac depression

____ 5. Used for stress incontinence; improves sphincter tone

____ 6. Constipation, dry mouth, pupil dilation, tachycardia

____ 7. Cardiac arrhythmias, nervousness, palpitations

____ 8. Sweating, flushing, GI distress, headache, visual disturbances

____ 9. Used for enuresis (with atropine); causes sphincter contraction

A. Anticholinergics

B. Beta-adrenergic blockers

C. Alpha adrenergics

D. Cholinergics

E. Alpha-adrenergic blockers

XVI. Match the definition on the left with the most appropriate term on the right.

____ 1. Loss of urine due to reflexive contraction   A.   Stress

____ 2. Loss of urine associated with a full bladder   B.   Functional

____ 3. Loss of urine during physical exertion   C.   Reflex

____ 4. Loss of urine that usually follows a strong desire to void   D.   Overflow

        E.   Urge

____ 5. Bladder functions normally but patient voids inappropriately

XVII. Match each drug classification on the left with the condition it can contribute to on the right. (Some drugs may contribute to more than one condition.)

____ 1. Alpha-adrenergic blockers   A.   Urinary incontinence

____ 2. Opiate agonists   B.   Urinary retention

____ 3. Antihistamines

____ 4. Antipsychotics

____ 5. Xanthines

____ 6. High-ceiling diuretics

____ 7. Anticholinergics

____ 8. Sedatives or hypnotics

____ 9. Sympathomimetics

____ 10. Antiparkinson agents

XVIII. Match the definition or description on the left with the most appropriate type of fecal incontinence on the right.

____ 1. Usually seen in dementia patients   A.   Anorectal

____ 2. Uncontrolled, frequent passage of small semi-soft stools; may be related to laxative dependence   B.   Neurogenic

        C.   Overflow

____ 3. Uncontrolled passage of stool several times a day; loss of anal reflex and sphincter tone   D.   Symptomatic

____ 4. Caused by constipation; fecal impaction may be present

____ 5. Formed stools are passed after meals; patients lack voluntary delay of defecation

____ 6. Incontinent stools, usually diarrhea; blood or mucus may be present in stools

____ 7. Result of colorectal disease

XIX. Choose the most appropriate answer.

1. Another word for urination is:
   A. mastication
   B. micturition
   C. parturition
   D. incontinence

2. The amount of urine remaining in the bladder after voiding is called the:
   A. urodynamic series
   B. clean catch
   C. voiding duration
   D. postvoid residual

3. Which treatment is NOT used for patients with reflex incontinence?
   A. cutaneous triggering
   B. tapping the suprapubic area
   C. stroking the inner thigh
   D. Credé's method

4. How much urine normally remains in the bladder after voiding?
   A. 50 ml or less
   B. 100 ml or less
   C. 200 ml or less
   D. 250 ml or less

5. If the bladder becomes overdistended, the patient with reflex incontinence may have a very serious reaction called:
   A. stress incontinence
   B. orthostatic hypotension
   C. autonomic dysreflexia
   D. tachycardia

6. Which is considered to be the last resort in the management of overflow incontinence?
   A. Credé's method
   B. Valsalva maneuver
   C. indwelling catheter
   D. anal stretch maneuver

7. When a person voids inappropriately due to an inability to get to the toilet, this is called:
   A. urge incontinence
   B. functional incontinence
   C. reflex incontinence
   D. stress incontinence

8. Stimuli that may encourage voiding include:
   A. decreasing the fluid intake to less than 2000 ml per day
   B. drinking caffeine and cola drinks
   C. pressing down on the abdomen
   D. stroking the inner thigh, pouring warm water over the perineum, and drinking water while on the toilet

9. The patient who is incontinent of urine is at risk for:
   A. urinary tract infection and urinary calculi (stones)
   B. upper respiratory infection and pelvic infection
   C. bradycardia and thrombophlebitis
   D. diarrhea and skin breakdown

10. People who often ignore or delay defecation tend to have:
    A. diarrhea
    B. constipation
    C. infection
    D. bleeding

11. The first step in the medical management of fecal overflow incontinence is to:
    A. treat the underlying medical condition
    B. use pelvic muscle exercise and biofeedback
    C. cleanse the colon, often with enemas and suppositories
    D. schedule toileting based on the patient's usual time of defecation

12. What type of incontinence is present in patients who do not voluntarily delay defecation?
    A. overflow
    B. anorectal
    C. neurogenic
    D. symptomatic

13. The treatment for fecal neurogenic incontinence is to:
    A. cleanse the colon, usually with enemas and suppositories
    B. treat the underlying medical condition
    C. schedule toileting based on the patient's usual time of defecation
    D. use pelvic muscle exercise and biofeedback

14. Fecal incontinence seen in colorectal disease with diarrhea in which blood or mucus may be seen in the stool is:
    A. neurogenic
    B. symptomatic
    C. anorectal
    D. overflow

15. Incontinence associated with nerve damage that causes the muscles of the pelvic floor to be weak is:
    A. symptomatic
    B. neurogenic
    C. anorectal
    D. overflow

Introductory Nursing Care of Adults

16. Causes of overflow fecal incontinence include:
    A. weak pelvic muscles
    B. colon or rectal disease
    C. loss of anal reflexes
    D. constipation in which the entire colon is full of fecal matter

17. Causes of anorectal fecal incontinence are:
    A. weak pelvic muscles, loss of anal reflexes
    B. constipation in which the entire colon is full of fecal matter
    C. colon or rectal disease
    D. fecal impaction

18. In order to prevent constipation, the patient with fecal incontinence is advised to consume:
    A. increased fluids and protein
    B. increased fluids and fiber
    C. decreased fluids and milk
    D. decreased fluids and protein

22

Loss, Death, and Dying

OBJECTIVES

1. Describe beliefs and practices related to death and dying.
2. Describe responses of patients and their families to terminal illness and death.
3. Identify nursing diagnoses that are appropriate for the terminally ill.
4. Identify nursing goals that are appropriate for the terminally ill.
5. Identify nursing interventions to meet the needs of terminally ill and dying patients.
6. Discuss the needs of the terminally ill patient's significant others.
7. Discuss the ways nurses can intervene to meet the needs of the terminally ill patient's significant others.
8. Explore the responses of the nurse who works with the terminally ill.
9. Explore the needs of the nurse who works with terminally ill patients.
10. Identify issues related to caring for the dying patient including advance directives, do not resuscitate decisions, brain death, organ donations, and pronouncement of death.

LEARNING ACTIVITIES

Match the definition on the left with the most appropriate term on the right.

____ 1. A wrap in which the body is placed after death for transport to the mortuary

____ 2. Written statement of a person's wishes regarding medical care

____ 3. A real or potential absence of someone or something that is valued

____ 4. Absence of cerebral cortex functioning

____ 5. Discoloration of the body after death caused by breakdown of red blood cells; usually in dependent areas of the body

____ 6. A defense mechanism in which the individual thinks and behaves as if not aware of an unpleasant reality

____ 7. Examination of a body after death to determine or confirm the cause of death

____ 8. Cooling of the body after death

____ 9. An emotional response to a loss

____ 10. Stiffening of the body after death

A. Livor mortis
B. Rigor mortis
C. Algor mortis
D. Denial
E. Grief
F. Shroud
G. Autopsy
H. Advance directive
I. Loss
J. Cerebral death

II.   Match the loss on the left with its most appropriate category on the right.

___ 1. Loss of dependence in young adulthood

___ 2. Hair loss

___ 3. Placement in nursing home with loss of home objects

___ 4. Getting a job

___ 5. Disabilities

___ 6. Separation from family when placed in nursing home

___ 7. Loss of family heirloom

___ 8. Children leave parents for school

___ 9. Radical surgery

___ 10. Loss of appointment calendar

___ 11. Pregnancy

___ 12. Death of family member

___ 13. Getting married and moving away from parents

___ 14. Increased dependence in old age

A.   Change of self image

B.   Loss of significant others

C.   Loss of possessions

D.   Developmental changes

III.   Match the definition on the left with the most appropriate term on the right.

___ 1. Grief that is helpful or that assists the person in accepting the reality of death

___ 2. Grief experienced after an actual loss or death occurs

___ 3. Grieving before a death actually occurs

___ 4. Grief that is prolonged, unresolved, or disruptive

A.   Reactive grief

B.   Dysfunctional grief

C.   Adaptive grief

D.   Anticipatory grief

IV.   Fill in the blanks.

1. According to Kübler-Ross, the five stages of dying are denial, anger, bargaining, depression, and

   _____.

2. Six physical symptoms of grief include tightness in the chest, shortness of breath, suffocation, weakness, tightening of abdomen, and _____

3. Three specific fears associated with dying are a fear of pain, fear of loneliness, and fear of_____

   _____.

4. Preceding death, the skin of the extremities becomes mottled and _____.

5. The last sense to remain intact during the death process is _____.

6. During the death process, the function that ceases first is _____.

7. Three examples of goals for anticipatory and dysfunctional grief are patient expression of feelings related to grief, acknowledgment of the impending loss, and behaviors that reflect progress in _____ _____.

8. Following death, in order to keep the mouth closed, the nurse should place a rolled towel under the _____.

9. The act that requires all institutions that participate with Medicare to provide written information to patients concerning their rights to accept or to refuse treatment is called the _____ _____.

10. Allowing the person to die without the interference of technology is referred to as _____ _____.

11. Allowing individuals to select someone to make health care decisions for them if they are unable to do so for themselves is referred to as _____.

V.   Match the definition or description on the left with the most appropriate stage of grieving on the right.

____ 1. Patient or family members may become angry or outraged with situations.

____ 2. Peaceful acknowledgment of the loss

____ 3. Patient realizes the loss is final and the situation cannot be altered; experiences sadness and grief

____ 4. Patient refuses to acknowledge the loss

____ 5. Patient wishes for more time to avoid the loss

____ 6. Patient expresses feelings that the loss is occurring as a punishment for past actions and may try to negotiate with a higher power for more time

____ 7. Protects the patient and family from the reality of the loss

A. Depression

B. Anger

C. Denial

D. Acceptance

E. Bargaining

VI. Match the definition or description on the left with the most appropriate cluster of grief on the right.

____ 1. Last stage of Martocchio's clusters of grief

____ 2. There may be a decreased interest in the future with decision making difficult

____ 3. Anger may be directed toward God, health care providers, survivors, and even the deceased

____ 4. Feelings of numbness, anger, sadness, or guilt; may include denial

____ 5. Survivors imitate behaviors unique to the deceased such as habits, traits, or goals

A. Reorganization and restitution

B. Yearning and protest

C. Shock and disbelief

D. Identification in bereavement

E. Anguish, disorganization, and despair

VII.   Match Kübler-Ross stages on the left with Martocchios's stages on the right.

____   1.   Depression

____   2.   Denial

____   3.   Acceptance

____   4.   Anger/bargaining

A.   Yearning and protest

B.   Anguish, disorganization and despair

C.   Shock and disbelief

D.   Reorganization and restitution

VIII.   Match the beliefs about death on the left with the most appropriate age range on the right.

____   1.   Sees death as inevitable

____   2.   Faces death of parents

____   3.   Examines death as it relates to various meaning, such as freedom from discomfort

____   4.   Death seen as future event

____   5.   Faces death of peers

____   6.   May experience death anxiety

A.   Young adulthood

B.   Middle adulthood

C.   Older adulthood

IX.   Match the definition or description on the left with the most appropriate state of awareness on the right.

____   1.   Patients and others involved freely discuss the impending death

____   2.   Patient and family know of a terminal prognosis but do not discuss the issue openly

____   3.   Patient and family recognize that patient is ill but do not understand severity of illness

A.   Mutual pretense

B.   Closed awareness

C.   Open awareness

X.   Match the actions on the left with the relevant fear on the right.

____   1.   Assure patient medication will be given promptly as needed

____   2.   Express worth of dying person's life

____   3.   Simple presence of person to provide support and comfort

____   4.   Discussion of pain relief measures

____   5.   Holding hands, touching, listening

____   6.   Provide consistent pain control

____   7.   Dying person reviews his life

A.   Fear of loneliness

B.   Fear of meaninglessness

C.   Fear of pain

XI. Match the definition on the left with the most appropriate term on the right.

___ 1.   The body's cooling after death

___ 2.   Discoloration in the skin after death

___ 3.   Stiffening of the body after death

A.   Rigor mortis

B.   Livor mortis

C.   Algor mortis

XII. For each goal related to anticipatory and dysfunctional grief below, supply the appropriate criterion for goal achievement.

1. Patient expression of feelings: _____.

2. Acknowledgment of the impending loss: _____.

3. Demonstration of behaviors that reflect progress in grief resolution: _____

_____.

XIII. List 2 nursing diagnoses that are frequently used during the grieving process.

1.

2.

XIV. In addition to the nursing diagnoses for grief listed for XIII, list 10 other nursing diagnoses related to dying patients and their families.

1.

2.

3.

4.

5.

6.

7.

8.

9.

10.

XV. Choose the most appropriate answer.

1. What happens to the pulse and blood pressure as they change preceding death?
   A.   Pulse quickens and blood pressure drops
   B.   Pulse quickens and blood pressure rises
   C.   Pulse slows and blood pressure drops
   D.   Pulse slows and blood pressure rises

2. Mouth breathing and the accumulation of mucus preceding death result in noisy, wet-sounding respirations called:
   A.   suffocation
   B.   death rattle
   C.   tightness in the chest
   D.   pneumonia

3. Livor mortis is generally most obvious in the:
   A.   skin in extremities
   B.   fingers and toes
   C.   face and chest
   D.   back and buttocks

4. Most states have replaced the idea of living wills with:
   A.   euthanasia acts
   B.   natural death acts
   C.   self-disclosure acts
   D.   DNR acts

The Patient with Cancer

OBJECTIVES

1. Explain the differences between benign and malignant tumors.
2. List the most common sites of cancer in men and women.
3. Describe measures to reduce the risk of cancer.
4. Define terms used to name and classify cancer.
5. List nursing responsibilities in the care of patients having diagnostic tests to detect possible cancer.
6. Explain the nursing care of patients undergoing each type of cancer therapy: surgery, radiation, chemotherapy, biological response modifiers.
7. Identify nursing needs of the terminally ill cancer patient and the family.

LEARNING ACTIVITIES

I. Match the definition on the left with the most appropriate term on the right.

___ 1. Tending to progress in virulence; has the characteristics of becoming increasingly undifferentiated, invasive of surrounding tissues, and colonizing distant sites

___ 2. A gene product that is normally suppressed in adult tissues but reappears in the presence of some types of cancer

___ 3. A substance that can cause cancer

___ 4. The use of radiation in the treatment of cancer and other diseases

___ 5. The transfer of cells from a primary site to a distant site

___ 6. Loss of hair

___ 7. An agent that inhibits the maturation or reproduction of malignant cells

___ 8. New growth; may be benign or malignant

___ 9. Use of chemicals to treat illness

___ 10. Not malignant

A. Radiotherapy

B. Benign

C. Chemotherapy

D. Metastasis

E. Neoplasm

F. Alopecia

G. Oncofetal antigen

H. Malignant

I. Antineoplastic

J. Carcinogen

II.   Fill in the blanks.

1. Cells that reproduce abnormally and in an uncontrolled manner form _____.

2. Tumors that do not spread to other parts of the body and that are relatively harmless are called _____.

3. Tumors found away from the original site of malignant cells are called _____.

4. Because the cells in the hair follicles are very sensitive to radiation, radiation of the head often produces

   _____.

5. Chemical agents specifically used to treat cancer are called _____.

6. The use of chemical agents in the treatment of disease is called _____.

7. A technique in which the drug is injected directly into an artery supplying the tumor is called

   _____.

8. The most dangerous side effect of antineoplastic drugs is _____.

9. The two most distressing side effects of antineoplastic drugs are _____ and

   _____.

10. The use of agents that work by promoting the natural defenses is called _____.

11. For bone marrow suppression, which may occur as a side effect of radiation therapy, the patient should

    _____.

12. The most common site of cancer in women is the _____.

13. The most common site of cancer in men is the _____.

14. Blood counts are usually ordered every week during radiation therapy to detect _____

    _____.

III.   Of the normal cells found in the following areas, check the 6 that are most sensitive to
       radiation:

_____	nail beds	_____	neck
_____	digestive and urinary tract linings	_____	feet
_____	heart lining	_____	testes
_____	forehead	_____	hair follicle
_____	lymph tissue	_____	bone marrow
_____	ovaries		

IV.   Check the 3 types of antineoplastic drugs that are frequently used in chemotherapy:

_____	diuretics	_____	antithyroid drugs
_____	bronchodilators	_____	antiemetics
_____	hormones	_____	sedatives
_____	antihistamines	_____	antihypertensives
_____	narcotics	_____	antitumor antibiotics
_____	alkylating agents	_____	hypnotics

V.   Check 3 major systemic side effects of antineoplastic drugs from the following list:

    _____   dry mouth   _____   constipation

    _____   bone marrow suppression   _____   dizziness

    _____   urinary retention   _____   alopecia

    _____   sedation   _____   electrolyte imbalance

    _____   nausea and vomiting   _____   tachycardia

VI. Check 2 actions of antineoplastic drugs:

    _____   compete with histamine receptors   _____   dilate blood vessels

    _____   depress the vomiting center in the brain   _____   depress the central nervous system

    _____   stimulate the vomiting center in the brain   _____   irritate the lining of the digestive tract

    _____   increase the excretion of water   _____   raise the pain threshold

VII. Check 4 common side effects of biological response modifiers (BRMs):

    _____   headache   _____   fever

    _____   hemoptysis   _____   fatigue

    _____   constipation   _____   hoarseness

    _____   dyspnea   _____   lesions of the skin

    _____   cough   _____   chills

VIII. Check 3 of the following that are side effects of phenothiazines (prochlorperazine [Compazine] and promethazine [Phenergan]):

    _____   nausea and vomiting   _____   electrolyte imbalance

    _____   sedation   _____   fluid volume depletion

    _____   nephrotoxicity   _____   tachycardia

    _____   ototoxicity   _____   hypotension

    _____   extrapyramidal symptoms

IX. Check 4 of the following signs and symptoms that are related to hypercalcemia:

    _____   tachycardia   _____   petechiae

    _____   cough   _____   confusion

    _____   cyanosis   _____   fluid volume excess

    _____   purpura   _____   nausea and vomiting

    _____   edema   _____   weakness

    _____   fatigue   _____   hemorrhage

X. Check 4 of the following signs and symptoms that are related to SIADH (syndrome of inappropriate antidiuretic hormone):

_____ nausea and vomiting   _____ hemorrhage

_____ cough   _____ petechiae

_____ cyanosis   _____ purpura

_____ water retention   _____ weakness

_____ hyponatremia

XI. Check 4 signs and symptoms that are related to DIC (disseminated intravascular coagulation):

_____ hyponatremia   _____ shock

_____ tachycardia   _____ petechiae

_____ hypertension   _____ edema

_____ cough   _____ ecchymoses

XII. Check 4 signs and symptoms that are related to SVCS (superior vena cava syndrome):

_____ shock   _____ dyspnea

_____ hyponatremia   _____ petechiae

_____ cough   _____ nausea and vomiting

_____ ecchymoses   _____ edema of face

_____ tachycardia

XIII. Check 5 of the following that are signs and symptoms of spinal cord compression:

_____ tachycardia   _____ dyspnea

_____ petechiae   _____ cough

_____ impaired bowel function   _____ weakness

_____ altered sensation   _____ ecchymoses

_____ distended neck   _____ hyponatremia

_____ intense pain   _____ nausea and vomiting

_____ impaired bladder function

XIV. List 4 ways to reduce the risk of developing cancer or to detect it in early stages.

1.

2.

3.

4.

XV. List 4 points to be covered in a public education program about cancer screening.

1.

2.

3.

4.

XVI. List the 7 warning signs of cancer.

1.

2.

3.

4.

5.

6.

7.

XVII. List 9 teaching points for the cancer patient undergoing MRI.

1.

2.

3.

4.

5.

6.

7.

8.

9.

XVIII. List 7 safety measures that are necessary to protect all visitors and nurses from excessive exposure to radiation.

1.

2.

3.

4.

5.

6.

7.

XIX. List two side effects that are common with *any* type of radiation therapy.

1.

2.

XX. List 3 examples of biological response modifiers (BRMs).

1.

2.

3.

XXI. List 3 nursing diagnoses in the diagnostic phase of patients with cancer and 3 appropriate goals.

1.   1.

2.   2.

3.   3.

XXII. List 5 key points in teaching the patient about external radiation therapy.

1.

2.

3.

4.

5.

XXIII. List 4 key points in teaching the patient about internal radiation therapy.

1.

2.

3.

4.

XXIV. List 3 reasons why most cancer patients are now told of their diagnoses.

1.

2.

3.

XXV. List 12 nursing diagnoses for patients having treatment for cancer.

1.

2.

3.

4.

5.

6.

7.

8.

9.

10.

11.

12.

XXVI.   List 12 goals of nursing care for the patient having therapy for cancer.

1.

2.

3.

4.

5.

6.

7.

8.

9.

10.

11.

12.

XXVII. List 7 nursing measures to manage nausea and vomiting.

1.

2.

3.

4.

5.

6.

7.

XXVIII.   List 6 groups of common known carcinogens.

1.

2.

3.

4.

5.

6.

XXIX.   List 4 things cancer patients should avoid if they experience skin redness and peeling as
side effects of radiation.

1.

2.

3.

4.

XXX. List 2 things that cancer patients who experience cystitis or cystalluria as side effects of radiation therapy should do for these conditions.

1.

2.

XXXI. A patient is receiving antineoplastic therapy. List interventions that the nurse needs to employ for (1) side effects of heart failure and (2) side effects of pneumonia.

1.

2.

XXXII. Match the definition or description on the left with the most appropriate term on the right.

___ 1. Tumors of the bone

___ 2. Tumors that develop from pigment cells in the skin

___ 3. Tumors that develop from fat tissue

___ 4. Tumors of cartilage

___ 5. Tumors that develop from smooth muscle tissue

___ 6. Tumors that develop from fibrous connective tissue

___ 7. Tumors found away from the original site of malignant cells

___ 8. Tumors that originate from tissues in the skin, glands, and linings, of the digestive, urinary, and respiratory tracts

___ 9. Tumors that arise from the blood-forming tissues

___ 10. Tumors that originate from bone, muscle, and other connective tissue

A. Chondrosarcomas

B. Fibromas

C. Melanomas

D. Metastatic growths

E. Osteosarcomas

F. Leiomyomas

G. Lipomas

H. Leukemias and lymphomas

I. Sarcomas

J. Carcinomas

XXXIII. Match the definition on the left with the most appropriate term on the right.

___ 1. There is limited spread of the cancer in the local area, usually to nearby lymph nodes.

___ 2. The malignant cells are confined to the tissue of origin. There is no invasion of other tissues.

___ 3. The cancer has metastasized to distant parts of the body.

___ 4. The tumor is larger or has spread from the site of origin into nearby tissues, or both. Regional lymph nodes are likely to be involved.

A. Stage I

B. Stage II

C. Stage III

D. Stage IV

XXIV. Match the definition or description on the left with the most appropriate term on the right.

____ 1. Removal of cells from living tissue for microscopic examination

____ 2. Nuclear scan that reveals patterns of tissue metabolism

____ 3. Useful for diagnosing tumors in the head or trunk

____ 4. Insertion of lighted tubes into hollow organs or body cavities

____ 5. Useful in diagnosing abnormalities of the central nervous system, spinal column, neck, bones, and joints

____ 6. Used to detect cancer cells in the cervix

A. Magnetic resonance imaging

B. Computed tomography

C. Endoscopy

D. Papanicolaou smear

E. Biopsy

F. Positron emission tomography

XXV. Match the effect on the left with the most appropriate drug on the right.

____ 1. Causes pulmonary inflammation and fibrosis

____ 2. Neurotoxicity resulting in numbness and tingling of extremities

____ 3. Toxic effects on the heart that may lead to heart failure

A. Vincristine (Oncovin)

B. Doxorubicin (Adriamycin)

C. Bleomycin (Blenoxane)

XXVI. Match the nursing diagnosis related to treatment of cancer on the right with its appropriate "related to" statement on the left.

____ 1. Multiple stressors, overwhelming threat to self

____ 2. Decreased salivation, inflammation (stomatitis, mucositis)

____ 3. Illness and therapy

____ 4. Effects and outcomes of treatment

____ 5. Loss of body part or altered appearance or function

____ 6. Decreased white blood cells, venous access devices

____ 7. Therapy, effects, and precautions

____ 8. Alopecia

____ 9. Side effects of therapy

____ 10. Anemia, effects of cancer

____ 11. Anorexia, nausea and vomiting

____ 12. Decreased activity, drug side effects

A. Altered oral mucous membranes

B. Altered family processes

C. Anxiety

D. Colonic constipation

E. Altered nutrition: less than body requirements

F. Dysfunctional grieving

G. High risk for infection

H. Fatigue

I. Ineffective individual coping

J. Body image disturbance

K. High risk for injury

L. Knowledge deficit

XXXVII.   Match the nursing diagnoses on the left with the evaluation criteria on the right.

____ 1. Dysfunctional grieving related to loss of body part or altered appearance or function

____ 2. Body image disturbance related to alopecia

____ 3. Ineffective individual coping related to multiple stressors or overwhelming threat to self

____ 4. Altered nutrition: less than body requirements related to anorexia, nausea, and vomiting

____ 5. Colonic constipation related to decreased activity or drug side effects

____ 6. Anxiety related to effects and outcomes of treatment

____ 7. Altered family processes related to illness and therapy

____ 8. High risk for injury related to side effects of therapy

____ 9. Knowledge deficit of therapy, effects, and precautions

____ 10. Altered oral mucous membranes related to decreased salivation or inflammation (stomatitis, mucositis)

____ 11. High risk for infection related to decreased white blood cells or venous access devices

____ 12. Fatigue related to anemia or effects of cancer

A. Family's reassignment of roles and responsibilities

B. Patient's statement of reduced anxiety and relaxed demeanor

C. Patient's discussion of feelings of loss and touching of affected parts

D. Patient's completion of essential activities without dyspnea or tachycardia

E. An intact skin and mucous membranes, an absence of bleeding, dyspnea, edema, diarrhea, and dysuria

F. Patient's demonstration of effective coping strategies

G. A bowel movement at least every 3 days

H. A stable body weight

I. Moist mucous membranes

J. A normal body temperature, an absence of purulent drainage

K. Patient's verbalization of content in the teaching plan

L. Patient's demonstration of acceptance or concealment of hair loss

XXXVIII. Match each test or procedure on the left to the potential cancer site on the right. (Some sites may be used more than once.)

____ 1. Counseling and checkup

____ 2. Mammography

____ 3. Papanicolaou test and pelvic examination

____ 4. Sigmoidoscopy

____ 5. Endometrial biopsy

____ 6. Digital rectal examination

____ 7. Prostate examination and prostate-specific antigen blood test

A. Endometrium

B. Colon, rectum

C. Cervix

D. Thyroid, testicles, ovaries, lymph nodes, mouth, skin

E. Prostate

F. Breast

XXIX. Indicate for each tumor characteristic on the left whether it refers to (A) benign or (B) malignant tumors.

___ 1. No metastasis

___ 2. Recurrence after removal common

___ 3. Tissue of origin not readily identifiable

___ 4. Usually rapid growth rate, but may be slow

___ 5. Usually no tissue destruction unless compression or obstruction occurs

___ 6. Invades surrounding tissues

___ 7. Usually slow growth rate

___ 8. Enlarges and expands, but does not usually invade surrounding tissues

___ 9. Can cause necrosis, ulceration, perforation

___ 10. Recurrence after removal unlikely

___ 11. Metastasizes

___ 12. Cells closely resemble those of tissue of origin

A. Benign

B. Malignant

L. Match each side effect of radiation therapy on the left with the appropriate nursing implications on the right.

___ 1. Pneumonitis

___ 2. Harm to embryo or fetus; sterility, impotence

___ 3. Cystitis, contracted bladder, crystalluria

___ 4. Partial or complete alopecia (hair loss); may be permanent; new hair may be different color and texture

___ 5. Suppressed production of red blood cells, white blood cells, and platelets

___ 6. Anorexia; inflammation and dryness of the mouth; decreased or altered sense of taste; dental caries; painful swallowing; nausea, vomiting; diarrhea

___ 7. Erythema (redness), desquamation (peeling); permanent darkening

A. Increase fluid intake. Have patient empty bladder often. Keep intake and output records.

B. Encourage coughing and deep breathing to prevent pneumonia. Use humidifier if ordered. Protect from respiratory infections.

C. Skin is easily injured. Avoid exposure to sun, trauma, harsh chemicals, or soaps. Until therapy is completed, no lotions or topical medications should be applied. Do not remove markings.

D. Small, frequent feedings; respect patient preferences; frequent oral hygiene; suggest artificial saliva; monitor weight to assess nutritional state. Encourage dental care; mouth care per protocol. Antacids and viscous lidocaine as ordered. Antiemetics as ordered; monitor intake. Antidiarrheals as ordered; perianal care.

E. Patient advised not to become pregnant during therapy or for specified time afterward. Physician may counsel male patient about banking sperm.

F. Schedule activities to prevent overtiring. Protect from infection. Protect from injury. Watch for excessive bruising or bleeding. Check results of blood tests. Report fever. Use soft toothbrush, electric razor.

G. Cover scalp with wig or scarf if patient desires. Refer to American Cancer Society for free hairpieces and help with styling and care.

XLI. Match each side effect of antineoplastic therapy on the left with the appropriate nursing implications on the right.

___ 1. Cardiomyopathy; heart failure

___ 2. Alopecia

___ 3. Harm to developing embryo or fetus. Sterility, impotence with some agents.

___ 4. Phlebitis at infusion site. Possible necrosis of surrounding tissue with extravasation.

___ 5. Numbness, tingling, loss of deep tendon reflexes

___ 6. Suppressed production of red blood cells, white blood cells, and platelets

___ 7. Lung inflammation, fibrosis

___ 8. Nausea and vomiting; anorexia; xerostomia; stomatitis; diarrhea, constipation

A. Protect affected areas from injury.

B. Monitor for dyspnea, edema, increasing pulse pressure. Request electrocardiograms as ordered.

C. Encourage turning, coughing, and deep breathing to prevent pneumonia. Use humidifier as ordered. Elevate head if dyspneic. Protect from respiratory infections. Monitor activity tolerance.

D. Monitor infusion carefully. Protect infusion site. Report signs of extravasations immediately.

E. Pregnancy discouraged while on therapy and for specified period thereafter. Physician may discuss banking sperm with male patients.

F. Give antiemetics as ordered; assess for dehydration; no fluids with meals; pleasant environment; respect food preferences. Small, frequent feedings; frequent oral hygiene; monitor weight; give supplements as ordered. Increase fluid intake; recommend artificial saliva, sugarless gum or hard candy, ice chips; moisten dry food. Encourage dental care; mouth care as ordered or per protocol; assess for lesions. Antidiarrheals as ordered; perianal care. Encourage fluids and high fiber foods, and exercise as tolerated; give laxatives, stool softeners, enemas as ordered.

G. Cover scalp with hairpiece, scarf, turban if patient wishes. Refer to American Cancer Society for free hairpieces and help with grooming.

H. Monitor blood test results. Allow rest. Prevent overtiring. Protect from infection. Report fever. Watch for excessive bruising or bleeding. Apply pressure to injection sites. Avoid rectal temperatures if white blood cell count is low. Use soft toothbrush and electric razor.

XLII. Match each side effect of biological response modifiers on the left with the appropriate nursing implications on the right.

____ 1. Serious arrhythmias, myocardial infarction

____ 2. Anaphylaxis with bronchial constriction. Pulmonary edema.

____ 3. Increased capillary permeability, pulmonary and dependent edema, hypotension

____ 4. Flu-like symptoms: fever, chills, muscle aches, severe fatigue, malaise, headaches, tachycardia

A. Assess for edema. Monitor blood pressure. Have patient change positions slowly; avoid prolonged standing, hot baths, and showers. For hypotension, give colloids or vasopressors as ordered.

B. Side effects may mask signs and symptoms of infection, so assess carefully. Give acetaminophen as ordered. Give meperidine as ordered for severe chills. Help patient plan for adequate rest.

C. Note signs of allergy: rash, wheezing, itching. For anaphylaxis, give epinephrine or dephenhydramine as ordered. Maintain airway. Assess lung for rales. Position for comfort (head elevated).

D. Monitor heart rate and rhythm. Report abnormal findings.

XLIII. Match the oncologic emergency on the left with the appropriate signs and symptoms in the middle and appropriate nursing care on the right.

____ 1. Syndrome of inappropriate antidiuretic hormone

____ 2. Hypercalcemia

____ 3. Spinal cord compression

____ 4. Superior vena cava syndrome

____ 5. Disseminated intravascular coagulation

A. Redness and edema of face, conjunctiva around eyes; distended neck and thoracic veins; dyspnea, cough, tachypnea, tachycardia, cyanosis progressing to increased intracranial pressure

B. Tumor in epidural space presses on spinal cord, causing intense pain, weakness, altered sensation in arms or legs, impaired bowel and bladder function

C. Water intoxication and dilutional hyponatremia due to water retention: nausea and vomiting, anorexia, weakness, lethargy at fist, followed by confusion, psychosis, loss of deep tendon reflexes, seizures, coma, and death

D. Normal clotting process is exaggerated, clotting factors are depleted. Early signs: petechiae, ecchymoses, prolonged bleeding from venipuncture. Late signs: signs of vascular obstruction, tachycardia, dyspnea, gastrointestinal bleeding, heart failure, and shock.

E. Fatigue, confusion, weakness, constipation, polyuria, hypertension, tachycardia, poor muscle tone. If untreated, renal failure, coma, cardiac dysrhythmias, or death can occur.

F. Avoid trauma. Handle gently. Give blood products and heparin as ordered. Monitor vital signs. Look for bleeding.

G. Explain and enforce fluid restriction. Monitor vital signs. Keep intake and output records. Do not give demeclocycline with food or dairy products.

H. Give analgesics as ordered. Assess for full bladder, constipation. Do neurologic checks on affected extremities.

I. Monitor fluid status. Give IV fluids and drugs as ordered. Monitor intake and output

J. Give medications as ordered. Elevate head and arms but not legs. Tell patient not to bend forward. Reassure patient that symptoms usually subside in 2–3 days.

Introductory Nursing Care of Adults

XLIV.   Choose the most appropriate answer.

1. The second most common cause of death in the United States is:
   A. heart disease
   B. emphysema
   C. cancer
   D. kidney disease

2. The type of invasion that involves the movement of cancer cells into adjoining tissue is:
   A. regional
   B. systemic
   C. localized
   D. centralized

3. Fibromas develop from which type of tissue:
   A. fat
   B. smooth muscle
   C. osseous
   D. fibrous connective

4. A patient whose primary tumor has grown and spread to regional lymph nodes but not to distant sites is staged:
   A. Tis, N2, M1
   B. T2, N1, M0
   C. T0, N3, M1
   D. T4, N0, M0

5. The recommended diet that may reduce the risk of some cancers is one that is:
   A. low fiber, fat, calories, and preservatives
   B. low fiber and preservatives; high fat and calories
   C. high fiber; low fat, calories, and preservatives
   D. high fiber, fat and calories; low preservatives

6. Postprocedure care for PET includes:
   A. taking vital signs
   B. forcing fluids
   C. keeping patient NPO
   D. coughing and deep breathing

7. The most common treatment for malignant tumors is:
   A. radiotherapy
   B. chemotherapy
   C. immunotherapy
   D. surgery

8. The use of ionizing radiation in the treatment of disease is called:
   A. surgery
   B. chemotherapy
   C. radiotherapy
   D. immunotherapy

9. Radiation has immediate and delayed effects on cells; the immediate effect is:
   A. cell death
   B. alteration of DNA, which impairs cell's ability to reproduce
   C. interruption of the clotting cascade
   D. cell starvation

10. What condition results from a deficiency of red blood cells?
    A. congestive heart failure
    B. kidney failure
    C. anemia
    D. diabetes mellitus

11. Signs and symptoms of internal bleeding include:
    A. decreased pulse
    B. restlessness
    C. increased urine output
    D. increased blood pressure

12. The patient with cancer therapy is offered what kind of diet?
    A. high protein, high calorie
    B. high protein, low calorie
    C. low protein, high calorie
    D. low protein, low calorie

CHAPTER

24

The Ostomy Patient

OBJECTIVES

1. List the indications for ostomy surgery to divert urine or feces.
2. Describe nursing interventions to prepare the patient for ostomy surgery.
3. Briefly explain the types of procedures used for fecal diversion.
4. Apply the nursing process in planning care for the patient with each of the following types of fecal diversion: ileostomy, continent ileostomy, ileoanal reservoir, and colostomy.
5. Briefly explain the types of procedures done for urinary diversion.
6. Apply the nursing process in planning care for the patient with each of the following types of urinary diversion: ureterostomy, ileal conduit, continent internal reservoir.
7. Discuss major topics and content to be included in teaching patients to learn to live with ostomies.

LEARNING ACTIVITIES

I.   Match the definition on the left with the most appropriate term on the right.

_____   1. Opening created to drain contents of an organ

_____   2. Surgically created opening in the kidney to drain urine

_____   3. Surgically created opening into the urinary bladder

_____   4. Surgical procedure that creates an opening into a body structure

_____   5. Capable of controlling natural impulses; in relation to an ostomy, able to retain feces or urine

_____   6. Surgically created opening in the ureter

_____   7. Downward displacement

_____   8. Communication or connection between two organs or parts of organs

_____   9. Surgically created opening in the ileum

_____   10. Surgically created opening in the colon

A. Anastomosis

B. Colostomy

C. Continent

D. Ileostomy

E. Nephrostomy

F. Ostomy

G. Prolapse

H. Stoma

I. Ureterostomy

J. Vesicostomy

II.   List 5 examples of ostomies of the digestive tract.

1.   4.

2.   5.

3.

III.   List one problem that may occur if the stoma site is too close to a bony prominence, preventing a good pouch seal.

1.

IV.   For the patient having ostomy surgery, list 1 goal and 2 interventions for each nursing diagnosis listed below.

	Nursing Goals	Nursing Interventions
1. Anxiety related to anticipated changes in body appearance and function	1.	1.
		2.
2. Knowledge deficit of what to expect postoperatively in relation to ostomy	1.	1.
		2.

V.   Ileostomy patients are NPO before and during surgery. Explain why the physician applies a temporary plastic pouch or a fluffy dressing in the operating room.

VI.   For the immediate postoperative ileostomy patient, list 1 appropriate nursing goal and 2 appropriate interventions for each nursing diagnosis listed below.
1.   High risk for fluid volume deficit related to nothing by mouth status, nasogastric suction, passage of liquid stool
2.   Impaired skin integrity related to stoma adhesive, fecal drainage
3.   Body image disturbance related to presence of stoma, altered body function
4.   Sexual dysfunction related to altered body structure and function
5.   Knowledge deficit of self-care with ostomy

A. Goals: B. Nursing interventions:

1.   1.

                                                       2.

2.   3.

                                                       4.

3.   5.

                                                       6.

4.   7.

                                                       8.

5.   9.

                                                       10.

VII. List 3 reasons why maintaining skin integrity is an ongoing problem for the patient with an intestinal ostomy.

1.

2.

3.

VIII. List nursing interventions to control odor for each of the areas listed below.

A. Foods in the diet (list 2)

1.

2.

B. Hygiene (list 3)

1.

2.

3.

IX. List 3 practical suggestions that may help patients with ileostomies resume sexual activity.

1.

2.

3.

X. List 9 topics to include in the teaching plan after ostomy surgery.

1.   6.

2.   7.

3.   8.

4.   9.

5.

XI. Fill in the appropriate response related to the following teaching points.

1. Activities: If the patient asks when normal activities can usually be resumed, the nurse answers:

_____

2. Bathing and showers: If the patient asks if it is all right to take a bath or shower with the appliance on, or should the patient take the appliance off first, how should the nurse respond?

_____

3. Clothing: if the patient asks if regular clothing can be worn, how should the nurse respond?

_____

4. Traveling: If the patient asks how to dispose of used supplies on a trip, how should the nurse respond?

_____

5. Traveling: If the patient asks if it is all right to eat everything on the trip, how should the nurse respond?

_____

XII. Patients with internal reservoirs must learn to strengthen perineal muscles in order to restore control of fecal elimination. Describe a recommended exercise that should be repeated 5 to 6 times four times daily.

XIII. What is the major complication that may be caused by colostomy irrigation?

XIV. List 2 ways the ureterostomy stoma differs from an intestinal stoma.

1.

2.

XV. Explain why ureterostomy pouch changes are usually done in the morning.

XVI. Explain why ureterostomy pouch care is treated as a clean rather than a sterile procedure.

XVII. List 6 complications that may occur in the early postoperative period following the ileal conduit procedure.

1.

2.

3.

4.

5.

6.

XVIII. Complete the statements on the left with the most appropriate term on the right.

_____ 1. Two examples of ostomies that are created to drain fecal matter from the intestines include colostomies and _____.

_____ 2. Two factors that must be considered in the placement of the stoma include ease of self-care and _____.

_____ 3. A temporary ostomy may be indicated following surgery or trauma, or when there is severe _____.

_____ 4. A registered nurse with specialized training who has passed a certification examination on ostomy care is called a(n) _____.

_____ 5. Three examples of stomas in the urinary tract are the ureterostomy, continent internal reservoirs, and _____.

A. Inflammation or infection

B. Secure pouch placement

C. Ileostomies

D. Enterostomal therapist

E. Ileal conduits

CHAPTER 24 THE OSTOMY PATIENT   203

XIX. Complete statements on the left with the most appropriate term on the right. Some terms may be used more than once, and some terms may not be used.

____ 1. When fecal matter is diverted from the colon, it may be liquid, semisolid, or formed; fecal matter in the ileum is _____.

____ 2. Following ileostomy surgery, the stoma is inspected for color and _____.

____ 3. The procedure that is required when the entire colon must be bypassed or removed is _____.

____ 4. Following ileostomy surgery, the base of the stoma is inspected for redness, purulent drainage, and _____.

____ 5. Following ileostomy surgery, a pale or bluish stoma may indicate poor _____.

____ 6. Following ileostomy surgery, the nurse should inform the physician if the color of the stoma is _____.

A. Ileostomy
B. Pale and blue
C. Circulation
D. Liquid
E. Red
F. Skin breakdown
G. Bleeding
H. Colostomy

XX. Complete the statements on the left with the most appropriate term on the right. Some terms may be used more than once, and some terms may not be used.

____ 1. If bowel obstruction occurs in the patient with an ileoanal reservoir, the patient is given intravenous fluids, placed on NPO status, and a nasogastric tube is inserted to _____.

____ 2. If the patient with an ileoanal reservoir develops abscesses or peritonitis, the infection is treated with _____.

____ 3. The patient with a continent ileostomy will have some dietary restrictions. Three dietary considerations include avoiding excessive gas, avoiding obstruction of the catheter, and maintaining a(n) _____.

____ 4. Three symptoms that a patient may experience if too much solution is used for colostomy irrigation of if the solution is too cold, are nausea, dizziness, and _____.

____ 5. Absence of drainage or patient complaints of a feeling of fullness in the pouch of continent ileostomy patients need to be reported, as these may be signs of _____.

____ 6. Scar tissue or strictures may cause obstruction of the ileoanal reservoir. Four signs and symptoms of small bowel obstruction are nausea and vomiting, decreased bowel sounds, a change in bowel pattern, and _____.

____ 7. Three major complications of the ileoanal reservoir are small bowel obstruction, leaking of suture lines leading to peritonitis, and _____.

A. Inflammation of the reservoir
B. Soft stool
C. Decompress the bowel
D. Abdominal distention
E. Anti-inflammatory drugs
F. Decrease anxiety
G. Inflammation of the bowel
H. Cramping
I. Antibiotics
J. Obstruction
K. Liquid stool

Introductory Nursing Care of Adults
Copyright © 1995 by W.B. Saunders Company. All rights reserved.

XXI. Complete the statements on the left with the appropriate term on the right. Some terms may be used more than once, and some terms may not be used.

_____ 1. An internal pouch created from a loop of ileum for storing fecal matter is called _____.

_____ 2. An opening in the colon through which fecal matter is eliminated is called a _____.

_____ 3. The two main complications of colostomy are prolapse and _____.

_____ 4. The two main causes of odor from an ileostomy that can be controlled are poor hygiene and _____.

_____ 5. Two serious consequences of urinary tract infections following ureterostomy include kidney damage and _____.

_____ 6. Yeast infections around the ureterostomy stoma may be treated with _____.

_____ 7. A type of medication that can be inserted into a colostomy stoma to stimulate evacuation is _____.

_____ 8. If odor is a problem with ureterostomy, the pouch can be soaked for 20–30 minutes in _____.

_____ 9. Complications experienced by patients with cutaneous ureterostomies include stenosis and _____.

_____ 10. Three contributing factors to prolapsed stoma include coughing or sneezing, a poorly attached stoma, and _____.

A. Urinary tract infections
B. Nystatin
C. Vinegar water
D. Ileostomy
E. Too small an abdominal opening
F. Continent ileostomy
G. Ureterostomy
H. Septicemia
I. Rectal suppository
J. Colostomy
K. Too large an abdominal opening
L. Stenosis
M. Lack of hand washing
N. Certain foods

XXII. For each of the following nursing diagnoses for the postoperative ileostomy patient, complete the related to section.

1. High risk for fluid volume deficit related to _____

2. Impaired skin integrity related to _____

3. Body image disturbance related to _____

4. Sexual dysfunction related to _____

5. Knowledge deficit related to _____

XXIII. Describe the signs and symptoms to observe in the postoperative ileostomy patient that would indicate electrolyte imbalances:

A. Mental status changes

1.

2.

B. Neuromuscular status changes

1.

2.

3.

C. Fluid volume changes

1.

2.

3.

XXIV.   List 4 food groups that patients with continent ileostomies should avoid, at least initially.

1.

2.

3.

4.

XXV.   Describe the signs and symptoms of peritonitis that occur in each of the following areas:

1. Pulse

2. Respiration

3. Temperature

4. Abdomen

5. WBC count

XXVI.   Complete the related to portion of the following nursing diagnoses for patients with internal reservoirs:

1. High risk for impaired skin integrity related to _____

2. Bowel incontinence related to _____

3. High risk for injury related to _____

XXVII.   Why should patients with ileostomies not be given timed-release capsules or enteric-coated pills?

XXVIII.   Since the stoma of an ileal or colonic conduit is intestinal mucosa, what color will it be?

XXIX.   Match the foods on the left with the type of stool they produce on the right.

____ 1. Boiled rice   A. Loose

____ 2. Fresh fruits   B. Thick

____ 3. Low-fat cheese

____ 4. Pasta

____ 5. Fresh vegetables

____ 6. Caffeine

XXX. Match the definition on the left with the most appropriate term on the right. Answers may be used more than once.

_____ 1. Urinary diversion method in which urine is stored and drained in a controlled fashion

_____ 2. Most common type of urinary diversion

_____ 3. Urinary diversion method in which the ureters are implanted into the sigmoid colon and urine drains into the colon and is eliminated through the rectum

_____ 4. A urinary drainage system made out of a portion of small intestine

_____ 5. The procedure in which one or both ureters are brought out through an opening in the abdomen

A. Cutaneous ureterostomy

B. Ileal conduit

C. Continent internal reservoir

D. Ureterosigmoidostomy

XXXI. For ureterostomy patients, match the 5 criteria for goal achievement on the right with the nursing goals on the left.

_____ 1. Unobstructed urine flow

_____ 2. Knowledge of self-care with ostomy

_____ 3. Absence of signs of infection

_____ 4. Normal skin around stoma

_____ 5. Adjustment in body image

A. Patient demonstration of proper demonstration of proper techniques of ostomy care

B. Patient acknowledging stoma

C. Intact, healed stoma base with no redness or edema

D. Balanced intake and output

E. Pulse, temperature, normal for patient

XXXII. Choose the most appropriate answer.

1. A colostomy is performed by bringing a loop of the intestine through the wall of the:
   A. bladder
   B. rectum
   C. abdomen
   D. stomach

2. The narrowing of the abdominal opening around the base of the stoma is called:
   A. prolapse
   B. stenosis
   C. hemorrhage
   D. infection

3. A nursing diagnosis for the colostomy patient is high risk for injury related to:
   A. hemorrhage or infection
   B. dyspnea or tachycardia
   C. hypotension or bradycardia
   D. prolapse or stenosis

4. If the nurse notices that the colostomy is not draining properly, the nurse:
   A. places a finger in the stoma to dilate it
   B. uses a larger catheter to irrigate
   C. informs the physician
   D. forces the catheter in 3 inches

5. The condition in which the kidney becomes swollen with urine, leading to serious kidney damage, is called:
   A. hydronephrosis
   B. pyelonephritis
   C. ileitis
   D. hydrocystitis

6. If the ileal conduit stoma turns gray or black, the physician should be notified immediately, as this may mean that:
   A. ureteral obstruction has occurred
   B. circulation is impaired
   C. wound infection is present
   D. prolapse has occurred

7. After bowel resection for the ileal conduit procedure, the nurse should expect:
   A. necrosis of the wound
   B. temporary ileus (absence of bowel activity)
   C. gray-black stoma
   D. ureteral calculi

8. In which procedure would the nurse expect to find mucus in the drainage?
   A. ureterostomy
   B. vesicostomy
   C. cystostomy
   D. ileal conduit

XXXIII. Using the figure below, label each type of colostomy (A–D) and indicate which type of drainage is passed by each (E–G). (Figure modified from Ignatavicius, D. D., & Bayne, M. V. [1991]. *Medical-surgical nursing: A nursing process approach* [p. 1384]. Philadelphia: W. B. Saunders.)

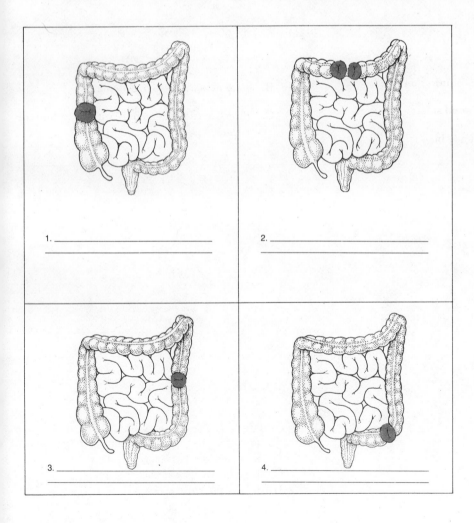

A. Descending colostomy
B. Ascending colostomy
C. Transverse colostomy
D. Sigmoid colostomy
E. Liquid to semisolid stool
F. Softly formed stool
G. Liquid material

1. _____
2. _____
3. _____
4. _____

Neurologic Disorders

OBJECTIVES

1. Identify common neurologic changes in the older person and the implications of these for nursing care.
2. Describe the diagnostic tests and procedures used to evaluate neurologic dysfunction and the nursing responsibilities associated with each.
3. Identify the uses, side effects, and nursing interventions associated with common drug therapies employed in patients with neurologic disorders.
4. Describe the signs and symptoms associated with increased intracranial pressure and the medical therapies used in its treatment.
5. List the components of the nursing assessment of the patient with a neurologic disorder.
6. Describe the pathophysiology, signs and symptoms, complications, and medical or surgical treatment for patients with selected neurologic disorders.
7. Apply the nursing process to plan care for the patient with a neurologic disorder.

LEARNING ACTIVITIES

I. Match the definition on the left with the most appropriate term on the right.

____ 1. Abnormal extension of the upper extremities with extension of the lower extremities; accompanies increased pressure on the entire cerebrum and the motor tract structures of the brain stem

____ 2. Biochemical messenger at nerve endings that stimulates an excitatory or inhibitory impulse

____ 3. A peculiar sensation that precedes a set of symptoms

____ 4. Weakness on one side of the body

____ 5. Abnormal flexion of the upper extremities with extension of the lower extremities; accompanies increased pressure on the frontal lobes

____ 6. Pain in a nerve or along the course of a nerve

____ 7. An abnormal sensation

____ 8. Inflammation of brain tissue

A. Aura
B. Automatism
C. Contralateral
D. Decerebrate posturing
E. Decorticate posturing
F. Encephalitis
G. Hemiparesis
H. Hemiplegia
I. Intracranial
J. Ipsilateral
K. Neuralgia
L. Neurotransmitter
M. Paresthesia
N. Postictal
O. Seizure

I. *Continues*

I. *Continued*

   ___   9. Aimless behavior performed without conscious control or knowledge

   ___   10. Affecting the same side

   ___   11. Paralysis on one side of the body

   ___   12. Affecting the opposite side

   ___   13. Within the skull

   ___   14. Convulsion; series of involuntary contractions of voluntary muscles

   ___   15. After a seizure

A. Aura

B. Automatism

C. Contralateral

D. Decerebrate posturing

E. Decorticate posturing

F. Encephalitis

G. Hemiparesis

H. Hemiplegra

I. Intracranial

J. Ipsilateral

K. Neuralgia

L. Neurotransmitter

M. Paresthesia

N. Postictal

O. Seizure

II.   Fill in the blanks.

1. Cerebrospinal fluid is composed primarily of water, glucose, sodium chloride, and _____.

2. The function of cerebrospinal fluid (CSF) is to act as a _____.

3. The spinal cord extends from the border of the first cervical vertebra to the level of the _____ _____.

4. Most older people retain normal cognition and behavior despite a decreasing number of nerve cells because _____.

5. Five areas the nurse should assess in patients with neurologic disorders include speech, behavior, coordination, alertness and _____.

6. Three assessments that the nurse should make following lumbar puncture include assessing numbness, tingling or pain in the extremities; drainage from the puncture site; and _____.

7. Three nursing interventions that may be done prior to a patient's EEG include a thorough shampoo, withholding medications such as anticonvulsants or tranquilizers, and restricting _____.

8. A neurotransmitter involved in motor function that is deficient in Parkinson's disease, causing loss of motor function, is _____.

I.   List 3 functions of the nervous system that relate to information received from the external
environment.

1.

2.

3.

V.   List 4 neurotransmitters.

1.   3.

2.   4.

.   List the 2 major subdivisions of the autonomic nervous system.

1.

2.

I.   List how the 4 parts of the nervous system listed below change with normal aging.

1. Nerve cells (number)

2. Brain (weight)

3. Ventricles (size)

4. Nerve tissues

II.   Briefly explain what happens to nerve cells when nerve tissue experiences hypoxia.

III.   Disturbances in glucose metabolism and electrolyte imbalances can lead to what 2 types of
deterioration in the nervous system?

1.

2.

X.   List 3 conditions involving accumulation of toxins that may result in neurologic
dysfunction.

1.

2.

3.

.   List normal characteristics of pupils that are noted in pupillary evaluation regarding the 3
areas below.

1. size _____

2. shape _____

3. reactivity _____

XI. List 5 common terms used to describe altered level of consciousness.

1.   4.

2.   5.

3.

XII. Explain why the examiner puts one finger on top of another when assessing upper arm strength by asking the patient to squeeze the examiner's fingers.

XIII. Explain why a hollow needle is inserted into the subarachnoid space at the level of the third lumbar vertebra.

XIV. In which position must the patient remain during a lumbar puncture?

XV. List 5 areas the nurse assesses in order to detect signs of increasing intracranial pressure so treatment can be initiated promptly.

1.   4.

2.   5.

3.

XVI. Explain why the level of consciousness is the most reliable indicator of mental status.

XVII. If there is a tumor in the right side of the brain, motor deficits will appear in what side of the body?

XVIII. Indicate the changes that occur in the 3 areas listed below as the 3 signs of Cushing's triad, which is generally associated with increased ICP.

1. blood pressure

2. pulse

3. pulse pressure

XIX. Indicate the medical treatment measures that are taken in each of the following 5 areas for patients with increased ICP.

1. positioning

2. hyperventilation

3. fluid restriction

4. mechanical drainage

5. drug therapy

X.   List 7 of the most common symptoms of MS.

1.   5.

2.   6.

3.   7.

4.

XI.   For each of the following 7 problems listed for patients with MS, list at least 2 nursing
      interventions.

1. Impaired physical mobility

2. Sensory perceptual alterations

3. Self-care deficit

4. Functional incontinence

5. High risk for infection

6. Ineffective individual coping

7. Knowledge deficit

XXII.   Complete the table below by filling in the appropriate "related to" statements and
        nursing goals for the patient with ALS.

Nursing Diagnosis	Related to:	Goals
Ineffective airway clearance		
Impaired physical mobility		participation in activities to maintain mobility
Altered nutrition: less than body requirements	dysphagia	
Impaired verbal communication		effective communication
Impaired skin integrity		
Anticipatory grieving	progressive, fatal disease	
Situational low self-esteem		
Altered family processes		

XXIII. List 5 nursing diagnoses for patients with trigeminal neuralgia.

1.

2.

3.

4.

5.

XXIV. Complete the statements on the left with the most appropriate term on the right. Some terms may be used more than once, and some terms may not be used.

___ 1. A control system that coordinates and regulates bodily functions is the _____.

___ 2. The functional unit of the nervous system is the _____.

___ 3. A branch of the nerve cell body that conducts impulses away from the cell body is the _____.

___ 4. A branch of the nerve cell body that conveys impulses toward the cell body is the _____.

___ 5. The white covering of nerve fibers that enhances conduction is called _____.

A. Dendrite

B. Nervous system

C. Neuron

D. Spinal cord

E. Axon

F. Myelin

G. Basal ganglia

XXV. Complete the statements on the left with the most appropriate term on the right. Some terms may be used more than once, and some terms may not be used.

___ 1. Neurons that transmit information from distal parts of the body toward the central nervous system are called afferent or _____ neurons.

___ 2. When an impulse reaches the end of its axon, a biochemical messenger is released called a(n) _____.

___ 3. Neurons that carry information from the central nervous system to the periphery are called efferent or _____ neurons.

___ 4. When the ions return to the resting state following nervous system stimulation, this process is called _____.

___ 5. At the point of nervous system stimulation, sodium and potassium ions are exchanged, resulting in a process called _____.

___ 6. Motor neurons are also called _____.

___ 7. Sensory neurons are also called _____.

___ 8. Impulses pass from one neuron to another across the _____.

A. Depolarization

B. Afferent

C. Neurotransmitter

D. Sensory

E. Efferent

F. Repolarization

G. Brain stem

H. Synapse

I. Interneurons

J. Motor

XXVI. Complete the statements on the left with the most appropriate term on the right. Some terms may be used more than once, and some terms may not be used.

____ 1. The brain and the spinal cord make up the _____.

____ 2. The nerves outside of the brain and spinal cord make up the _____.

____ 3. The part of the brain that is divided in right and left hemispheres is the _____.

____ 4. Cerebral spinal fluid is produced in the _____.

____ 5. There are 31 pairs of _____ nerve roots.

____ 6. There are 12 pairs of _____ nerves in the peripheral nervous system.

____ 7. Part of the peripheral nervous system that helps maintain homeostasis for the body is the _____.

____ 8. The involuntary nervous system that controls activities of the viscera, smooth muscles, cardiac muscle, and glands is the _____.

A. Cerebrum

B. Autonomic nervous system

C. Spinal

D. Cerebellum

E. Ventricles

F. Peripheral nervous system

G. Sympathetic nervous system

H. Cranial

I. Central nervous system

J. Subarachnoid space

XXVII. In each of the physical examination areas on the left indicate the possible age-related change by matching with a term on the right. Some terms may be used more than once, and some terms may not be used.

____ 1. Pupil of the eye

____ 2. Pupillary response to light

____ 3. Tracking movement of eyes

____ 4. Reflexes

____ 5. Achilles tendon jerk

____ 6. Reaction time

A. Slower

B. Decrease(s)

C. Remain(s) intact

D. Larger

E. Faster

F. May be absent

G. Smooth

H. Increase(s)

I. Jerky

J. Smaller

XXVIII. Complete the statements on the left with the most appropriate term on the right. Some terms may be used more than once, and some terms may not be used.

____ 1. Decreased responsiveness accompanied by lack of spontaneous motor activity is _____.

____ 2. A patient who cannot be aroused even by powerful stimuli is _____.

____ 3. The most accurate and reliable indicator of neurologic status is the _____.

____ 4. Excessive drowsiness is _____.

____ 5. If a patient is stuporous but can be aroused, the patient is _____.

____ 6. Unnatural drowsiness or sleepiness is _____.

A. Agitation

B. Level of consciousness

C. Combativeness

D. Somnolence

E. Neuromuscular response

F. Lethargy

G. Comatose

H. Pupillary evaluation

I. Semicomatose

J. Stupor

XXIX. Complete the statements on the left with the most appropriate term on the right. Some terms may be used more than once, and some terms may not be used.

____ 1. Two pupillary changes that may indicate neurologic deterioration include changes in equality or _____.

____ 2. Temperature is monitored in patients with neurologic disorders to detect increases that may be associated with impaired thermoregulation or _____.

____ 3. Parts of the brain that influence coordination and balance are the cerebral cortex and the _____.

____ 4. An unconscious, involuntary response that is entirely mediated at the level of the spinal cord is a _____.

____ 5. An invasive procedure used to detect CNS infections, tumors, or hydrocephalus is _____.

____ 6. A graphic representation of electrical activity in brain cells is _____.

____ 7. A study of the response of peripheral motor and sensory nerves to electrical stimuli is _____.

____ 8. A test useful in detecting tumors by depicting the pattern of distribution of a radioactive isotope injected intravenously is _____.

A. Electroencephalogram

B. Brain scan

C. Magnetic resonance imaging

D. Infection

E. Color

F. Reactivity

G. Electromyography

H. Lumbar puncture

I. Spinal cord

J. Reflex

K. Cerebellum

L. Pneumoencephalography

XXX.   Complete the statements on the left with the most appropriate term on the right. Some terms may be used more than once, and some terms may not be used.

____ 1. A diagnostic test that permits visualization of the cerebral blood vessels is _____.

____ 2. A radiologic test that creates images of intracranial structures by placing the patient's head in the scanner with a circular frame surrounding the head is _____.

____ 3. A noninvasive examination that involves placing the patient in a strong magnetic field to produce images is _____.

____ 4. A procedure in which gas is injected into the lumbar subarachnoid space and then radiographic views are taken to outline the cerebral ventricles is _____.

A.   CT scan

B.   Lumbar puncture

C.   Pneumoencephalography

D.   Brain scan

E.   Cerebral angiography

F.   MRI

XXXI.   Complete the statements on the left with the most appropriate term on the right. Some terms may be used more than once, and some terms may not be used.

____ 1. The most common type of pain is _____.

____ 2. Inflammation of the coverings of the brain and spinal cord caused by either viral or bacterial organisms is called _____.

____ 3. Inflammation of brain tissue usually caused by a virus is _____.

____ 4. A rapidly progressing disease that affects the motor component of the peripheral nervous system is _____.

____ 5. A progressive degenerative disorder that results in an eventual loss of coordination and control over involuntary motor movement is _____.

A.   Meningitis

B.   Parkinson's disease

C.   Seizure disorder

D.   Cerebral palsy

E.   Guillain-Barré syndrome

F.   Headache

G.   Encephalitis

XXXII. Complete the statements on the left with the most appropriate term on the right. Some terms may be used more than once, and some terms may not be used.

____ 1. The amount of acetylcholine available at the neuromuscular junction is reduced in _____.

____ 2. A chronic progressive degenerative disease that attacks the protective myelin sheath around axons and disrupts motor pathways of the CNS is _____.

____ 3. A degenerative neurologic disease that is also known as Lou Gehrig's disease is _____.

____ 4. Young adults have the highest rate of incidence, with women affected more frequently than men, in _____.

____ 5. A disease that affects males more than females, striking most often between 40 and 70 years of age, is _____.

____ 6. An inherited degenerative neurologic disorder that begins in middle adulthood with abnormal movements is _____.

____ 7. A chronic, progressive disease in which there is a defect at the neuromuscular junction, where electrical impulses are transmitted to muscle tissue, is _____.

A. ALS

B. Huntington's disease

C. Parkinson's disease

D. Myasthenia gravis

E. MS

F. Cerebral palsy

G. Guillain-Barré syndrome

XXXIII. Indicate whether the following responses are controlled by the (A) sympathetic or (B) parasympathetic nervous system.

____ 1. Bronchial dilation

____ 2. Pupil constriction

____ 3. Increased gut peristalsis and tone in lumen

____ 4. Decreased rate and force of cardiac contractions

____ 5. Pupil dilation

____ 6. Bronchial constriction

____ 7. Decreased gut peristalsis and tone in lumen

____ 8. Increased rate and force of cardiac contractions

____ 9. Flight or fight response

____ 10. Mediates rest response

A. Sympathetic

B. Parasympathetic

XXXIV. Match the parts of the brain on the right with the corresponding dysfunctions on the left. Some brain parts may be used more than once, and some may not be used.

____ 1. Loss of steady gait

____ 2. Dysfunction occurs on the same side as the offending lesion

____ 3. Motor dysfunction on the opposite side from the lesion

____ 4. Loss of steady, balanced posture

A. Cerebellum

B. Hypothalamus

C. Cerebral cortex

D. Spinal cord

XXXV. Match the diagnostic test on the right with the appropriate intervention or description on the left. Some diagnostic tests may be used more than once, and some tests may not be used.

____ 1. People who are confused or claustrophobic may require mild sedation before this test.

____ 2. A shampoo is done before the test and medications, such as anticonvulsants and stimulants, are withheld 24 to 48 hours before the test.

____ 3. The patient is told to expect to lie still on a stretcher while the dye is injected and radiographs taken of the head.

____ 4. The patient is kept flat and log-rolled for up to 48 hours.

____ 5. A cannula is usually inserted into the femoral artery and a catheter advanced to the carotid or vertebral arteries.

____ 6. Needle electrodes are placed on several points over a nerve and muscles supplied by the nerve.

____ 7. Infusion pumps cannot be placed in the room where this test is done, so IV sites must be converted to heparin locks before this test.

____ 8. Encourage fluid intake following the procedure to minimize headache.

____ 9. The nurse informs the radiologist about any allergies to iodine, shellfish, or contrast media.

____ 10. Patient must remain on one side in a knee-to-chest position.

____ 11. Potassium chloride is given 2 hours before the isotope is given for this test to prevent excessive isotope uptake.

____ 12. Because air, blood, bone, tissue and CSF have varying densities, they appear in various shades of gray in this test.

____ 13. A contrast dye is injected, followed by a series of radiographs.

____ 14. The nurse tells the patient to expect to hear noises like a muffled drumbeat while in the machine.

A. Brain scan

B. Lumbar puncture

C. Magnetic resonance imaging

D. Pneumoencephalography

E. CT scan

F. Cerebral angiography

G. Electromyography

H. Pupillary evaluation

I. Electroencephalogram

XXXVI. Match the definition or description on the left with the most appropriate term on the right.

____ 1. Surgery that requires opening the skull

____ 2. Excision of a segment of the skull

____ 3. Procedure done to repair a skull defect

A. Cranioplasty

B. Craniotomy

C. Craniectomy

XXXVII. Match the definition on the left with the most appropriate term on the right. Some terms may be used more than once, and some terms may not be used.

____ 1. Term used to describe deficits on the opposite side from the brain injury

____ 2. Weakness on one side

____ 3. Paralysis on one side

____ 4. Patient exhibits abnormal flexion of upper extremities with extension of lower extremities

____ 5. Patient exhibits extended lower extremities and extended upper extremities

A. Hemiplegia

B. Ipsilateral

C. Decerebrate posturing

D. Hemiparesis

E. Paraplegia

F. Decorticate posturing

G. Contralateral

H. Babinski's reflex

XXXVIII. Match the definition on the left with the most appropriate term on the right. Some terms may be used more than once, and some terms may not be used.

____ 1. Lacerations, contusions, abrasions, and hematomas

____ 2. Head trauma in which there is no visible injury to the skull or brain

____ 3. Head trauma in which there is actual bruising and bleeding in the brain tissue

____ 4. A collection of blood, usually clotted, that may be classified as subdural or epidural

____ 5. Injuries resulting form sharp objects that penetrate the skull and brain tissue

A. Contusion(s)

B. Seizure(s)

C. Scalp injuries

D. Penetrating injuries

E. Amnesia

F. Hematoma

G. Concussion

H. Fixed pupils

XXXIX. Match all nursing diagnoses for patients with meningitis on the left with their "related to" statements on the right.

____ 1. Altered cerebral tissue perfusion

____ 2. Ineffective breathing pattern

____ 3. Pain

____ 4. High risk for injury

____ 5. Fluid volume deficit

____ 6. High risk for disuse syndrome

A. Confusion, seizures

B. Irritation of the meninges

C. Bedrest

D. Intracranial pressure

E. Vomiting and fever

F. Depression of the respiratory center

XL. Match the descriptions of symptoms of Parkinson's disease on the left with the most appropriate terms on the right. Some terms may be used more than once, and some may not be used.

____ 1. Trembling, shaking type of movement usu-ally seen in upper extremities

____ 2. Stiffness

____ 3. Extremely slow movements

____ 4. Movement of thumb against fingertips

A. Bradykinesia

B. Tremor

C. Bradycardia

D. Rigidity

E. Pill rolling

F. Dementia

XLI. Match the uses of drugs on the left with names of drugs used for multiple sclerosis on the right.

____ 1. Anti-inflammatory drug used during period of exacerbation

____ 2. Anti-inflammatory drug used to encourage remission

____ 3. Drug used to decrease the frequency of recur-rent neurologic episodes in relapsing-remit-ting MS

____ 4. Drug used to treat the spasticity experienced by MS patients

A. Betaseron

B. Prednisone

C. Baclofen

D. ACTH

XLII. Match the nursing diagnoses for patients with multiple sclerosis on the left with appropriate goals on the right.

_____ 1. Impaired physical mobility

_____ 2. Sensory-perceptual alterations

_____ 3. Self-care deficit

_____ 4. Functional incontinence

_____ 5. High risk for infection

_____ 6. Ineffective individual coping

_____ 7. Knowledge deficit of disease

A. Patient knowledge of disease, treatment, and self-care

B. Absence of infection

C. Continued mobility

D. Adaptation to changes in physical function

E. Absence of injury associated with impaired sensation

F. Regular bladder elimination

G. Achievement of self-care

XLIII. Match the definition on the left with the most appropriate neurologic disease on the right. Some diseases may be used more than once, and some may not be used.

_____ 1. A disease characterized by intense pain along nerve lines in the face

_____ 2. A disease characterized by multiple tumors of peripheral, spinal, and cranial nerves

_____ 3. Acute paralysis of the seventh cranial nerve

_____ 4. Paralysis associated with a loss in motor coordination caused by cerebral damage

_____ 5. Progressive muscle weakness, fatigue, pain, and respiratory problems years after the initial infection, illness, and recovery

A. Myasthenia gravis

B. Neurofibromatosis

C. Cerebral palsy

D. Bell's palsy

E. Parkinson's disease

F. Postpolio syndrome

G. Trigeminal neuralgia

H. Multiple sclerosis

XLIV. Match the description on the left with the most appropriate type of cerebral palsy (CP) on the right.

_____ 1. Overall exaggerated reflexes and muscle spasms

_____ 2. Random, purposeless movement with extreme muscle tone

_____ 3. Characterized by poor balance, uncoordinated staggering gait, and speech or vision defects

A. Athetoid CP

B. Spastic paralysis

C. Ataxic CP

XLV. Choose the most appropriate answer.

1. In order to minimize headache following a lumbar puncture, what should be increased?
   A. calcium
   B. fluid intake
   C. potassium
   D. ambulation

2. The family should be advised that a craniotomy can take as long as:
   A. 2 hours
   B. 6 hours
   C. 12 hours
   D. 24 hours

3. As ICP increases and perfusion is reduced, oxygen delivery to cerebral tissue is:
   A. increased
   B. bypassed
   C. reduced
   D. stopped

4. Classic pupillary changes are seen in increasing ICP. Sometimes a "blown pupil" is observed, which means that the pupil:
   A. is dilated
   B. is pinpoint
   C. reacts to light
   D. is unequal

5. The pupils may become dilated and fixed as ICP rises due to pressure on the:
   A. oculomotor nerve
   B. cerebellum
   C. hypothalamus
   D. optic nerve

6. The primary route for venous outflow from the brain is the:
   A. carotid artery
   B. subclavian vein
   C. jugular vein
   D. inferior vena cava

7. A type of headache in which the pain is usually unilateral and has a warning is called:
   A. cluster
   B. migraine
   C. tension
   D. sinus

8. Seizure activity involves a large number of hyperactive neurons that use excessive:
   A. calcium and vitamin D
   B. potassium and chloride
   C. sodium and iron
   D. oxygen and glucose

9. Management of bacterial meningitis revolves around prompt recognition and treatment with:
   A. corticosteroids
   B. antihistamines
   C. anticholinergics
   D. antimicrobials

10. One common source of anxiety for many patients with Guillain-Barré syndrome is impaired:
    A. communication
    B. self-esteem
    C. circulation
    D. elimination

11. In order to reduce the symptoms of Parkinson's disease, L-dopa given with carbidopa (Sineret) crosses the blood-brain barrier and is converted to:
    A. epinephrine
    B. dopamine
    C. norepinephrine
    D. acetylcholine

12. Trigeminal neuralgia is characterized by:
    A. hypotension
    B. tachycardia
    C. infection
    D. intense pain

13. In myasthenia gravis, rapid improvement of muscle strength after administration of Tensilon indicates an underlying:
    A. hypertensive crisis
    B. adrenergic crisis
    C. myasthenic crisis
    D. cholinergic crisis

Cerebrovascular Accident

OBJECTIVES

1. Explain the risk factors for cerebrovascular accident (CVA).
2. Identify the four types of CVA.
3. Describe the pathophysiology, signs and symptoms, and medical treatment for each type of CVA.
4. Describe the neurologic deficits that may result from CVA.
5. Explain tests and procedures used to diagnose a CVA.
6. Explain nursing responsibilities for patients having those tests and procedures.
7. List data to be included in the nursing assessment of the CVA patient.
8. Identify nursing diagnoses, goals, and interventions during the acute and the rehabilitation phases for the patient who has had a CVA.
9. Specify criteria used to evaluate the outcomes of nursing care for the CVA patient.
10. Identify resources for the CVA patient and family.

LEARNING ACTIVITIES

1. Match the definition on the left with the most appropriate term on the right.

___ 1. Inability to speak clearly due to neurologic damage that impairs normal muscle control

___ 2. Between the arachnoid and pia mater layers of the membranes covering the brain

___ 3. Drooping of the upper eyelid

___ 4. Difficulty initiating speech

___ 5. Neurologic deficits that last less than 24 hours; caused by diminished cerebral blood flow

___ 6. Double vision

___ 7. The inability to understand words or the inability to respond with words, or both.

___ 8. Loss of half the field of vision; loss is on the side opposite the brain lesion

___ 9. Partial inability to initiate coordinated voluntary motor acts

___ 10. Ability to speak clearly but without meaning

___ 11. Within the cerebrum

___ 12. Difficulty swallowing

___ 13. Inability to comprehend words

___ 14. Paralysis of one side of the body

A. Intracerebral

B. Hemiplegia

C. Nonfluent aphasia

D. Dyspraxia

E. Dysarthria

F. Ptosis

G. Subarachnoid

H. Homonymous hemianopsia

I. Fluent aphasia

J. Receptive aphasia

K. Transient ischemic attack

L. Aphasia

M. Dysphagia

N. Diplopia

II. Complete the statements on the left with the most appropriate term on the right. Some terms may be used more than once, and some terms may not be used.

____ 1. The part of the brain that controls the left side of the body is the _____.

____ 2. The part of the brain that controls the right side of the body is the _____.

____ 3. The part of the brain that controls vital, basic functions including respiration, heart rate, and consciousness is the _____.

____ 4. The part of the brain that coordinates movement, balance, and posture is the _____.

____ 5. The circulatory system in the cerebrum is called the _____.

____ 6. The part of the brain that controls analytic mental processes such as language ability, mathematics, and reasoning powers is the

_____.

____ 7. The part of the brain that includes the midbrain, pons, and medulla is the _____.

____ 8. The part of the brain that controls emotional and artistic tendencies is the _____.

A. Cerebellum

B. Brain stem

C. Spinal cord

D. Cerebrovascular system

E. Right hemisphere

F. Cerebrum

G. Left hemisphere

III. Complete the statements on the left with the most appropriate term on the right. Some terms may be used more than once, and some terms may not be used.

____ 1. An important warning condition for a possible later stroke is _____.

____ 2. A buildup of fatty deposits in the blood vessels is called _____.

____ 3. The common name for cerebrovascular accident is _____.

____ 4. A temporary neurologic deficit caused by impairment of cerebral blood flow is

_____.

____ 5. A swooshing noise in a clogged carotid artery that can be auscultated in diagnosing a TIA is

_____.

____ 6. Opening an obstructed blood vessel, and removing the plaque from a patient with TIA is called _____.

A. Bruit

B. TIA

C. Angioplasty

D. Stroke

E. Endarterectomy

F. Atherosclerosis

. Complete the statement on the left with the most appropriate term on the right. Some terms may not be used.

___ 1. Three factors that create problems related to physical mobility for the stroke patient include dyspraxia, visual field disturbances, and _____.	A. Aspiration
	B. Injury
	C. Homonymous hemianopsia
___ 2. Two causes of thick secretions being retained in the respiratory tract following CVA are immobility and _____.	D. Edema
	E. Oxygenation
___ 3. Dysphagia may result in airway obstruction or pneumonia due to _____.	F. Hypertension
	G. Urinary tract infection
___ 4. Patients who see only half the field of vision following a stroke have _____.	H. Dehydration
	I. Hemiplegia
___ 5. The most frequent cause of death following a stroke is _____.	J. Diplopia
	K. Dysphagia
___ 6. Dehydration in patients following a stroke may result in signs and symptoms of constipation, skin dryness, and _____.	L. Pneumonia
___ 7. A priority immediately after a stroke is _____.	
___ 8. A sensory-perceptual problem in a patient with a stroke is _____.	
___ 9. The patient who does not feel pressure or pain due to lost sensation following a stroke is susceptible to _____.	

Match the nursing diagnosis of patients with CVA on the left with the most appropriate "related to" statement on the right.

___ 1. High risk for injury	A. dysphagia, inability to feed self, inability to chew
___ 2. Fluid volume deficit	
___ 3. Fluid volume excess	B. impaired cough reflex, altered consciousness, impaired swallowing
___ 4. Altered nutrition: less than body requirements	C. inadequate intake, excessive diuresis
___ 5. Altered family processes	D. weakness, paralysis, spasticity, impaired balance
___ 6. Ineffective airway clearance	E. seizure activity, confusion, motor impairment
___ 7. Impaired verbal communication	F. overhydration
___ 8. Impaired physical mobility	G. disruption of family roles and functions
	H. aphasia

VI. Match the uses of drugs on the left with the drugs for stroke treatment on the right.

___ 1. Treat cerebral edema

___ 2. New treatment for subarachnoid hemorrhage which dilates and prevents spasms in cerebral blood vessels

___ 3. Reduce intracranial pressure by reducing cerebral inflammation

___ 4. Prevent strokes caused by thrombi

___ 5. Used experimentally to dissolve clots that cause acute ischemic stroke

___ 6. Used to treat seizures, if seizures are present with stroke

___ 7. Used to break up clots

A. Anticonvulsants, such as phenytoin and phenobarbital

B. Antithrombotic agents, such as aspirin, and dipyridamole

C. Osmotic diuretics, such as mannitol

D. Streptokinase

E. Calcium channel blockers, such as nimodipine

F. Tissue plasminogen activator (TPA)

G. Corticosteroids

VII. List 3 reasons why nutritional status may be compromised in the stroke patient.

1.

2.

3.

VIII. List 5 areas of medical treatment for patients with CVA.

1.

2.

3.

4.

5.

IX. The nursing assessment enables the nurse to recognize risk factors for CVA and to identify nursing care needs. List 8 important areas of data to assess in the review of systems.

1.

2.

3.

4.

5.

6.

7.

8.

X. List 2 behaviors that are characteristic of patients with aphasia.

1.

2.

XI. Signs and symptoms of stroke depend on the type, location, and extent of brain injury. List 7 common signs and symptoms of an embolic stroke.

1.

2.

3.

4.

5.

6.

7.

XII. List 5 sensory perceptual problems in the stroke patient.

1.

2.

3.

4.

5.

XIII. List 4 communication techniques the nurse should use when working with stroke patients who have impaired verbal communication.

1.

2.

3.

4.

XIV. List 4 factors that contribute to skin breakdown in patients with strokes.

1.

2.

3.

4.

XV. List 2 problems that usually occur with hemiplegia, beyond motor problems, making physical mobility more difficult.

1.

2.

XVI. List 6 measures to reduce the risk of stroke.

1.   4.

2.   5.

3.   6.

XVII. List the 2 biggest risk factors for CVA.

1.

2.

XVIII. Choose the most appropriate answer.

1. A folded layer of nerve cells that covers each hemi-sphere of the brain is called the:
   A. cerebellum
   B. cerebrum
   C. gyrus
   D. cortex

2. One of the most important needs of the acute stroke patient is to be turned and repositioned at least every:
   A. 2 hours
   B. 4 hours
   C. 8 hours
   D. 12 hours

3. Turning and repositioning the stroke patient will reduce the incidence of:
   A. hypertension
   B. skin breakdown
   C. headache
   D. cerebral edema

CHAPTER

27

Spinal Cord Injury

OBJECTIVES

1. Explain the impact of spinal cord injury.
2. Describe the diagnostic tests used to evaluate spinal cord injuries and related nursing responsibilities.
3. Explain the physical effects of spinal cord injury.
4. Describe the medical and surgical treatment during the acute phase of spinal cord injury.
5. List the data to be included in the nursing assessment of the patient with a spinal cord injury.
6. Identify nursing diagnoses, goals, and interventions for the patient with spinal cord injury.
7. Describe the nursing care for the patient having a laminectomy.
8. State the goals of rehabilitation for the patient with spinal cord injury.

LEARNING ACTIVITIES

I.   Match the definition on the left with the most appropriate term on the right.

____ 1. Loss of motor and sensory function in all four extremities due to damage to the spinal cord

____ 2. Soft, in relation to muscle, lacking tone

____ 3. Abnormally exaggerated response of the autonomic nervous system to a stimulus

____ 4. Loss of motor and sensory function due to damage to the spinal cord that spares the upper extremities but, depending on the level of the damage, affects the trunk, pelvis, and lower extremities

____ 5. Increased muscle tone, characterized by sudden, involuntary muscle spasms

____ 6. Area of skin supplied by sensory nerve fibers from a single posterior spinal root

____ 7. Surrounded with a sheath

A.   Paraplegia

B.   Myelinated

C.   Quadriplegia

D.   Dermatome

E.   Flaccid

F.   Spastic

G.   Autonomic dysreflexia

II. Complete the statements on the left with the most appropriate term on the right. Some terms may be used more than once, and some terms may not be used.

_____ 1. The first 7 vertebrae of the vertebral column are called _____.

_____ 2. The body part that passes through the opening in the center of each vertebral arch is the _____.

_____ 3. Each vertebral body is separated from the next vertebra by the _____.

_____ 4. The posterior portion of each vertebra is called the _____.

_____ 5. The spinal cord extends from the brain stem to the level of the _____.

_____ 6. The outermost layer of the meninges, which covers the spinal cord, is the _____.

_____ 7. The innermost layer of the meninges, which directly covers the spinal cord, is the _____.

_____ 8. The middle layer of the meninges, which contains the cerebrospinal fluid (CSF), is the _____.

_____ 9. Motor and sensory information from the spinal cord to the brain is carried through _____.

_____ 10. Motor and sensory information from the brain to the spinal cord is carried through _____.

A. Third lumbar vertebra

B. Intervertebral disk

C. Pia mater

D. Spinal cord

E. Descending tracts

F. Dura mater

G. Cerebrospinal fluid

H. Ascending tracts

I. Cervical

J. Arch

K. Second lumbar vertebra

L. Arachnoid

III. Complete the statements on the left with the most appropriate term on the right. Some terms may be used more than once, and some terms may not be used.

_____ 1. The function of the spinal cord that occurs when a sensory stimulus enters the spinal cord and is immediately switched to an outgoing motor neuron is called _____.

_____ 2. The function of the spinal cord that is concerned with transferring information from the spinal cord to the brain, then from the brain back down the cord and out to effector muscles is called _____.

_____ 3. Information is conveyed to and from the external environment to the brain and spinal cord via the _____.

_____ 4. The twelve nerves that arise from the brain stem and are part of the PNS are called _____.

_____ 5. The 31 pairs of nerves that arise from the spinal cord and travel between the vertebrae to muscles and visceral organs are called _____.

A. Relay

B. Cranial nerves

C. Ascending tract

D. Reflexive

E. Spinal nerves

F. Thoracic nerves

G. Peripheral nervous system

IV. Complete the statements on the left with the appropriate diagnostic test on the right. Some terms may be used more than once, and some terms may not be used.

___ 1. A noninvasive procedure that allows visualization of the spinal cord, including bony vertebrae and the spinal nerves is _____.

___ 2. The nurse tells the patients to expect to hear a humming sound as the radio waves are turned on and off during the _____.

___ 3. The patient must have no metal materials or equipment on when entering this test, called _____.

___ 4. A visualization of the spinal cord and vertebrae through the injection of a radiopaque dye directly into the subarachnoid space of the spinal cord is called _____.

___ 5. A noninvasive procedure, not involving radiation, in which the patient is moved through a magnetic field and then subjected to short bursts of radio waves, is called _____.

___ 6. A puncture between L-3 and L-4 is necessary to produce the _____.

A.   MRI

B.   CT scan

C.   Electroencephalography

D.   Myelogram

E.   Electromyography

V. Complete the statements on the left with the most appropriate term on the right. Some terms may be used more than once, and some terms may not be used.

___ 1. As spinal shock begins to subside and reflex activity returns, the patient is at risk for _____.

___ 2. Cervical injuries below the level of C-4 spare the diaphragm, but can involve the impairment of the _____.

___ 3. An immediate, transient response to injury in which reflex activity below the level of the injury temporarily ceases is called _____.

___ 4. A very serious and potentially dangerous problem for the spinal cord–injured patient, which is described as an exaggerated response of the autonomic nervous system in patients whose injury is at or above the T-6 level, is called _____.

___ 5. Increased muscle tone is called _____.

___ 6. When the abdomen becomes distended and bowel sounds are absent, peristalsis has ceased, a condition called _____.

A.   Spinal shock

B.   Respiratory arrest

C.   Autonomic dysreflexia

D.   Spasticity

E.   Flaccidity

F.   Intercostal muscles

G.   Ileus

H.   Coma

Introductory Nursing Care of Adults

VI. Complete the statements on the left with the most appropriate term on the right. Some terms may be used more than once, and some terms may not be used.

____ 1. When the patient is ready to tackle the work of rehabilitation, the stage is _____.

____ 2. When the patient is in emotional shock and may express a desire to die, the stage is _____.

____ 3. When the patient is ready to begin to plan for the future, the stage is _____.

____ 4. When the patient begins to face the injury and deal with it realistically, the stage is _____.

____ 5. When the patient becomes aware of the devastating changes that have taken place, the stage is _____.

____ 6. The stage marked by depression and withdrawal as the patient considers the implications of the injury is _____.

A. Impact

B. Denial

C. Acknowledgment

D. Retreat

E. Reconstruction

F. Remediation

VII. Complete the statements on the left with the most appropriate term on the right. Some terms may be used more than once, and some terms may not be used.

____ 1. Removal of all or part of the posterior arch of the vertebra is called _____.

____ 2. The placement of a piece of donor bone, commonly taken from the hip, into the area between the involved vertebrae is called _____.

____ 3. The determination of sensory loss is best described by the use of a _____.

____ 4. This surgical procedure that is done to alleviate compression on the cord or spinal nerves is called _____.

A. Dermatome chart

B. Immobilization

C. Spinal fusion

D. Proprioception

E. Laminectomy

F. Traction

VIII. Explain why high cervical injuries may result in immediate death.

IX. If a patient with a high cervical injury is fortunate enough to receive immediate attention and rapid transport to a skilled facility, what medical treatment will be instituted right away?

X.   List 3 actions that elicit spastic activity in the spinal cord–injured patient.

  1.

  2.

  3.

XI.   Explain why the spinal cord–injured patient may have difficulty maintaining body
       temperature within a normal range.

XII.   Explain why most spinal cord–injured patients can maintain bowel function.

XIII. List 2 factors which contribute to problems with the integumentary system of the spinal
       cord–injured patient.

  1.

  2.

XIV.   List the 3 major medical goals for the spinal cord–injured patient.

  1.

  2.

  3.

XV.   Explain why the traditional head-tilt–chin-lift method of opening the airway is
       inappropriate in spinal cord–injured patients.

XVI.   List 3 reasons why postoperative immobilization of the area following laminectomy is
       necessary.

  1.

  2.

  3.

XVII. During the acute phase of spinal cord injury, list 5 areas that the nurse monitors.

1.

2.

3.

4.

5.

XVIII. List 3 aspects of the medical management of ileus.

1.

2.

3.

XIX. Match the nursing diagnoses on the left with the "related to" statements on the right.

_____ 1. High risk for infection

_____ 2. Sensory perceptual alterations (kinesthetic, tactile)

_____ 3. Ineffective thermoregulation

_____ 4. Self-care deficit (feeding, dressing, grooming)

_____ 5. Altered sexuality patterns

_____ 6. Dysreflexia

_____ 7. High risk for disuse syndrome

_____ 8. Bowel incontinence

_____ 9. Altered urinary elimination

_____ 10. Hopelessness

_____ 11. Ineffective breathing patterns

_____ 12. High risk for injury

A. Sensory motor impairment

B. Altered body function

C. Involuntary muscle spasms

D. Skeletal traction pins

E. Overwhelming losses

F. Neurologic impairment

G. Altered sensory transmission

H. Impaired conduction of impulses

I. Bladder or bowel distention

J. Pathologic or prescribed immobility

K. Spinal cord trauma

XX.   Choose the most appropriate answer.

1. The halo device is used to provide immobilization and alignment of the:
   A.   cervical vertebrae
   B.   thoracic vertebrae
   C.   lumbar vertebrae
   D.   sacral vertebrae

2. For the patient maintained in cervical traction while on a conventional bed, position changes must be accomplished by:
   A.   assisted ambulation
   B.   range of motion exercises
   C.   log rolling
   D.   grasping the muscles

3. Which of the following is a medical emergency and requires immediate intervention in patients with spinal cord injury?
   A.   elevated temperature
   B.   hypotension
   C.   autonomic dysreflexia (AD)
   D.   increased respirations

4. Prompt intervention following autonomic dysreflexia (AD), which is a medical emergency, must be directed toward the severe:
   A.   hypertension
   B.   hypotension
   C.   infection
   D.   lung compromise

5. Patients with tongs are maintained on:
   A.   bedrest with ambulation three times a day
   B.   isolation precautions
   C.   high-roughage diets
   D.   strict bedrest

6. When the patient has spasticity, nursing management is directed toward the prevention of contractures and:
   A.   infection
   B.   muscle atrophy
   C.   dyspnea
   D.   heart failure

7. During the time of flaccid paralysis, the nurse must be diligent in performing:
   A.   active range of motion exercises
   B.   passive range of motion exercises
   C.   cough and deep-breathing exercises
   D.   early ambulation

8. Following an ileus, the patient will be given oral fluids and food when:
   A.   the swallow reflex returns
   B.   the patient is no longer anorexic
   C.   bladder continence returns
   D.   peristalsis returns

9. Utilizing the Grading Scale for Muscle Strength, the nurse would score a finding of no movement with total paralysis as:
   A.   0
   B.   1
   C.   3
   D.   5

10. Utilizing the Grading Scale for Muscle Strength, the nurse would score a finding of full active range of motion against gravity and resistance as:
   A.   1
   B.   2
   C.   3
   D.   5

Acute Respiratory Disorders

OBJECTIVES

1. Identify data to be collected in the nursing assessment of the patient with a respiratory disorder.
2. Identify the nursing implications of age-related changes in the respiratory system.
3. Describe diagnostic tests or procedures for respiratory disorders and nursing interventions.
4. Explain nursing care of patients receiving therapeutic treatments for respiratory disorders.
5. For selected respiratory disorders, describe the pathophysiology, signs and symptoms, complications, diagnostic measures, and medical treatment.
6. Apply the nursing process to plan care for the patient who has an acute respiratory disorder.

LEARNING ACTIVITIES

I.   Match the definition on the left with the most appropriate term on the right.

_____   1. Dry, rattling sound caused by partial bronchial obstruction

_____   2. Rapid respiratory rate

_____   3. Accumulation of air in the pleural cavity that results in complete or partial collapse of a lung

_____   4. Low oxygen level

_____   5. Movement of air in and out of the lungs

_____   6. Thickened and dried; often used to describe pulmonary secretions

_____   7. Rales; abnormal lung sounds heard on auscultation

_____   8. Difficulty breathing when lying down

_____   9. Accumulation of blood in the pleural space

_____ 10. Low level of oxygen in the blood

_____ 11. Blood flow

_____ 12. Collapsed lung or part of a lung

_____ 13. Difficulty breathing

_____ 14. Excess carbon dioxide in the blood

A.   Atelectasis

B.   Crackles

C.   Dyspnea

D.   Hemothorax

E.   Hypercapnia

F.   Hypoxemia

G.   Hypoxia

H.   Inspissated

I.   Orthopnea

J.   Perfusion

K.   Pneumothorax

L.   Rhonchus

M.   Tachypnea

N.   Ventilation

II.   List 3 characteristics of the right bronchus which explain why foreign bodies from the trachea enter the right bronchus.

1.

2.

3.

III. List 3 changes occurring with aging in the pharynx and the larynx.

1.

2.

3.

IV.   Why is it necessary to assess Homans's sign in a patient with respiratory problems?

V.   List 4 purposes of pulmonary function tests.

1.

2.

3.

4.

VI.   List 6 reasons why older persons may experience difficulty with respiration.

1.

2.

3.

4.

5.

6.

VII. List 5 consequences of aging changes which result in difficulties with respiration.

1.

2.

3.

4.

5.

VIII. Explain why culture and sensitivity specimens should be collected before antimicrobial therapy is begun.

X. List 5 points to be included in teaching patients to cough and deep breathe.

1.

2.

3.

4.

5.

. Explain why smoking is not allowed when a patient is receiving oxygen therapy.

I. List 2 reasons for using inflatable cuffs.

1.

2.

II. List 3 ways PEEP works.

1.

2.

3.

III. Explain the purpose of chest tubes.

IV. List 3 nursing diagnoses specific to the patient who has had a thoracotomy.

1.

2.

3.

V. List 3 nursing goals for the patient who has had a thoracotomy.

1.

2.

3.

VI. List the 3 criteria for evaluating the outcomes of nursing interventions for the patient who has had a thoracotomy.

1.

2.

3.

XVII. List 2 symptoms which patients who have had thoracotomies must report to the physician, if these symptoms occur when the patients return home.

1.

2.

XVIII. List 6 points of instruction that the nurse should explain to patients with colds in order to reduce the risk of spreading the cold or acquiring secondary bacterial infections.

1.

2.

3.

4.

5.

6.

XIX. List 5 signs or symptoms about which the patient with a cold should notify the physician.

1.

2.

3.

4.

5.

XX. List 4 causes of nosocomial pneumonia.

1.

2.

3.

4.

XXI. List 7 nursing diagnoses for the patient with a respiratory disorder.

1.

2.

3.

4.

5.

6.

7.

XXII. List 7 nursing goals for the patient with pneumonia.

1.

2.

3.

4.

5.

6.

7.

XIII. List 1 reason why patients with pneumonia should be placed in a semi-Fowler's position.

1.

XIV. List 4 signs and symptoms of fluid volume deficit which may be present in patients with pneumonia.

1.   3.

2.   4.

XV. List 2 reasons why patients with pneumonia may lose excess fluid.

1.

2.

XVI. List 2 reasons why patients with pneumonia may have inadequate fluid intake.

1.

2.

XVII. List 7 criteria for evaluating the effectiveness of nursing interventions for patients with pneumonia.

1.   5.

2.   6.

3.   7.

4.

XVIII. List 3 nursing diagnoses for patients with pleurisy.

1.

2.

3.

XIX. List 5 complications of chest trauma for which patients at risk.

1.   4.

2.   5.

3.

XX. List 11 signs and symptoms of chest injury.

1.   7.

2.   8.

3.   9.

4.   10.

5.   11.

6.

XXXI. List 10 signs and symptoms of pneumothorax.

1.   6.

2.   7.

3.   8.

4.   9.

5.   10.

XXXII. For the patient with pneumothorax, complete the following table, listing at least 2
interventions for each nursing diagnosis.

Nursing Diagnoses	Goals	Interventions	Criteria for Evaluation
1. Ineffective breathing patterns related to decreased lung expansion			
2. Fear related to dyspnea			
3. High risk for decreased cardiac output related to mediastinal shift			
4. Pain related to trauma, altered pressure in chest cavity or chest tube			
5. High risk for infection related to traumatic injury or chest tube insertion			
6. Knowledge deficit of condition and treatment			

XXXIII. List 5 signs and symptoms of rib fractures.

1.

2.

3.

4.

5.

XXXIV. List 1 nursing diagnosis, 1 nursing goal, 5 nursing interventions, and 3 criteria for evaluation of the patient with fractured ribs.

Nursing Diagnosis   Goal

1.   1.

Interventions   Criteria for Evaluation

1.   1.

2.   2.

3.   3.

4.

5.

XXXV. List 5 signs and symptoms of flail chest.

1.

2.

3.

4.

5.

XXXVI. In the table below, list 3 nursing diagnoses, 3 nursing goals, 1 nursing intervention, and 5 criteria for evaluation of interventions for the patient with flail chest.

Nursing Diagnoses	Goals	Interventions	Criteria for Evaluation
1.	1.	1.	1.
2.	2.		2.
3.	3.		3.
			4.
			5.

XXXVII. List 5 signs and symptoms of PE (pulmonary embolus).

1.

2.

3.

4.

5.

XXXVIII. In the table below, for the 4 nursing diagnoses provided, list 4 goals, nursing interventions for each diagnosis, and 4 criteria for evaluation of interventions for the patient with *pulmonary embolus*.

Nursing Diagnoses	Goals	Interventions	Criteria for Evaluation
1. Altered cardio-pulmonary tissue perfusion related to interruption of blood flow to the alveoli	1.	1.	1.
2. Anxiety related to dyspnea or fear of death	2.	2.	2.
3. High risk for injury related to anticoagulant therapy	3.	3.	3.
4. Knowledge deficit of PE, treatment, prevention, and self-care	4.	4.	4.

XXXIX. For each of the following conditions of adult respiratory distress syndrome listed on the left, list the resulting condition that occurs in the patient.

1. Lung compliance decreases, leading to

2. Fluid shifts into the interstitial spaces in the lungs and into alveoli, causing

3. Production of pulmonary surfactant decreases, leading to

XL. List 6 signs and symptoms of ARDS (adult respiratory distress syndrome).

1.

2.

3.

4.

5.

6.

XLI. Fill in the blanks.

1. The correct order for the passage of air into the lungs is the nose, pharynx, trachea, and the _____.

2. Dust particles and bacteria are filtered from the air by the mucous membranes and _____.

3. A structure that serves as a passage for both the respiratory and digestive systems is the _____.

4. The structure that prevents aspiration of food into the trachea is the _____.

Introductory Nursing Care of Adults

5. Sound is produced when air from the lungs causes a rapid, repeated opening and closing of the _____.

6. The windpipe is the _____.

7. The exchange of oxygen and carbon dioxide takes place in the _____.

8. The air moves from the larynx to the trachea, bronchi, bronchioles, and _____.

9. The lungs are located in the _____ body cavity.

10. The thoracic cavity is separated from the abdominal cavity by the _____.

11. Each lung is covered by a membrane called the _____.

12. Four factors that interfere with accurate measurement of the oximeter include hypotension, hypothermia, vasoconstriction, and _____.

13. Three complications of bronchograms include pneumonia, delayed hypersensitivity reaction, and

    _____.

14. Four indications for performing a thoracentesis include the removal of pleural fluid, blood, or air, and to

    _____.

15. Four complications of thoracentesis include air embolism, hemothorax, pneumothorax, and

    _____.

16. Two purposes of teaching pursed lip breathing to patients with chronic lung diseases include inhibiting airway collapse and _____.

17. Four complications of oxygen therapy include hypoventilation, toxicity, atelectasis, and _____

    _____.

18. Four reasons why IPPB treatments are not being used as often as they used to be are: (1) they are not as effective as incentive spirometry and hand-held nebulizers, (2) they are more expensive, (3) they may cause tension pneumothorax in patients with COPD, and (4) they may cause _____

    _____.

19. Four types of artificial airways include oral airways, nasal airways, endotracheal tubes, and

    _____.

20. Three common purposes for doing thoracic surgery include: (1) evaluation of chest trauma, (2) removal of tumors and cysts, and (3) _____.

21. Three reasons why atelectasis may occur in the postthoracotomy patient include: (1) effects of anesthesia, which impairs ciliary motion, (2) drugs that dry secretions, and (3) _____.

22. Common complaints associated with respiratory disorders are cough, pain, and _____.

23. The normal respiratory rate is _____.

24. Flaring of the nares is a common sign of _____.

25. The structure that separates the nares is the nasal _____.

26. When the nurse observes breathing pattern and effort, the rise and fall of the chest should be regular and

    _____.

27. The sputum originates in the _____.

28. An indication of bacterial infection is sputum that is thick, foul-smelling, and _____.

29. The insertion of a large-bore needle through the chest wall into the pleural space is called

    _____.

30. After a thoracentesis, the patient is positioned on the _____ .

31. Observations a nurse should make following thoracentesis include uneven chest movement, respiratory distress, and _____ .

32. Improving oxygen and carbon dioxide exchange in the lungs by removing excessive mucous secretions is the goal of _____ .

33. When suctioning patients, each suction pass should not exceed _____ .

34. Equipment that creates water vapor to raise the relative humidity of inspired gas to 100% is called

_____ .

35. An instrument used to deliver aerosol therapy is called _____ .

36. Symptoms of adverse effects of oxygen therapy include lethargy and _____ .

37. Exposure to 100% oxygen can cause _____ .

38. Agents that liquefy secretions are called _____ .

39. IPPB treatments promote _____ .

40. The surgical opening of the chest wall is called _____ .

41. The removal of an entire lung is called _____ .

42. The removal of ribs is called _____ .

43. After a thoracotomy, the patient is at risk for pneumonia and _____ .

44. Fluids are encouraged in the postthoracotomy patient, because good hydration _____

_____ .

45. The insertion of an endoscope through a small thoracic incision for surgical purposes is called

_____ .

46. Drugs used to treat respiratory disorders which increase the size of the lumen of bronchi are called

_____ .

47. Drugs that cause constriction of nasal blood vessels and reduce the swelling of mucous membranes are called

_____ .

48. Side effects of decongestants include systemic vasoconstriction and _____ .

49. Decongestants should be avoided in patients with heart disease and _____ .

50. Drugs that suppress the cough reflex are called _____ .

51. Drugs that should be given to persons with a nonproductive cough that keeps them awake are called

_____ .

52. Over-the-counter medications that are frequently used to dry nasal secretions are called _____

_____ .

53. Drugs that thin respiratory secretions so they are more readily mobilized and cleared from the airways are called

_____ .

54. Antibiotics are used to treat _____ .

55. Drugs that relax smooth muscle in the bronchial airways and blood vessels are called _____

_____ .

56. The primary drawback to most bronchodilators is the tendency to cause cardiac stimulation and _____ _____.

57. Anti-inflammatory drugs used to treat asthma are called _____.

58. Inflammation of the pleura that causes pain with breathing is called _____.

59. A condition of collapsed alveoli is called _____.

60. The accumulation of excess carbon dioxide in the blood is called _____.

61. When the level of oxygen in the blood is low, this is referred to as _____.

62. Signs of hypoxemia include restlessness, tachycardia, and _____.

63. Immediate care of a person with a chest injury is directed at _____.

64. Emboli are usually blood clots, but may be fat, air, tumors, bone marrow, amniotic fluid, or _____.

65. When a portion of a pulmonary blood vessel is occluded by an embolus, the patient is said to have _____.

66. Most pulmonary emboli originate in the deep veins of the pelvis or _____.

XLII. Match the definition or description on the left with the most appropriate term on the right.

____ 1. Provide(s) a passageway for air going to and from the lungs; split into left and right

____ 2. Where the exchange of oxygen and carbon dioxide takes place

____ 3. A 4- to 5-inch tube from the larynx into the bronchi

____ 4. The space between the folds of the vocal cords

____ 5. Act(s) like a lid to help prevent aspiration of food into the trachea

____ 6. Wave(s) back and forth about 12 times a second to help the mucus clean the air

A.   Trachea
B.   Cilia
C.   Glottis
D.   Bronchi
E.   Epiglottis
F.   Alveoli

XLIII. Match the definition or description on the left with the most appropriate term on the right.

____ 1. Membrane covering each lung

____ 2. Large sheet of muscle

____ 3. Area within the chest wall that holds the lungs

A.   diaphragm
B.   thoracic cavity
C.   pleura

XLIV. Match the definition or description on the left with the most appropriate term on the right.

_____ 1. Process of air entering into the lungs   A.   Inspiration

_____ 2. Process of air leaving the lungs   B.   Expiration

_____ 3. Active movement of muscles

_____ 4. Chest wall enlarges

_____ 5. Passive process

_____ 6. Muscles relax

_____ 7. Chest returns to normal size

XLV. Match the definition on the left with the most appropriate term on the right.

_____ 1. Difficulty with breathing in a lying position   A.   Dyspnea

_____ 2. Temporary interruption in normal breathing pattern when no air movement occurs   B.   Orthopnea

    C.   Apnea

_____ 3. Difficulty breathing, or shortness of breath

XLVI. Match each diagnostic procedure on the left with appropriate nursing implications on the right. (Some nursing implications may be used more than once.)

_____ 1. CT scan   A.   Tell patient not to move or cough during procedure to prevent damage to pleural tissue

_____ 2. Bronchogram

_____ 3. Thoracentesis   B.   Advise patient not to smoke or eat for 4 to 6 hours before test.

_____ 4. MRI

_____ 5. Pulmonary function tests   C.   Determine whether patient is allergic to iodine

    D.   Tell patients not to wear metal

XLVII. Match the definition or description on the left with the most appropriate term on the right.

_____ 1. Tube used with a surgically created opening through the neck into the trachea   A.   Endotracheal tube

    B.   Nasal airway

_____ 2. Curved tube used to maintain an airway temporarily   C.   Tracheostomy tube

    D.   Oral airway

_____ 3. Soft rubber tube inserted through the nose and extended to the base of the tongue

_____ 4. Long tube inserted through the mouth or nose into the trachea

XLVIII. Match the definition or description on the left with the most appropriate term on the right.

_____ 1. Humidifier raises the relative humidity of inspired gas to:

_____ 2. Maximum time for each suction pass

_____ 3. Delivers warm water vapor directly into the air

_____ 4. Delivers humidified aerosol through large tubing

_____ 5. Possible result of exposure to 100% oxygen

_____ 6. Goal is to improve oxygen and carbon dioxide exchange in the lungs

_____ 7. Percentage of oxygen in air in the atmosphere

_____ 8. Adverse effect of oxygen therapy

_____ 9. Percussion generally done for this amount of time

_____ 10. Possible result of IPPB

A. Suctioning

B. 10 seconds

C. 20–30 seconds

D. Humidifier

E. Nebulizer

F. 21%

G. 100%

H. Bradypnea

I. Retinal injury

J. Tension pneumorax

IL. Match the definition or description on the left with the most appropriate term on the right.

_____ 1. Suppress the cough reflex

_____ 2. Dry up nasal secretions

_____ 3. Relax smooth muscle in the bronchial airways and blood vessels

_____ 4. Side effect of antihistamines

_____ 5. Used to prevent acute asthma attacks, but not to stop them after they've started

_____ 6. Side effect of bronchodilators

_____ 7. Cause constriction of nasal blood vessels, reduce swelling of mucous membranes

_____ 8. Anti-inflammatory drugs that can be used in the treatment of asthma

_____ 9. Thin respiratory secretions so they are more readily mobilized

_____ 10. Possible side effects of antimicrobials

_____ 11. Possible side effect of decongestants

_____ 12. Antibiotics are used for treatment of _____

A. Decongestants

B. Hypertension

C. Allergic responses

D. Antitussives

E. Expectorants

F. Antihistamines

G. Drowsiness

H. Mast cell stabilizers

I. Bacterial infections

J. Bronchodilators

K. CNS stimulation

L. Corticosteroids

L. Match the definition or description on the left with the most appropriate term on the right.

_____ 1. Surgical opening of the chest

_____ 2. Removal of an entire lung

_____ 3. Good hydration after thoracotomy

_____ 4. Stripping of the membrane that covers the visceral pleura

_____ 5. Agents that liquefy secretions

_____ 6. Performed by inserting an endoscope through a small thoracic incision

_____ 7. IPPB promotes this

_____ 8. Removal of ribs

_____ 9. Preset amount of oxygenated air delivered during each ventilator breath

_____ 10. Collapsed alveoli

A. Mucolytics

B. Productive cough

C. Tidal volume

D. Thoracotomy

E. Pneumonectomy

F. Thoracoplasty

G. Atelectasis

H. Thins secretions

I. Decortication

J. Thoracoscopy

LI. Match the definition or description on the left with the most appropriate term on the right.

_____ 1. Low level of oxygen in the blood

_____ 2. Potentially fatal complication of open pneumothorax

_____ 3. Accumulation of fluid between the pleura that encases the lungs and the pleura that lines the thoracic cavity

_____ 4. Potentially fatal complication of tension pneumothorax

_____ 5. Air repeatedly enters the pleural space with inspiration, causing the pressure to rise and the affected lung to collapse

_____ 6. Inflammation of the pleura that causes pain with breathing

_____ 7. Results from a chest wound that allows air to move in and out freely with inspiration and expiration

_____ 8. Possible sign of hypoxemia

_____ 9. Excess carbon dioxide accumulates in the blood

A. Pleurisy

B. Pleural effusion

C. Hypercapnia

D. Hypoxemia

E. Tachypnea

F. Tension pneumothorax

G. Open pneumothorax

H. Mediastinal shift

I. Mediastinal flutter

LII. Choose the most appropriate answer.

1. If the air is not moistened in the nasal cavity, what is destroyed?
   A. cilia
   B. mucus
   C. cartilage
   D. blood cells

2. One of the most frequently used methods for respiratory screening and diagnosis is the:
   A. lung scan
   B. fluroscopy
   C. chest radiograph
   D. MRI

3. An examination that gives information about the speed and degree of lung expansion and structural defects in the bronchial tree is:
   A. lung scan
   B. fluoroscopy
   C. chest radiograph
   D. MRI

4. A test to assess lung ventilation and lung perfusion is the:
   A. lung scan
   B. fluoroscopy
   C. chest radiograph
   D. MRI

5. The mucous membrane lining of the lower respiratory tract responds to acute inflammation by increasing the production of:
   A. blood cells
   B. secretions
   C. hormones
   D. neurons

6. A test done to determine the presence of the bacteria that cause tuberculosis is:
   A. MRI
   B. the lung scan
   C. spirometry
   D. the acid-fast test

7. A test done to determine the presence of malignant cells is:
   A. the acid-fast test
   B. the lung scan
   C. sputum cytology
   D. spirometry

8. Chest physiotherapy should be performed:
   A. 8 times each day
   B. after meals
   C. before meals
   D. at bedtime

9. The technique of positioning the patient to facilitate gravitational movement of respiratory secretions toward the bronchi and trachea for expectoration is:
   A. postural drainage
   B. chest percussion
   C. chest vibration
   D. clapping

10. If excessive secretions that the patient cannot expectorate accumulate in the oral or nasal airway, what may be required?
    A. spirometry
    B. lung scan
    C. MRI
    D. suctioning

11. Humidity is necessary in the respiratory tract to prevent secretions from becoming:
    A. inspissated
    B. moist
    C. wet
    D. warm

12. With simple oxygen masks for patients, flow rates from the flowmeter should be adjusted to:
    A. 1 to 6 liters/min.
    B. 6 to 10 liters/min.
    C. 10 to 12 liters/min.
    D. 15 to 20 liters/min.

13. Ventilators are most commonly required for patients with:
    A. oxygen toxicity
    B. tachycardia
    C. hypoxemia
    D. hyperventilation

14. The preset amount of oxygenated air delivered during each ventilator breath is called the:
    A. vital capacity
    B. nebulizing dose
    C. tidal volume
    D. respiratory rate

15. The total number of breaths delivered per minute is called the:
    A. oxygen level setting
    B. tidal volume setting
    C. pressure setting
    D. respiratory rate setting

16. What is prescribed to keep the pressure in the lungs above the atmospheric pressure at the end of expiration?
    A. oxygen level setting
    B. tidal volume setting
    C. positive end-expiratory pressure (PEEP)
    D. negative inspiratory pressure

Introductory Nursing Care of Adults

17. A drug used to prevent acute asthma attacks but that is not useful in stopping an attack once it has begin is called:
   A.   mast cell stabilizer
   B.   antitussive
   C.   expectorant
   D.   antihistamine

Chronic Respiratory Disorders

OBJECTIVES

1. Identify examples of chronic obstructive and restrictive pulmonary diseases.
2. Explain the relationship between cigarette smoking and chronic respiratory disorders.
3. For selected chronic respiratory disorders, describe the pathophysiology, signs and symptoms, complications, diagnostic measures, and medical treatment.
4. Apply the nursing process to plan care for the patient who has a chronic respiratory disorder.

LEARNING ACTIVITIES

I. Match the definition on the left with the most appropriate term on the right.

___ 1. Right-sided heart failure associated with pulmonary disease

___ 2. One of many occupational diseases caused by inhalation of particles of industrial substances

___ 3. Permanent dilation of a portion of the bronchi or bronchioles

___ 4. A collection of inflammatory cells commonly surrounded by fibrotic tissue that represents a chronic inflammatory response to infectious or noninfectious agents

___ 5. A condition characterized by episodes of bronchospasm that causes wheezing and dyspnea

___ 6. Abnormal accumulation of air in body tissue; in the lung, a disorder characterized by loss of lung elasticity with trapping of air, retained carbon dioxide, and dyspnea

___ 7. Inflammation of the lung

___ 8. Placement of a radiation source in the body to treat a malignancy

___ 9. Bronchial inflammation

___ 10. Interstitial fibrosis caused by inhalation of asbestos fibers

A. Granuloma

B. Asthma

C. Brachytherapy

D. Pneumoconiosis

E. Asbestosis

F. Bronchiectasis

G. Pneumonitis

H. Bronchitis

I. Cor pulmonale

J. Emphysema

Ii. Complete the statements on the left with the most appropriate term on the right. Some terms may be used more than once, and some terms may not be used.

___ 1. Chronic obstructive pulmonary disease (COPD) is characterized as varying combinations of asthma, chronic bronchitis, and _____.

___ 2. Constriction of the airways is called _____.

___ 3. Severe, persistent bronchospasm is called _____.

___ 4. Bronchial inflammation characterized by increased production of mucus and chronic cough that persist for at least 3 months of the year for 2 consecutive years is called _____.

___ 5. A degenerative nonreversible disease characterized by the breakdown of the alveolar walls distal to the terminal bronchioles is _____.

___ 6. The term used to describe right-sided heart failure secondary to pulmonary disease is _____.

A. Cor pulmonale
B. Acute bronchitis
C. Emphysema
D. Congestive heart failure
E. Bronchospasm
F. Status asthmaticus
G. Chronic bronchitis
H. Status epilepticus

III. Complete the statements on the left with the most appropriate term on the right. Some terms may be used more than once, and some terms may not be used.

___ 1. An abnormal dilation and distortion on the bronchi and bronchioles that is usually confined to one lung lobe or segment is _____.

___ 2. A hereditary disorder that is characterized by dysfunction of the exocrine glands and the production of thick, tenacious mucus is _____.

___ 3. An infection spread by droplets emitted by infected people during coughing, laughing, sneezing, and singing is _____.

A. Chronic bronchitis
B. Cystic fibrosis
C. Sarcoidosis
D. Tuberculosis
E. Bronchiectasis

. Complete the statements on the left with the most appropriate term on the right. Some
terms may be used more than once, and some terms may not be used.

___ 1. The leading cause of lung cancer is
_____.

___ 2. Four types of lung surgery procedures include a wedge resection, segmental resection,
pneumonectomy, and _____.

___ 3. The four warning signs of lung cancer are
recurring pneumonia, chest pain, persistent
cough, and _____.

___ 4. The four major types of lung cancer are small
cell (oat cell) carcinoma, adenocarcinoma,
large cell carcinoma and _____.

A.   Hemoptysis

B.   Squamous cell carcinoma

C.   Fever

D.   Lobectomy

E.   Bronchitis

F.   Cigarette smoking

List 2 effects that occur when an asthma patient comes in contact with an allergen; the
antibodies cause chemical mediators to be released, which have what effect on the
bronchial smooth muscle and the airways?

1.

2.

I. List 5 complications that may occur if status asthmaticus is not corrected.

1.   4.

2.   5.

3.

II. List 5 classifications of drugs that may be used to prevent acute asthma attacks.

1.   4.

2.   5.

3.

III. List 10 signs and symptoms of impending respiratory failure to watch for with patients
experiencing impaired gas exchange.

1.   6.

2.   7.

3.   8.

4.   9.

5.   10.

IX.   List 8 factors that may lead to complications for patients with emphysema.

1.   5.

2.   6.

3.   7.

4.   8.

X.   Explain why the red blood cell count is typically elevated in patients with chronic hypoxemia.

XI.   List 2 goals of medical treatment of patients with COPD.

1.

2.

XII.   In the treatment of COPD, the initial liter flow of oxygen is usually 1 to 3 liters per minute. Why are high levels of oxygen not administered to COPD patients?

XIII.   Tuberculosis was a leading cause of death in the United States until effective drugs became available in the 1940s and 1950s. The incidence declined until 1986, when the numbers of reported cases began to rise. List 3 reasons for the recent rise.

1.

2.

3.

XIV.   List 4 diagnostic tests that are done to confirm the diagnosis of tuberculosis.

1.

2.

3.

4.

XV.   List 7 examples of offending substances that may lead to occupational lung diseases.

1.

2.

3.

4.

5.

6.

7.

VI. Match the definition on the left with the most appropriate term on the right. Some terms may be used more than once, and some terms may not be used.

___ 1. The patient's ability to inhale or to exhale by force.

___ 2. Vital capacity, inspiratory capacity, expiratory reserve volume, residual volume, and total lung capacity

___ 3. Measurement of the ability of gases to diffuse across the alveolar capillary membrane.

A. Airflow limitation

B. Lung volumes

C. Airway dynamics

D. Diffusing capacity

E. Osmosis

VII. Indicate whether the following characteristics are related to (A) intrinsic or (B) extrinsic asthma.

___ 1. Asthmatic symptoms are caused by the release of acetylcholine in response to parasympathetic stimulation

___ 2. Atopic or allergic asthma

___ 3. Characterized by hypersensitivity to molds, animal dander, and pollens

___ 4. Patients respond to nonimmunologic stimuli such as infection, cold air, and exercise

___ 5. External antigens cause an antigen-antibody reaction in the sensitive patient

___ 6. Nonatopic or nonallergic asthma

A. Intrinsic

B. Extrinsic

VIII. Match the nursing diagnoses for patients with bronchial asthma on the left with the "related to" statement on the right.

___ 1. Ineffective breathing patterns

___ 2. Impaired gas exchange

___ 3. Anxiety

A. Bronchospasm, air trapping, increased secretions

B. Air trapping

C. Perceived threat of suffocation, hypoxemia

XIX. Match the signs and symptoms on the left with the respective conditions on the right.

___ 1. Productive cough, exertional dyspnea, and wheezing

___ 2. Cough, night sweats, chest pain and tightness, fatigue, anorexia

___ 3. Dyspnea on exertion; may display use of accessory muscles of respiration; barrel chest

A. Emphysema

B. Chronic bronchitis

C. Tuberculosis

XX. Match the nursing diagnoses for patients with COPD on the left with the "related to" statements on the right.

___ 1. Impaired gas exchange

___ 2. Ineffective airway clearance

___ 3. Anxiety

___ 4. Altered nutrition: less than body requirements

___ 5. High risk for infection

___ 6. Activity intolerance

___ 7. Decreased cardiac output

A. decreased ciliary action, increased secretions, weak cough

B. alveolar destruction, bronchospasm, air trapping

C. anorexia, dyspnea

D. right-sided heart failure

E. increased secretions, weak cough

F. inability to meet oxygen needs

G. hypoxemia

XXI. For each sign on the left, indicate whether it will (A) increase or (B) decrease when inadequate oxygenation is present.

___ 1. Respiratory rate

___ 2. pH level

___ 3. $PaCO_2$ level

___ 4. Heart rate

A. Increases

B. Decreases

XXII. Choose the most appropriate answer.

1. The basic pathology with asthma is the narrowing of the bronchi or bronchioles as a result of:
   A. dilated smooth muscle around the airways
   B. contracted smooth muscle around the airways
   C. rapid, shallow respirations
   D. slow, deep respirations

2. The opening of the airways decreases in size in patients with asthma due to contracted smooth muscle and:
   A. redness
   B. increased temperature
   C. infection
   D. inflammation

3. A serious complication of bronchoconstriction is:
   A. hypoxemia
   B. hypotension
   C. drowsiness
   D. headache

4. Signs and symptoms of an asthma attack include dyspnea, productive cough, and :
   A. tachycardia
   B. bradycardia
   C. slow respirations
   D. apnea

5. The best position for patients with bronchial asthma is:
   A. supine
   B. prone
   C. side-lying
   D. Fowler's

6. Findings that should be reported to the physician if they occur in patients with impaired gas exchange include:
   A. PaO_2 decreases, pH increases
   B. PaO_2 increases, pH increases
   C. PaO_2 decreases, $PaCO_2$ increases
   D. PaO_2 increases, $PaCO_2$ increases

7. A nasal cannula is preferred over a face mask because the mask may increase the patient's feeling of:
   A. insecurity
   B. safety
   C. suffocation
   D. self-esteem

8. In patients with emphysema, the lungs often become hyperinflated, causing the diaphragm to flatten and increasing the reliance on:
   A. coughing and deep breathing exercises
   B. accessory muscles for breathing
   C. extra fluids to thin secretions
   D. increased heart rate

9. The most serious complications of chronic obstructive pulmonary disease are respiratory failure and:
   A. kidney failure
   B. heart failure
   C. brain hemorrhage
   D. paralytic ileus

10. The term *blue bloater* is used to describe patients with:
    A. advanced emphysema
    B. pneumonia
    C. adult respiratory distress syndrome
    D. advanced chronic bronchitis

11. The term *pink puffer* is used describe patients with emphysema because skin color is apt to be normal due to:
    A. normal arterial blood gases
    B. unlabored respirations
    C. barrel chest formation
    D. normal body temperature

12. The most reliable diagnostic tests for COPD are:
    A. chest radiograph
    B. MRI
    C. pulmonary function tests
    D. CBC (complete blood count)

13. Drugs that are ordered to decrease airway resistance and the work of breathing for patients with COPD are called:
    A. vasoconstrictors
    B. diuretics
    C. calcium channel blockers
    D. bronchodilators

14. The preferred route of administration of drugs for patients with COPD is by:
    A. mouth
    B. inhalation
    C. intramuscular injection
    D. intravenous injection

15. During the physical examination of patients with COPD, the nurse observes the neck for:
    A. edema
    B. distended veins
    C. enlarged lymph nodes
    D. cyanosis

16. Because good hydration helps to thin secretions in patients with impaired gas exchange, what is the recommended daily fluid intake?
    A. 600–800 ml
    B. 1000–1500 ml
    C. 2500–3000 ml
    D. 4000–5000 ml

17. The feeling of not being able to breathe is frightening; in addition, feelings of restlessness and anxiety are increased in the asthma patient due to decreased:
    A. arterial oxygen
    B. arterial carbon dioxide
    C. heart rate
    D. respiratory rate

18. During the physical examination of patients with COPD, the shape of the thorax is inspected for the classic:
    A. pink color
    B. blue tinge
    C. pulmonary edema
    D. barrel chest

19. The patient with COPD is monitored for signs and symptoms of airway obstruction, which include tachycardia, abnormal breath sounds, and:
    A. headache
    B. oliguria
    C. constipation
    D. dyspnea

20. Patients with COPD are encouraged to drink extra fluids each day in order to:
    A. improve urinary output
    B. increase circulation
    C. liquefy secretions
    D. prevent kidney stones

21. The work of breathing is increased with COPD, which in turn increases the patient's:
    A. caloric requirements
    B. requirements for calcium
    C. requirements for sodium
    D. dietary roughage requirements

22. The recommended diet for the patient who is dyspneic is a soft diet with:
    A. three large meals
    B. low-protein emphasis
    C. low-calorie emphasis
    D. frequent small meals

23. During hospitalization of the COPD patient, the nurse must attempt to schedule treatments, meals, and exercise so that the patient has time to rest. If the patient becomes excessively dyspneic or develops tachycardia during activity, the patient should:
    A. increase the activity slowly
    B. stop the activity
    C. sit down briefly and resume activity
    D. drink a full glass of water

24. Patients with chronic bronchitis and emphysema are at risk for heart failure and decreased cardiac output; the nurse monitors for signs of heart failure, which include increasing dyspnea, dependent edema, and:
    A. bradycardia
    B. tachycardia
    C. increased urine output
    D. dehydration

25. A persistent, productive cough with bloody sputum (hemoptysis) is a common symptom of:
    A. emphysema
    B. cystic fibrosis
    C. sinusitis
    D. tuberculosis

26. The most common preventive drug therapy for tuberculosis is:
    A. streptomycin
    B. isoniazid
    C. gamma globulin
    D. aminophylline

27. The patient who is thought to have active tuberculosis is isolated at first. Which of the following is NOT necessary related to the care of the patient?
    A. good hand washing
    B. wearing masks
    C. wearing gowns
    D. universal precautions

Hematologic and Lymphatic Disorders

OBJECTIVES

1. Identify data to be collected when assessing a patient with a disorder of the hematologic or lymphatic system.
2. Describe tests and procedures used to diagnose disorders of the hematologic or lymphatic system and nursing considerations for each.
3. Describe nursing care for patients undergoing common therapeutic measures for disorders of the hematologic or lymphatic system.
4. Describe the pathophysiology, signs and symptoms, complications, and medical or surgical treatment for selected disorders of the hematologic or lymphatic system.
5. Write a nursing care plan for a patient with a disorder of the hematologic or lymphatic system.
6. Identify measures the nurse can take to reduce the risk of disorders of the hematologic or lymphatic system and to detect problems early.

LEARNING ACTIVITIES

I.   Match the definition on the left with the most appropriate term on the right.

____ 1. Person with type AB positive blood who can receive transfusions with any type of blood because all the common antigens (A,B and Rh) are present in the blood

____ 2. A purplish skin lesion resulting from blood leaking outside the blood vessels

____ 3. A deficiency in the number of red blood cells, hemoglobin, or both in the blood

____ 4. A small (1–3mm) red or reddish-purple spot on the skin resulting from blood capillaries breaking and leaking small amounts of blood into the tissues

____ 5. Actions taken to help protect patients with low white blood cell counts from infection

____ 6. Person with type O negative blood who can donate blood to anyone because none of the common antigens are present in the blood

____ 7. Cancer of the white blood cells in which the bone marrow produces too many immature white blood cells

____ 8. Red or reddish-purple skin lesions 3 mm or more in size that result from blood leaking outside of the blood vessels

____ 9. Cancer of the lymph system

A.   Anemia

B.   Compromised host precautions

C.   Ecchymosis

D.   Leukemia

E.   Lymphoma

F.   Petechia

G.   Purpura

H.   Universal donor

I.   Universal recipient

II. List 6 nursing actions for the patient who is anemic (the patient with a hematocrit less than 30 and/or a hemoglobin less than 10).

1.

2.

3.

4.

5.

6.

III. List 10 nursing actions for the patient who is neutropenic (compromised host precautions).

1.

2.

3.

4.

5.

6.

7.

8.

9.

10.

IV. List 7 nursing actions for patients who are thrombocytopenic.

1.

2.

3.

4.

5.

6.

7.

V. List 5 nursing diagnoses and 5 goals for the patient in sickle cell crisis.

1.   1.

2.   2.

3.   3.

4.   4.

5.   5.

VI. List 5 nursing diagnoses and 7 nursing goals for the patient with acute leukemia.

1.   1.

2.   2.

3.   3.

4.   4.

5.   5.

                                        6.

                                        7.

VII. List 3 nursing diagnoses for patients with hemophilia.

1.

2.

3.

VIII. List the 5 major types of white blood cells.

1.   4.

2.   5.

3.

IX. List 6 symptoms of a patient with a low hematocrit who would probably need a blood transfusion.

1.   4.

2.   5.

3.   6.

X. Fill in the blanks.

1. Four types of blood transfusion reactions include hemolytic, allergic, febrile, and _____

_____.

2. The four components of blood are red blood cells, white blood cells, platelets, and _____.

XI. Match the definition or description on the left with the most appropriate term on the right.

____ 1. Protect the body from infections   A. bone marrow

____ 2. Erythrocytes   B. clotting factors

____ 3. Straw-colored fluid that is mainly water   C. hematocrit

____ 4. Spongy center of the bones   D. hemoglobin

____ 5. Total number of erythrocytes in a cubic millimeter of blood   E. plasma

                                                   F. platelets

____ 6. Thromboplastin, prothrombin, fibrinogen   G. red blood cells

____ 7. Percentage of red blood cells in whole blood   H. red blood cell count

____ 8. Thrombocytes   I. white blood cells

____ 9. Carries the oxygen in the blood

XII. Match the definition or description on the left with the most appropriate term on the right.

___ 1. Decrease in blood pressure of 15–20 points from lying to standing; increase in pulse of 10–20 points from lying to standing

___ 2. Individual with type O negative blood

___ 3. Nurse with a master's degree who specializes in the care of patients with cancer

___ 4. Individual with type AB positive blood

___ 5. Actions taken to help protect patients with low white blood cell counts from infection

A. compromised host precautions

B. oncology clinical nurse specialist

C. orthostatic vital sign changes

D. universal recipient

E. universal donor

XIII. Match the blood test on the left with its appropriate range of normal values on the right.

___ 1. Normal RBC

___ 2. Normal hematocrit

___ 3. Normal hemoglobin

___ 4. Normal WBC

___ 5. Normal platelets

A. 5000 to 10,000

B. 3.6 to 5.4 million/liter

C. 150,000 to 350,000

D. 12 to 17.5 gm/dl

E. 37 to 54%

XIV. Match the test/study on the left with the appropriate patient preparation on the right.

___ 1. Urine protein electrophoresis

___ 2. Stool cultures

___ 3. Sputum cultures

___ 4. Blood tests (such as CBC, PT/PTT)

___ 5. Urine cultures

___ 6. Blood cultures

___ 7. Bleeding time

A. Blood culture results are evaluated at 48 and 72 hr. Tell the patient not to expect any final results for 3 to 4 days.

B. Give the patient a sterile cup. Have the patient collect sputum next time he or she coughs. Caution the patient not to collect saliva. Sputum comes from the lungs with coughing. Send the specimen to the laboratory immediately.

C. Have the patient defecate into a clean bedpan or other container. Using a sterile tongue blade, collect a specimen in a sterile container. Send the specimen to the laboratory immediately. Some tests must be done while the specimen is still warm.

D. Choose the correct blood tubes to collect the blood in. Tell the patient he or she will feel a needle stick as the needle goes through the skin.

E. Tell the patient a blood pressure cuff is placed above the elbow and pumped up to 40 mm Hg. A puncture is made on a cleaned area of the forearm. A stop watch is started. The wound is blotted with filter paper every 30 sec until all the bleeding has stopped. The time is noted.

F. Have the patient void into the toilet. Mark the time. Have the patient collect all urine for the next 24 hours. The container should be kept on ice. Exactly 24 hr after the starting time, have the patient void for the last time and submit the entire 24-hr collection to the laboratory.

G. Give the patient wipes and a sterile container. have the patient clean around the meatus of the urethra. Tell the patient to urinate a small amount into the toilet and stop. Then tell the patient to collect a urine specimen. Send the specimen to the laboratory immediately.

XV. Match each test/study on the left with its purpose/procedure on the right.

___ 1. Urine protein electrophoresis

___ 2. Sputum cultures

___ 3. Bleeding time

___ 4. Stool cultures

___ 5. Blood tests

___ 6. Urine cultures

___ 7. Blood cultures

A. Measures the time it takes for the platelet plug to form.

B. Detects and identifies microorganisms in the urine. The specimen can normally be collected by the patient. If the patient is unable to collect the specimen, the physician may request a straight catheterization to collect the specimen. Follow the procedures for catheterizing a patient.

C. Measures various blood components. Different blood tests are collected in different laboratory tubes containing specific reagents or no reagents at all. Usually the tubes have color-coded tops. Be sure and collect the blood in the blood tube specific for the blood test ordered. Usually each institution's laboratory publishes a manual identifying what colored tube to use for each blood test.

D. Performs an electrophoresis on the urine to detect abnormal amounts of protein.

E. Detects and identifies microorganisms in the stool.

F. Detects and identifies microorganisms in the blood. The vein is prepared with betadine and allowed to dry. Do not touch the site. The tops of the blood culture bottles are prepared with betadine and allowed to dry. Usually there is one anaerobic culture bottle and one aerobic culture bottle. Ten ml of blood are drawn and 5 ml are placed in each culture bottle. Send the specimen to the laboratory immediately.

G. Detects and identifies microorganisms in the sputum.

XVI. Match each test/study on the left with the appropriate patient preparation on the right.

____ 1. Spleen sonogram or ultrasound

____ 2. Bone marrow biopsy

____ 3. Spleen scan

____ 4. Lymphangiogram (LAG)

A. Explain the purpose and procedure to the patient. A permit must be signed. No fasting is necessary. Some local discomfort may be experienced as the local anesthesia is injected to numb the top of the foot. Incisions may be blue stained from the dye. The procedure takes approximately 3 hr. The patient returns to Diagnostic Radiology 12–24 hr later for more radiographs.

B. Explain the purpose and procedure to the patient. No fasting is necessary. An intravenous line must be in place to inject the dye. The procedure takes approximately 80 min.

C. Explain the purpose and procedure to the patient. The patient should fast from food 12 hr before the examination. Water is permitted. The procedure will take approximately 30–45 min.

D. Explain the purpose and procedure to the patient. A permit must be signed. No fasting is necessary. Some local discomfort may be experienced as the local anesthesia is injected before the Jameshedi needle is inserted. The patient usually feels pressure as the Jameshedi needle is inserted into the bone and a momentary sharp pain down the leg as the bone marrow fluid is aspirated. The procedure takes approximately 30 min.

XVII. Match the blood component on the left with the indications for its use in the center and its usual amount on the right.

____ 1. Platelets

____ 2. Cryoprecipitate

____ 3. Packed red blood cells

____ 4. Fresh frozen plasma

A. Clotting deficiencies, hemophilia, for rapid reversal of warfarin (Coumadin), with massive red blood cell transfusions

B. Symptoms from a low hematocrit or hemoglobin such as shortness of breath, tachycardia, decreased blood pressure, chest pain, lightheadedness, or fatigue

C. Hemophilia A

D. Bleeding from thrombocytopenia

E. 10 ml/bag; usually 10 bags are pooled together

F. 60 ml/pack; usually four to six packs are pooled together

G. 200–280 ml/unit

H. 250–300 ml/unit

XVIII. Match each test/study on the left with its purpose/procedure on the right.

____ 1. Lymphangiogram (LAG)

____ 2. Spleen sonogram

____ 3. Spleen scan

____ 4. Bone marrow biopsy

A. Used to estimate the size of the spleen. The patient lies on the back in the Ultrasound Department. A gel or lubricant that acts as a conductor is applied to the left upper quadrant of the abdomen. A technician moves a handheld transducer over the area while watching a screen and recording the ultrasound echoes from the spleen.

B. Used to evaluate how well the bone marrow is making red blood cells, white blood cells, and platelets. The patient is positioned on an examining table according to the location of the bone marrow biopsy. The most common site is the posterior lilac crest, although the anterior crest, sternum, and tibia are also potential sites. The selected site is prepared and draped as for a minor surgical procedure. A local anesthetic is injected. A Jameshedi needle is forced into the bone marrow. Bone marrow fluid is aspirated and a core biopsy taken through and with the Jameshedi needle. The needle is removed and a pressure dressing applied to the site. A laboratory technician must be present during the procedure to immediately fix and stain the specimens. Sometimes a short-acting anesthetic such as midazolam (Versed) is used to sedate the patient during the procedure.

C. Evaluates the anatomy of the lymphatic vessels and nodes. The patient is taken to Diagnostic Radiology, where a 1–2 incision is made on the dorsum of each foot. The lymphatic vessels are cannulated and dye is injected. Several radiographs are taken as the dye moves up the extremity. The patient returns to Diagnostic Radiology 12–24 hr later for more radiographs of the lymph nodes and higher lymphatic channels.

D. Used to evaluate the size as well as the function of the spleen. In the Nuclear Medicine Department, a radioactive dye is injected into a vein. The amount of dye taken up by the spleen is measured by a machine 20–60 min after the dye is infected.

XIX. Match the drug on the left with its action in the center and the appropriate nursing interventions. (Some actions may be used more than once.)

___ 1. Corticosteroids

___ 2. Vitamin B_{12}

___ 3. Ferrous sulfate

___ 4. Epoetin alfa

___ 5. Iron dextran

A. Iron replacement

B. Vitamin replacement

C. Stimulates the bone marrow to produce red blood cells

D. Immunosuppressive

G. Intramuscular injection. Must be given every month the rest of the person's life.

H. Have the patient take the drug with food but not with milk, eggs, or caffeinated drinks because the milk and caffeine inhibit drug absorption. If the patient is taking liquid iron, dilute the drug and administer through a straw to prevent the drug from staining the teeth.

I. May be given by intravenous or subcutaneous injection. Patient is usually treated three times per week until the hematocrit is 30–33.

J. Give these drugs with meals. An H_2–receptor antagonist such as ranitidine (Zantac) may be prescribed to decrease gastric acid production. If the patient takes these drugs for an extended period of time, the drug should not be stopped abruptly. Instead, the drug dose should be gradually decreased over time under a physician's direction.

K. Test dose before starting treatment. Give intramuscular injections only in the upper, outer quadrant of the buttock using the Z-track technique.

XX. Choose the most appropriate answer.

1. Red blood cells are called.
   A. erythrocytes
   B. lymphocytes
   C. thrombocytes
   D. neutrophils

2. A condition in which there are too many blood cells is called:
   A. anemia
   B. Hodgkin's disease
   C. lymphoma
   D. polycythemia vera

3. The treatment for acquired hemolytic anemia is:
   A. vitamin B$_{12}$ injections
   B. ferrous sulfate and high-iron diet
   C. iron dextran and high-carbohydrate diet
   D. corticosteroids and transfusions

4. The treatment for aplastic anemia is:
   A. Vitamin B$_{12}$ injections
   B. ferrous sulfate and high-iron diet
   C. iron dextran and high-carbohydrate diet
   D. transfusions, antibiotics, and corticosteroids

5. Sickle cell crisis results in:
   A. headache and hypertension
   B. obstructed blood flow and severe pain
   C. dyspnea and tachycardia
   D. urinary retention and oliguria

6. Treatment for sickle cell crisis includes:
   A. ferrous sulfate and high-iron diet
   B. iron dextran and high-carbohydrate diet
   C. aggressive intravenous hydration and IV Demerol
   D. corticosteroids and transfusions

7. The acute leukemias are initially treated with high doses of:
   A. radiation
   B. chemotherapy
   C. corticosteroids
   D. iron sulfate

8. Bone marrow transplants are administered to patients through:
   A. intravenous lines
   B. surgery
   C. nasogastric tubes
   D. blood transfusions

9. Compromised host precautions can be discontinued and a regular diet eaten when the:
   A. erythrocyte count is above 4 million
   B. lymphocyte count is above 5000
   C. neutrophil count is above 1000
   D. thrombocyte count is above 100,000

10. Physicians try not to prescribe platelet transfusions for patients unless the:
    A. neutrophil count is below 2000
    B. erythrocyte count is below 3.5 million
    C. leukocyte count is below 10,000
    D. platelet count is below 20,000

11. Anemia is defined as a hematocrit below:
    A. 30 and hemoglobin below 10
    B. 35 and hemoglobin below 15
    C. 40 and hemoglobin below 20
    D. 45 and hemoglobin below 25

12. Inflammation of the mucous membranes is called:
    A. anemia
    B. thrombocytopenia
    C. stomatitis
    D. leukemia

13. A cancer of the bone marrow that causes abnormal levels of blood proteins and weakened areas of the bones is:
    A. lymphoma
    B. Hodgkin's disease
    C. multiple myeloma
    D. anemia

14. The diagnosis of lymphoma is made with a:
    A. complete blood count
    B. urine analysis of proteins
    C. lymph node biopsy
    D. leukocyte count

15. The treatment for thrombocytopenia is:
    A. antibiotics and transfusions
    B. corticosteroids, platelets, and fresh frozen plasma
    C. anticoagulants, beta blockers, antipyretics, and whole blood
    D. anticholinergics, platelets, and barbiturates

16. The main symptom of hemophilia is:
    A. infection
    B. headache
    C. bleeding
    D. anemia

17. How many times larger is the hematocrit than the hemoglobin count?
    A. 2 times
    B. 3 times
    C. 4 times
    D. 10 times

18. White blood cells are called:
    A. erythrocytes
    B. thrombocytes
    C. leukocytes
    D. platelets

19. The normal life span of a white blood cell is:
    A. 2 hours
    B. 12 hours
    C. 60 days
    D. 120 days

20. A "shift to the left" refers to the bone marrow production of large numbers of:
    A. neutrophils
    B. eosinophils
    C. erythrocytes
    D. thrombocytes

21. Plasma is made primarily of:
    A. water
    B. red blood cells
    C. white blood cells
    D. platelets

22. The function of lymph nodes is to act as a:
    A. pump
    B. valve
    C. filter
    D. resevoir

23. The spleen is located in the:
    A. lower left quadrant of the abdomen
    B. lower right quadrant of the abdomen
    C. upper right quadrant of the abdomen
    D. upper left quadrant of the abdomen

24. Functions of the spleen include storage of red blood cells, destruction of old red blood cells, and:
    A. storage of platelets
    B. forming blood clots
    C. production of antibodies
    D. production of red blood cells

25. If a patient is having a planned splenectomy for Hodgkin's disease, patients should receive a:
    A. hepatitis B vaccine
    B. blood transfusion
    C. platelet transfusion
    D. Pneumovax vaccine

26. The cells responsible for the humoral immune response are the:
    A. B lymphocytes
    B. T lymphocytes
    C. erythrocytes
    D. thrombocytes

27. The cells responsible for the cellular immune response are:
    A. B lymphocytes
    B. T lymphocytes
    C. erythrocytes
    D. platelets

28. Red or reddish-purple spots that are the result of blood vessels breaking and that are 3 mm or larger are:
    A. petechiae
    B. purpura
    C. ecchymoses
    D. nodes

29. Patients with low red blood cell counts may have:
    A. bradycardia
    B. hypotension
    C. bleeding problems
    D. tachycardia

30. If a patient is orthostatic and TILT positive, what should be increased?
    A. carbohydrates
    B. fluids
    C. fiber
    D. vitamins

31. A bone marrow biopsy is often done to diagnose:
    A. Hodgkin's disease
    B. anemia
    C. liver disease
    D. leukemia

32. LAG (lymphangiogram) is done as part of the staging work-up for:
    A. leukemia
    B. anemia
    C. liver disease
    D. Hodgkin's disease

33. The universal donor blood is type:
    A. O negative
    B. A negative
    C. AB positive
    D. B positive

34. The universal recipient is type:
    A. O negative
    B. A negative
    C. AB positive
    D. B positive

35. Once blood is picked up from the blood bank, the transfusion should be started within:
    A. 5 minutes
    B. 30 minutes
    C. 1 hour
    D. 6 hours

36. Platelets are generally administered when a patient's platelet count drops below:
    A. 10,000
    B. 20,000
    C. 150,000
    D. 300,000

37. If platelets are ordered before a procedure such as a lumbar puncture or endoscopy to prevent postprocedure bleeding, the platelets should be administered:
    A. one week before the procedure
    B. one day before the procedure
    C. 6 hours before the procedure
    D. immediately before the procedure

. Once treatment starts, the greatest risks to patients
with lymphoma are:
A. tachycardia and palpitations
B. urinary retention and oliguria
C. nausea and vomiting
D. infection and bleeding

. The treatment for hemophilia is:
A. plasma and cryoprecipitate transfusions
B. red blood cell and antibiotic transfusions
C. white blood cell and potassium transfusions
D. platelets and anticoagulant transfusions

. Symptoms of thrombocytopenia include:
A. fatigue and pallor
B. petechiae and purpura
C. nausea and vomiting
D. tachycardia and palpitations

41. Treatment for thrombocytopenia includes:
A. red blood cell transfusions and iron
B. white blood cell transfusions and antibiotics
C. corticosteroids and platelet transfusions
D. cryoprecipitate transfusions and anticon-
vulsants

42. The condition in which a person has too few platelets
circulating in the blood is called:
A. leukemia
B. anemia
C. lymphoma
D. thrombocytopenia

XI. Label the parts of the lymphatic system.

A.

B.

C.

D.

E.

F.

G.

H.

I.

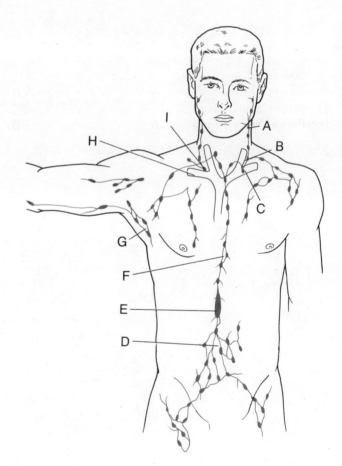

Cardiac Disorders

OBJECTIVES

1. Label the major parts of the heart.
2. Explain the physiology of cardiac function.
3. Explain the nursing considerations for patients having diagnostic procedures to detect or evaluate cardiac disorders.
4. Identify nursing implications for common therapeutic measures, including drug, diet, or oxygen therapy; pacemakers and cardioverters; cardiac surgery; and cardiopulmonary resuscitation.
5. For selected cardiac disorders, explain the pathophysiology, risk factors, signs and symptoms, complications, and treatment.
6. List the data to be obtained in assessing the patient with a cardiac disorder.
7. Apply the nursing process to develop a plan of care for patients with cardiac disorders.

LEARNING ACTIVITIES

Match the definition on the left with the most appropriate term on the right.

___ 1. Slow heart rate, usually defined as fewer than 60 beats per minute

___ 2. Rapid heart rate, usually defined as greater than 100 beats per minute

___ 3. Abnormal thickening and hardening of the arterial walls caused by fat and fibrin deposits

___ 4. Obstruction of a blood vessel with a blood clot transported through the blood stream

___ 5. A sound heard on auscultation; in the heart, it indicates turbulent blood flow across heart valves

___ 6. Abnormal thickening and hardening of the arterial walls

___ 7. The amount of blood in the left ventricle at the end of diastole; the pressure generated at the end of diastole

___ 8. Disturbance of rhythm; arrhythmia

___ 9. Study of the movement of blood and the forces that affect it

A. Murmur

B. Thromboembolism

C. Hemodynamics

D. Regurgitation

E. Syncope

F. Atherosclerosis

G. Bradycardia

H. Perfusion

I. Preload

J. Infarct

K. Palpitation

L. Tachycardia

M. Afterload

N. Arteriosclerosis

O. Dysrhythmia

I. Continues

I. *Continued*

____ 10. A heartbeat that is strong, rapid, or irregular enough that the person is aware of it

____ 11. Fainting

____ 12. The amount of resistance the left ventricle must generate to open the aortic valve

____ 13. Backward flow

____ 14. An area of ischemic necrosis caused by disruption of circulation

____ 15. Passage of blood through the vessels of an organ

A. Murmur
B. Thromboembolism
C. Hemodynamics
D. Regurgitation
E. Syncope
F. Atherosclerosis
G. Bradycardia
H. Perfusion
I. Preload
J. Infarct
K. Palpitation
L. Tachycardia
M. Afterload
N. Arteriosclerosis
O. Dysrhythmia

II. Match the definition on the left with the most appropriate term on the right.

____ 1. The delivery of an electric shock to the myocardium to restore normal sinus rhythm

____ 2. The percentage of ventricular end-diastolic volume ejected with each contraction of the left ventricle

____ 3. The ability of a cell to respond to an electrochemical stimulus

____ 4. The amount of blood (measured in liters) ejected by each ventricle per minute

____ 5. Adaptations made by the heart and circulation to maintain normal cardiac output

____ 6. The ability of a cell to generate an impulse without external stimulation

____ 7. Capacity for shortening in response to stimuli

____ 8. Enlargement of existing cells resulting in increased size of an organ or tissue

____ 9. A wall that divides a body cavity

____ 10. Termination of fibrillation, usually by electric shock

____ 11. Contraction phase of the cardiac cycle

____ 12. The ability of the cell to transmit electrical impulses rapidly and efficiently to distant regions of the heart

____ 13. Formation of a blood clot

____ 14. Relaxation phase of the cardiac cycle

A. Cardiac output
B. Systole
C. Conductivity
D. Ejection fraction
E. Compensation
F. Defibrillation
G. Contractility
H. Cardioversion
I. Diastole
J. Hypertrophy
K. Excitability
L. Thrombosis
M. Septum
N. Automaticity

III. Match the definition on the left with the most appropriate term on the right.

____ 1. Cup-shaped structure; semilunar heart valves have three cusps

____ 2. Capable of preventing the formation of blood clots

____ 3. Sudden difficulty breathing when asleep

____ 4. Shortness of breath

____ 5. Accessory, side branch

____ 6. Difficulty breathing in a supine position

____ 7. Wet with excessive perspiration

____ 8. Referring to the pointed end of a structure

A. Paroxysmal nocturnal dyspnea

B. Collateral

C. Cusp

D. Orthopnea

E. Anticoagulant

F. Apical

G. Dyspnea

H. Diaphoretic

IV. What is the main function of the cardiovascular system?

V. List the 3 layers of cardiac muscle tissue from the inside to the outside.

1.

2.

3.

VI. List 2 purposes of the 4 valves found in the heart.

1.

2.

VII. Trace the route of an impulse through the electrical conduction system of the heart, beginning with the SA node and ending with the Purkinje fibers.

1. SA node

2.

3.

4.

5. Purkinje fibers

VIII. List 3 effects of sympathetic stimulation on the heart.

1. Heart rate _____

2. Speed of conduction through the AV node _____

3. Contractions _____

IX. List 3 factors that affect vascular resistance.

1.

2.

3.

X. Indicate the changes in the areas below as a result of age-related changes.

1. Heart muscle connective tissue density _____

2. Elasticity _____

3. Cardiac contractility _____

4. Valves _____

5. Emptying of chambers _____

6. Number of pacemaker cells in the SA node _____

7. Number of nerve fibers in ventricles _____

8. Aging heart's response to stress _____

XI. Indicate how blood vessels change in the areas below in the elderly.

1. Elasticity _____

2. Systolic blood pressure _____

3. Pulse pressure _____

4. Veins _____

XII. The pain of heart problems may radiate or be referred to other areas. List 3 areas to which pain may radiate, as described by patients with cardiac conditions.

1.

2.

3.

XIII. Indicate the nursing interventions or patient teaching which should be done in the areas listed below for patients who have undergone cardiac catheterization.

1. Puncture site _____

2. Vital signs _____

3. Cannula insertion site _____

4. Peripheral pulses _____

5. Ambulation _____

6. Fluids _____

7. Diet _____

8. Complications _____

XIV. List the 2 invasive catheters that have been developed to assess the pressures within the heart and the lungs.

1.

2.

XV. Indicate how the following factors affect cardiac output.

1. Stress _____

2. Myocardial infarction _____

3. Bradycardia _____

4. Tachycardia _____

XVI. List 4 words that patients with angina use to describe the anginal pain.

1.

2.

3.

4.

XVII. List 3 reasons related to the characteristics below why an angioplasty may be a preferred treatment over bypass surgery.

1. Type of anesthesia _____

2. Invasiveness _____

3. Recovery time _____

XVIII. Indicate the findings the nurse would expect to observe in patients with mitral stenosis regarding the areas listed below.

1. Heart rate _____

2. Respirations _____

3. Pulse pressure _____

4. Jugular vein _____

5. Auscultated lung sounds _____

6. Sound of murmur _____

XIX. List 4 causes or reasons why the nurse may observe fluid volume excess in patients with mitral stenosis or congestive heart failure.

1.

2.

3.

4.

XX. What is the name of the procedure where a catheter is passed through a peripheral artery into the occluded coronary artery and a balloon at the tip of the catheter is inflated to dilate the artery?

XXI. Match the characteristics on the left with the correct heart chamber on the right. Some chambers may be used more than once; some may not be used.

____ 1. Contains the highest pressure in the heart

____ 2. Receives blood through the tricuspid valve

____ 3. Cone-shaped, has the thickest muscle mass of the four chambers

____ 4. Receives blood saturated with oxygen from the four pulmonary veins

____ 5. Receives blood from inferior and superior vena cava

A. Right atrium (RA)

B. Right ventricle (RV)

C. Left atrium (LA)

D. Left ventricle (LV)

XXII. Complete the statements on the left with the most appropriate term on the right. Some terms may be used more than once, and some terms may not be used.

____ 1. These vessels carry blood to the lungs where they release carbon dioxide as waste and are resaturated with oxygen _____.

____ 2. These vessels carry blood saturated with oxygen to the left atrium _____.

____ 3. An apical pulse is taken by auscultating the heartbeat at this location _____.

____ 4. Blood is received from the LA into the LV through the _____.

____ 5. This valve is located between the RA and the RV _____.

A. Semilunar valve

B. Pulmonary veins

C. Mitral valve

D. Coronary artery

E. Tricuspid valve

F. Pulmonary arteries

G. Apex

XXIII. Indicate whether the following factors (A) increase or (B) decrease the following categories.

____ 1. Dehydration, hemorrhage, and venous vasodilation _____ preload.

____ 2. Increased venous return to the heart and overhydration _____ preload.

____ 3. Catecholamines _____ contractility.

____ 4. Acidosis and beta blockers _____ contractility

____ 5. Vasodilation _____ afterload.

____ 6. Hypertension, vasoconstriction, and aortic stenosis _____ afterload.

A. Increases

B. Decreases

Introductory Nursing Care of Adults

XXIV. Match the definition on the left with the most appropriate diagnostic test or procedure on the right. Some terms may be used more than once, and some may not be used.

___ 1. An ambulatory ECG that provides continuous monitoring

___ 2. A transducer is used that picks up sound waves and converts them to electrical impulses

___ 3. A high resolution, three-dimensional image of the heart; cardiac tissue is imaged without lung or bone interference

___ 4. An exercise tolerance test that is a recording of an individual's cardiovascular response during a measured exercise challenge

___ 5. Study of electrical activity of the heart

___ 6. A procedure in which a catheter is advanced into the heart chambers or coronary arteries under fluoroscopy

___ 7. Test that may determine pressures in the RA, RV and pulmonary artery

___ 8. Electrodes placed on the surface of the skin pick up the electrical impulses of the heart

___ 9. The patient ambulates on a treadmill or a stationary bicycle while connected to a monitor

___ 10. Heart sonogram that is a visualization and recording of the size, shape, position, and behavior of the heart's internal structures

A. Stress test

B. Cardiac catheterization

C. EEG

D. Echocardiogram

E. ECG

F. MRI

G. Holter monitor

XXV. Match the definition on the left with the most appropriate term on the right. Some terms may be used more than once, and some may not be used.

___ 1. A test that determines the body's ability to maintain the acid-base balance

___ 2. A test to measure a blood lipid that is produced by the liver and is used to form bile salts for the digestion of fats and to form some hormones

___ 3. In addition to LDL cholesterol, these lipids are a major contributor to coronary artery disease

A. Triglycerides

B. Erythrocyte sedimentation rate

C. Cardiac enzymes

D. Cholesterol level

E. Pulse oximetry

F. Arterial blood gases

XXVI. Match the descriptions of complications of coronary artery disease on the left with the terms on the right. Some terms may be used more than once, and some may not be used.

___	1. Disturbances in heart rhythm	A. Ventricular rupture
___	2. When the injured left ventricle is unable to meet the body's circulatory demands	B. Mitral stenosis
___	3. The most frequent cause of death after an AMI; marked by hypotension and decreasing alertness	C. Dysrhythmias
		D. Hemorrhage
___	4. When clots form in the injured heart chambers, they may break loose and travel to the lung	E. Cardiogenic shock
		F. Thromboembolism
		G. Cardiac failure
___	5. A fatal complication in which weakened areas of the ventricular wall bulge and burst	

XXVII. Complete the statements on the left with the most appropriate term on the right. Some terms may be used more than once, and some terms may not be used.

___	1. When the ventricles fail as pumps and the heart is unable to meet the metabolic demands of the body, this is called _____.	A. Catecholamines
		B. Ventricular hypertrophy
___	2. A term used to describe the cardiac and circulatory adjustments that maintain or restore cardiac output to normal is _____.	C. Acute myocardial infarction
		D. Renal compensation
___	3. The sympathetic nervous system responds to decreased cardiac output and blood pressure by releasing _____.	E. Hepatic compensation
		F. Compensation
___	4. A response to decreased cardiac output, in which the renin-angiotensin mechanism is initiated, is called _____	G. Congestive heart failure
___	5. Enlargement of the ventricular myocardium that results from strain is called _____.	

XXVIII. Complete the statements on the left with the most appropriate term on the right. Some terms may be used more than once, and some terms may not be used.

___	1. The narrowing of the opening in the valve that impedes blood flow from the left atrium into the left ventricle is called _____.	A. Tricuspid stenosis
		B. Commissurotomy
___	2. The leading cause of mitral stenosis is _____.	C. Angioplasty
		D. Mitral stenosis
___	3. In patients with mitral stenosis, the chamber of the heart that dilates to accommodate the amount of blood not ejected is the _____.	E. Heart murmur
		F. Rheumatic heart disease
___	4. Excision of parts of the leaflets of the mitral valve to enlarge the opening is called _____.	G. Left ventricle
		H. Left atrium
___	5. When collecting data for the assessment of the patient with mitral stenosis, the nurse takes the vital signs and auscultates for _____.	I. Right ventricle

Introductory Nursing Care of Adults

XXIX. Match the definition on the left with the most appropriate term on the right. Some terms may be used more than once, and some may not be used.

____ 1. Ability of cardiac muscle fibers to shorten when stimulated

____ 2. Amount of pressure the LV must generate to open the aortic valve; affects the rate of contraction

____ 3. Cell's ability to transmit electric impulses rapidly and efficiently to distant regions of the heart

____ 4. Inotropy that is affected by biochemical changes

____ 5. Cell's capacity to generate an impulse without external stimulation

____ 6. Amount of blood in the LV at the end of diastole; the pressure generated at end diastole

____ 7. Cell's capacity to respond to an electrochemical stimulus

A. Excitability

B. Automaticity

C. Preload

D. Repolarization

E. Afterload

F. Conductivity

G. Ejection fraction

H. Contractility

XXX. Match the characteristics of laboratory tests on the left with the most appropriate test on the right. Some terms may be used more than once, and some may not be used.

____ 1. Indicates the body's ability to defend itself against infection and inflammation

____ 2. Determines ability of the blood to carry oxygen from the lungs to the tissues and carbon dioxide from the tissues to the lung

____ 3. Percentage of packed RBCs in the total sample of whole blood

____ 4. Measurement of main component of the RBCs whose function is to transport oxygen to the cells

____ 5. Measurement of formed elements in the blood needed for coagulation

____ 6. The rate of settlement of RBCs in unclotted blood, which detects tissue necrosis

____ 7. Measurement of enzymes that are released when heart cells die as a result of damage

A. Lipid profile

B. Erythrocyte sedimentation rate

C. Hematocrit

D. WBC

E. Arterial blood gases

F. RBC

G. Hemoglobin

H. Cardiac enzymes

I. Platelets

XXXI. Match the uses of cardiac drugs on the left with the type of drug on the right. Some types may be used more than once, and some may not be used.

   ____ 1. Used to treat fluid retention, often experienced by patients with heart problems

   ____ 2. Used to prevent clot formation

   ____ 3. Used after a myocardial infarction to prevent strokes

   ____ 4. Used to destroy clots that have already formed

   ____ 5. Used for patients having a myocardial infarction who experience severe chest pain, if pain persists after they have taken nitroglycerine

A. Antidysrhythmics

B. Thrombolytic agents

C. Anticoagulants

D. Anticholinergics

E. Antiplatelet agents

F. Diuretics

G. Analgesics

H. Vasodilators

XXXII. Match the names of drugs used for cardiac disorders on the left with their classifications on the right. Some classifications may be used more than once, and some may not be used.

   ____ 1. Nitroglycerine

   ____ 2. Aspirin and Persantine

   ____ 3. Heparin and warfarin (Coumadin)

   ____ 4. Morphine and meperidine hydrochloride (Demerol)

   ____ 5. Furosemide (Lasix) and hydrochlorothiazide (Esidrix, HCTZ, and Oretic)

   ____ 6. Streptokinase, urokinase, and tissue plasminogen activator

A. Anticholinergics

B. Vasodilators

C. Narcotic analgesics

D. Antiplatelet agents

E. Antidysrhythmics

F. Diuretics

G. Antithrombolytic agents

H. Anticoagulants

XXXIII. Match the nursing diagnoses for the postoperative cardiac surgery patient with the most appropriate "related to" statements on the right.

   ____ 1. Ineffective thermoregulation

   ____ 2. Decreased cardiac output

   ____ 3. High risk for infection

A. Altered skin integrity

B. Cooling during surgery

C. Fluid loss or decreased fluid intake

XXXIV. Match the ECG changes on the left with the features of acute myocardial infarction on the right.

___ 1. The T wave is inverted

___ 2. There is ST segment elevation

___ 3. A significant Q wave is present; the Q wave is greater than one third the height of the R wave

A. Ischemia

B. Infarction

C. Injury

XXXV. Match the uses of AMI drug therapy on the left with the specific drug on the right. Some drugs may be used more than once, and some may not be used.

___ 1. Used for chest pain

___ 2. Administered IV or into the coronary arteries to dissolve thrombi

___ 3. Following the administration of the anti-thrombolytics, this drug is administered to prevent further clot formation

___ 4. Administered for ventricular tachycardia

___ 5. Increases myocardial contractility and decreases the heart rate

A. Lasix

B. Streptokinase

C. Digitalis

D. Morphine sulfate

E. Atropine sulfate

F. Lidocaine

G. Heparin

XXXVI. Match the nursing diagnoses for patients with coronary artery disease on the left with the "related to" statement on the right.

___ 1. Anxiety

___ 2. Pain

___ 3. Decreased cardiac output

A. Dysrhythmia

B. Feeling of impending doom

C. Lack of oxygen to the myocardium

XXXVII. For the signs and symptoms of congestive heart failure on the left, indicate whether they are indicative of (A) right-sided or (B) left-sided failure.

___ 1. Dependent edema

___ 2. Decreasing BP readings

___ 3. Increased central venous pressure

___ 4. Anxious, pale and tachycardic

___ 5. Jugular vein distention

___ 6. Abdominal engorgement

___ 7. Crackles, wheezes, dyspnea, and cough

A. Right-sided

B. Left-sided

XXXVIII. Match the actions of drugs used to treat CHF on the left with drug classifications on the right. Some classifications may be used more than once, and some may not be used.

____ 1. Improve(s) pump function by increasing con-tractility and decreasing heart rate

____ 2. Decrease(s) circulating fluid volume and decrease(s) preload

____ 3. Decrease(s) anxiety, dilate(s) the vasculature, and reduce(s) myocardial consumption in the acute stage

A. Heparin

B. Morphine

C. Diuretics

D. Streptokinase

E. Cardiac glycosides or inotropic agents, such as digoxin

XXXIX. Complete the statements on the left with the most appropriate term on the right. Some terms may be used more than once, and some terms may not be used.

____ 1. The narrowing of the opening in the mitral valve that impedes blood flow from the left atrium into the left ventricle is called _____.

____ 2. When one or both of the mitral valve leaflets become rigid and shorten, preventing com-plete closure of the valve, this condition is called _____.

____ 3. When one or both of the mitral valve leaflets enlarge and protrude into the left atrium during systole, this condition is called _____.

____ 4. When the aortic valve cusps become fibrotic and calcify, this condition is called _____.

____ 5. Fibrosis and thickening of the aortic valve cusps may progress until the valves no longer maintain undirectional flow; this condition is called _____.

A. Tricuspid stenosis

B. Aortic stenosis

C. Mitral stenosis

D. Aortic insufficiency

E. Tricuspid insufficiency

F. Mitral insufficiency

G. Mitral valve prolapse

XL. Match the nursing diagnoses for patients with CHF on the left with the "related to" statements on the right.

____ 1. Fluid volume excess

____ 2. Impaired gas exchange

____ 3. Anxiety

____ 4. Decreased cardiac output

A. Decreased pulmonary perfusion

B. Mechanical failure

C. Ineffective cardiac pumping

D. Edema and inability to breathe

XLI. Choose the most appropriate answer.

1. A hollow muscular pump located in the mediastinum is the:
   A. lung
   B. sternum
   C. thorax
   D. heart

2. The oxygen saturation in the LV is:
   A. 20–30%
   B. 40–50%
   C. 60–70%
   D. 95–98%

3. Which valves are open during systole and closed during diastole?
   A. semilunar valves
   B. atrioventricular valves
   C. tricuspid valves
   D. mitral valves

4. The first branches of the systemic circulation are the:
   A. subclavian arteries
   B. coronary arteries
   C. carotid arteries
   D. brachial arteries

5. The ventricles contract when the electrical impulse reaches the:
   A. SA node
   B. AV node
   C. Purkinje fibers
   D. bundle of His

6. The contraction phase of the cardiac cycle is known as:
   A. diastole
   B. pacemaker
   C. systole
   D. tachycardia

7. Stroke volume, the amount of blood ejected with each ventricular contraction, depends on myocardial:
   A. contractility
   B. excitability
   C. conductivity
   D. automaticity

8. If the valves of the heart do not close properly, the patient is said to have:
   A. infarction
   B. murmur
   C. necrosis
   D. tachycardia

9. The only ways to increase oxygen supply to the myocardium are to administer supplemental oxygen and to increase coronary blood flow by:
   A. coronary artery vasoconstriction
   B. increased myocardial contraction
   C. coronary artery vasodilation
   D. decreased myocardial contraction

10. Thrombophlebitis and varicosities are more common in:
    A. adolescents
    B. young adults
    C. middle-aged people
    D. older people

11. Because the cardiovascular system adapts more slowly to changes in position in the elderly, what is more likely to occur?
    A. tachycardia
    B. bradycardia
    C. postural hypotension
    D. headache

12. In asking cardiac patients about their diets, the nurse should especially record information about what 2 areas of intake?
    A. calcium and vitamin D
    B. salt and fat
    C. protein and iron
    D. vitamin C and vitamin E

13. A noninvasive measure of cardiac output is:
    A. cardiac catheterization
    B. pulse pressure
    C. angioplasty
    D. blood gas measurement

14. The sound produced by turbulent blood flow across the valves is called a:
    A. heart murmur
    B. ventricular gallop
    C. atrial gallop
    D. orthopnea

15. A common diagnostic test that measures the electrical activity of the heart is the:
    A. CT scan
    B. echocardiogram
    C. ECG
    D. phonocardiogram

16. A normal ECG finding is documented as a normal:
    A. tachycardia
    B. sinus rhythm
    C. bradycardia
    D. ventricular gallop

17. The stress test must be stopped immediately if which of the following symptoms occur?
    A. angina and falling blood pressure
    B. increased heart rate and increasing respirations
    C. diaphoresis and thirst
    D. slower respirations and hunger

18. The normal cardiac output is:
    A. 1–3 liters/minute
    B. 4–8 liters/minute
    C. 10–13 liters/minute
    D. 15–20 liters/hour

19. Patients with acute myocardial infarction often exhibit:
    A. respiratory acidosis
    B. respiratory alkalosis
    C. metabolic acidosis
    D. metabolic alkalosis

20. A noninvasive measurement of arterial oxygen saturation is:
    A. blood pressure
    B. blood gases
    C. central catheter
    D. pulse oximetry

21. What type of diet is generally recommended for cardiac patients?
    A. low-fat, high-protein
    B. low-fat, high-fiber
    C. high-fat, low protein
    D. high-fat, low-fiber

22. If fluid retention accompanies the cardiac problem, the physician may order restriction of:
    A. potassium
    B. sodium
    C. fats
    D. calcium

23. What do patients taking diuretics such as furosemide need to include in their diets?
    A. sodium
    B. calcium
    C. fiber
    D. potassium

24. The purpose of temporary and permanent pacemakers is to improve cardiac output and tissue perfusion by restoring regular:
    A. rhythm
    B. pulse pressure
    C. blood pressure
    D. stroke volume

25. The delivery of a synchronized shock to terminate atrial or ventricular tachydysrhythmias is called:
    A. pacemaker
    B. cardiac catheterization
    C. angioplasty
    D. cardioversion

26. During open-heart surgery, the patients's core temperature is reduced to decrease the body's need for:
    A. oxygen
    B. sodium
    C. potassium
    D. ATP

27. Nicotine, hypertension, and obesity are risk factors for:
    A. pneumonia
    B. coronary artery disease
    C. kidney disease
    D. brain tumor

28. The most frequent symptom of CAD, which represents lack of oxygen to tissues, is:
    A. fever
    B. cyanosis
    C. indigestion
    D. pain

29. The substernal pain resulting from lack of oxygen to the myocardium is called:
    A. heartburn
    B. dyspnea
    C. pleurisy
    D. angina pectoris

30. Modifiable risk factors for acute myocardial infarction include hypertension, obesity, and:
    A. diabetes mellitus
    B. male gender
    C. smoking
    D. family history

31. What drugs are used to decrease coronary artery spasm and myocardial oxygen demand for patients with CAD?
    A. diuretics
    B. analgesics
    C. calcium channel blockers
    D. antiplatelet agents

32. Early symptoms of congestive heart failure as a complication of AMI include dyspnea, restlessness, and:
    A. increased temperature
    B. increasing heart rate
    C. headache
    D. cyanosis

33. Cardiogenic shock is marked by cool, moist skin; oliguria; decreasing alertness; and:
    A. hypotension
    B. increased temperature
    C. headache
    D. cyanosis

34. Which drug is administered to dilate coronary arteries and increase blood flow to the damaged area?
    A. nitroglycerine
    B. furosemide
    C. Persantine
    D. streptokinase

35. Which veins are generally used in coronary artery bypass surgery as grafts to the coronary arteries?
    A. subclavian
    B. femoral
    C. jugular
    D. saphenous

36. Which of the following signs of fluid volume excess in patients with CAD should be reported to the physician if the nurse observes them?
    A. rales and cough
    B. pain relief
    C. reduced anxiety
    D. increased fluid intake

37. When angiotensin I is converted to angiotensin II, this mechanism causes vasoconstriction and triggers the release of:
    A. antidiuretic hormone
    B. thyroxine
    C. epinephrine
    D. aldosterone

38. The recommended position for patients with CHF in order to decrease cardiac workload and increase oxygenation to the myocardium is:
    A. side-lying
    B. prone
    C. semi-Fowler's
    D. supine

39. The most common adverse effects of diuretic therapy for patients with CHF are:
    A. hypertension and tachycardia
    B. fluid and electrolyte disturbances
    C. headache and oliguria
    D. confusion and weakness

40. A common finding in patients with CHF is:
    A. fluid volume deficit
    B. hypoxia
    C. dehydration
    D. hypotension

41. Drugs that may be given to patients with CHF who have decreased cardiac output include diuretics, vasodilators, and:
    A. inotropics
    B. anticonvulsants
    C. antihistamines
    D. cholinergics

42. The most common site for organisms to accumulate in patients with infective endocarditis is the:
    A. mitral valve
    B. tricuspid valve
    C. aortic valve
    D. pulmonic valve

43. Symptoms of endocarditis include weight loss, malaise, and:
    A. oliguria
    B. hypertension
    C. fever
    D. convulsions

44. An important diagnostic test for patients with endocarditis is the:
    A. RBC count
    B. WBC count
    C. hematocrit
    D. hemoglobin

45. The main drugs used for endocarditis are:
    A. cardiac glycosides
    B. diuretics
    C. calcium channel blockers
    D. antimicrobials

46. The main symptom of pericarditis is:
    A. chest pain
    B. headache
    C. hypertension
    D. indigestion

47. The patient with pericarditis is treated with analgesics, anti-inflammatory agents, antibiotics, and:
    A. diuretics
    B. anticonvulsants
    C. antipyretics
    D. anticholinergics

48. When an assessment is done on the patient with pericarditis, the nurse auscultates for pericardial:
    A. wheezes
    B. crackles
    C. murmur
    D. friction rub

49. Disease of the heart muscle that generally has an unknown cause and leads to heart failure is called:
    A. myocardial infarction
    B. congestive heart failure
    C. cardiomyopathy
    D. pericarditis

50. Which of the following heart conditions has a high incidence of sudden death?
    A. cardiomyopathy
    B. pericarditis
    C. endocarditis
    D. congestive heart failure

51. Lifelong medications that must be given to patients with heart transplants include:
    A. antihistamines
    B. analgesics
    C. antimicrobials
    D. immunosuppressive medications

52. The two major valve problems of the heart are insufficiency and:
    A. inflammation
    B. stenosis
    C. emboli
    D. hemorrhage

53. Heparin dosage for patients with cardiac disorders is adjusted according the patient's:
    A. hemoglobin
    B. WBC count
    C. partial thromboplastin time
    D. hematocrit

54. Diuretics such as furosemide and hydrochlorothiazide may cause hypokalemia, which can lead to:
    A. hypertension
    B. dysrhythmias
    C. edema
    D. hemorrhage

55. Before each dose of digitalis, the apical pulse i counted for 1 full minute; the drug is withheld and th physician notified if the pulse is below:
    A. 60
    B. 70
    C. 72
    D. 80

56. Elderly people are more susceptible to adverse drug effects because they:
    A. metabolize drugs more quickly
    B. have decreased elasticity of vessels
    C. excrete drugs more slowly
    D. are hypersensitive to more drugs

57. Patients taking immunosuppressive drugs to preven rejection of transplanted tissue have reduced:
    A. circulation
    B. resistance to infection
    C. metabolism of drugs
    D. red blood cell count

58. Antidysrhythmic drugs are used to treat dysrhyth mias and restore normal:
    A. sinus tachycardia
    B. sinus bradycardia
    C. sinus rhythm
    D. atrioventricular block

59. A major part of treatment for persons with hear disease is the reduction of dietary fat and:
    A. sugar
    B. protein
    C. cholesterol
    D. vitamin E

LII.   In Figure 31–2 below, label the parts (A–M) of the heart.

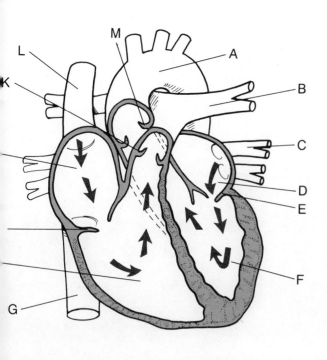

A.

B.

C.

D.

E.

F.

G.

H.

I.

J.

K.

L.

M.

XLIII.   In Figure 31–4 below, label the parts (A–E) of the conduction system of the heart.

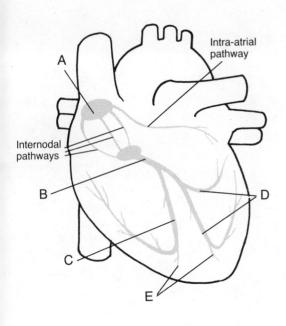

A.

B.

C.

D.

E.

Peripheral Vascular Disorders

OBJECTIVES

1. Identify specific anatomic and physiologic factors that affect the peripheral blood supply and tissue oxygenation.
2. Indicate appropriate parameters for assessing a patient with peripheral vascular involvement.
3. Discuss tests and procedures that aid in the determination of peripheral vascular involvement and the nursing considerations for each.
4. State the pathophysiology, signs and symptoms, complications, and medical or surgical treatments for selected peripheral vascular disorders.
5. Use the nursing process to plan care for patients with peripheral vascular disorders.

LEARNING ACTIVITIES

I.   Match the definition on the left with the most appropriate term on the right.

____	1. Sudden obstruction of an artery by a floating clot or foreign material	A.	Bruit
____	2. An abnormal sensation	B.	Thrombophlebitis
____	3. Concentration of the blood	C.	Thrombosis
____	4. Development of venous thrombi in the presence of venous inflammation	D.	Phlebothrombosis
____	5. Deficient blood flow due to obstruction or constriction of blood vessels	E.	Embolism
		F.	Vasoconstriction
____	6. Increase in blood vessel diameter	G.	Paresthesia
____	7. A murmur heard by auscultation	H.	Viscosity
____	8. Development of venous thrombi without venous inflammation	I.	Ischemia
____	9. Decrease in blood vessel diameter	J.	Phlebitis
____	10. Coolness in an area of the body due to decreased blood flow	K.	Hemoconcentration
		L.	Poikilothermia
____	11. Resistance to flow related to the friction between two components; thickness	M.	Vasodilation
____	12. Development or presence of a thrombus		
____	13. Inflammation of a vein		

II. Match the definition or description on the left with the most appropriate term on the right. Some terms may be used more than once, and some may not be used.

___ 1. Vessels that return blood to the heart

___ 2. The two main trunks of these vessels are the thoracic duct and the right lymphatic duct

___ 3. Thick-walled, elastic structures

___ 4. Equipped with valves that aid in the transportation of blood against gravity

___ 5. Formed by a single layer of endothelial cells

___ 6. Vessels that carry blood away from the heart

___ 7. Transfer of oxygen and nutrients between the blood and the tissue cells occurs here

___ 8. Thin-walled vessels that collect and drain fluid from the peripheral tissues and transport the fluid to the venous system

A. Veins

B. Valves

C. Leaflets

D. Capillaries

E. Lymph vessels

F. Arteries

G. Lymph nodes

III. Indicate whether each of the factors on the left (A) increases or (B) decreases peripheral resistance.

___ 1. Sympathetic nervous system stimulation

___ 2. Epinephrine

___ 3. Angiotensin

___ 4. Viscous blood

___ 5. Heat

___ 6. Cold

A. Increases

B. Decreases

IV. Match the definition or description on the left with the most appropriate term on the right. Some terms may be used more than once, and some may not be used.

___ 1. Patients notice the relief of pain when the extremity is dangled in a dependent position

___ 2. A decrease in arterial perfusion to an area that is aggravated by exercise

___ 3. The identification of an area of decreased temperature located at an ischemic site

___ 4. Reflects the presence of a severe arterial occlusion

___ 5. Development of paleness over an area of reduced blood supply

___ 6. Exercise is a precipitating factor

___ 7. An abnormality with the sensation of touch

___ 8. Burning pain in the foot area when hydrostatic pressure in the extremity is lost

___ 9. Pain is described as a feeling of tightness, burning, fatigue, aching, or cramping

A. Paresthesia

B. Poikilothermy

C. Paralysis

D. Rest pain

E. Pallor

F. Intermittent claudication

G. Pulselessness

Introductory Nursing Care of Adults

V. Match the definition or description on the left with the most appropriate term on the right. Some terms may be used more than once, and some may not be used.

____ 1. A test to evaluate the pain response in the calf area to determine venous thrombosis is _____.

____ 2. A test used to determine the patency of the ulnar and radial artery is _____.

____ 3. When blood flowing through the arteries sounds like turbulent, fast-moving fluid, these sounds are called _____.

____ 4. Brown pigmentation sites with flaky skin over the edematous areas of the ankles are described as _____.

A. Bruits
B. Babinski reflex
C. Allen's sign
D. Moro reflex
E. Homans's sign
F. Stasis dermatitis

VI. Complete the statements on the left with the most appropriate term on the right. Some terms may be used more than once, and some terms may not be used.

____ 1. A noninvasive, inexpensive, diagnostic tool in which sound waves are directed toward the artery or vein being tested is _____.

____ 2. A noninvasive examination that measures the blood volume and graphs changes in the flow of blood is _____.

____ 3. The segmental limb pressure test and pulse volume measurement test are examples of _____.

____ 4. An invasive procedure that requires the injection of dye into the vascular system is called _____.

A. MRI
B. Pressure measurement
C. ECG
D. Angiography
E. Doppler ultrasound
F. Plethysmography

VII. Complete the statements on the left with the most appropriate term on the right. Some terms may be used more than once, and some terms may not be used.

____ 1. An infrequently used procedure that involves the injection of a chemical that irritates the venous endothelium for patients with varicose veins is called _____.

____ 2. A procedure that is done to relieve arterial stenosis in people who are poor surgical risks is _____.

____ 3. A procedure used primarily for varicose veins is called _____.

____ 4. An incision into the obstructed vessel to strip away emboli and atherosclerotic plaque followed by surgical closure of the vessel is called _____.

____ 5. The excision of the sympathetic ganglia that is used for patients with intermittent claudication is called _____.

____ 6. The removal of a blood clot located in a large vessel is called _____.

A. Sympathectomy
B. Percutaneous transluminal angioplasty
C. Thermotherapy
D. Embolectomy
E. Sclerotherapy
F. Intermittent pneumatic compression
G. Vein ligation and stripping
H. Endarterectomy

VIII. Complete the statements relating to signs and symptoms of deep vein thrombosis on the left with the most appropriate term on the right. Some terms may be used more than once, and some terms may not be used.

___ 1. The affected extremity may display _____.

___ 2. Superficial veins are _____.

___ 3. The affected area of compromise may display _____.

___ 4. Homans's sign is _____.

A. Warmth and tenderness
B. Negative
C. Coolness
D. Prominent
E. Positive
F. Edema or swelling
G. Lack of sensation

IX. Match the nursing diagnosis on the left for patients with thrombosis with the appropriate "related to" statements on the right.

___ 1. Impaired skin integrity

___ 2. Pain

___ 3. Activity intolerance

___ 4. Altered tissue perfusion

A. Impaired circulation and tissue ischemia
B. Venous stasis
C. Impaired peripheral circulation
D. Leg pain or swelling

X. Complete the statements on the left with the most appropriate term on the right. Some terms may be used more than once, and some terms may not be used.

___ 1. The cardinal signs and symptoms of Raynaud's disease include chronically cold hands, numbness, tingling, and _____.

___ 2. The most common infectious agent involved with lymphangitis is _____.

___ 3. The most common sites for plaque formation and resulting occlusion in peripheral arterial occlusive disease are the distal superficial femoral arteries and the _____.

___ 4. An acute inflammation of the lymphatic channels is called _____.

___ 5. The goals of the medical treatment plan for Raynaud's disease are to prevent pain and to promote _____.

___ 6. Controllable risk factors for peripheral arterial occlusive disease include hyperlipidemia, diabetes mellitus, hypertension, cigarette smoking, and _____

___ 7. A dilated segment of an artery caused by weakness and stretching of the arterial wall is called _____.

___ 8. A small tear in the intima that permits blood to escape into the space between the intima and the media is called _____.

A. Varicosities
B. Lymphangitis
C. Aneurysm
D. Hemolytic streptococcus
E. Abdominal aorta
F. Arteriosclerosis
G. Vena cava
H. Raynaud's disease
I. Redness
J. Aortic dissection
K. Vasodilation
L. Intermittent claudication
M. Popliteal arteries
N. Pallor
O. Stress

___ 9. The hallmark sign of peripheral arterial occlusive disease is _____.

___ 10. Varicose veins are referred to as _____.

___ 11. The most common cause of aneurysms is _____.

___ 12. An intermittent arteriolar vasoconstriction that affects the hands primarily is _____.

___ 13. The most common site of aneurysm formation is the _____.

A. Varicosities
B. Lymphangitis
C. Aneurysm
D. Hemolytic streptococcus
E. Abdominal aorta
F. Arteriosclerosis
G. Vena cava
H. Raynaud's disease
I. Redness
J. Aortic dissection
K. Vasodilation
L. Intermittent claudication
M. Popliteal arteries
N. Pallor
O. Stress

XI. List 8 factors that increase the risk of peripheral vascular disease.

1.   5.
2.   6.
3.   7.
4.   8.

XII. List 2 factors that affect circulating blood flow by increasing or decreasing the blood flow.

1.

2.

XIII. List the 6 classical P's characteristic of peripheral vascular disease.

1.   4.
2.   5.
3.   6.

XIV. Describe the changes that may occur in the following areas when the circulation is compromised to the peripheral area.

1. Nails

2. Skin appearance

3. Temperature

4. Muscles

5. Affected extremity

XV. List 3 areas that are evaluated by palpation.

1.

2.

3.

XVI. Name the two types of angiography, which are classified by the vessels examined during the procedure.

1. Radiographs of arteries following injection of dye into the vascular system

2. Radiographs of veins following injection of dye into the vascular system

XVII. List 4 risks associated with angiography, which is done to confirm the diagnosis of peripheral vascular disease.

1.

2.

3.

4.

XVIII. Following angiography, the nurse should observe the patient for what 4 complications?

1.

2.

3.

4.

XIX. List 6 goals for the treatment plan for patients with peripheral vascular disease.

1.

2.

3.

4.

5.

6.

XX. List 7 therapeutic measures for patients with peripheral vascular disease.

1.

2.

3.

4.

5.

6.

7.

XXI.   List a very effective and simple exercise that promotes venous return.

XXII.   List a type of exercise that is effective in the management of PVD and that allows gravity to fill and empty the blood vessels.

XXIII.   List the actions to be taken for pain management in patients with peripheral vascular disease for the following types of pain.

1. Pain related to intermittent claudication:

2. Pain due to immobility and disease process:

3. Pain caused by wearing girdles, belts and tight pantyhose:

XXIV.   Explain why care must be taken when using heat on patients with peripheral vascular disease.

XXV.   List 4 classifications of drugs that are used in the general management of peripheral vascular disease to improve peripheral circulation.

1.

2.

3.

4.

XXVI.   List the 2 primary anticoagulants.

1. Oral route:

2. Parenteral route:

XXVII. List the antidotes for the following anticoagulants.

1. Heparin:

2. Warfarin sodium:

XXVIII. List 7 risk factors that may predispose a person for the development of a thrombus.

1.

2.

3.

4.

5.

6.

7.

XXIX. The possibility of developing a pulmonary embolus during the treatment of thrombosis is an ever-present concern; list 6 nursing interventions the nurse can implement to improve the gas exchange of the patient who has a pulmonary embolism.

1.

2.

3.

4.

5.

6.

XXX. List 6 signs and symptoms of tissues that do not have adequate blood supply.

1.

2.

3.

4.

5.

6.

XXXI. List 4 complications of aneurysms.

1.

2.

3.

4.

XXXII. Choose the most appropriate answer.

1. Any interruption of the blood flow to the distal regions of the body, as occurs in peripheral vascular disease, results in:
   A. kidney failure
   B. cardiac shock
   C. dyspnea
   D. hypoxia

2. The three layers of arteries, arterioles, and veins are called the intima, media, and:
   A. arachnoid
   B. adventitia
   C. dura mater
   D. pleura

3. The nervous system that acts on the smooth muscles of vessels, resulting in dilation and constriction of the artery walls, is the:
   A. autonomic
   B. somatic
   C. central
   D. cranial

4. The sympathetic nervous system acts on the musculature of the veins to stimulate:
   A. vasodilation
   B. vasoconstriction
   C. tachycardia
   D. bradycardia

5. The resistance within the vascular system is controlled by factors that regulate the:
   A. heart rate
   B. number of blood vessels
   C. diameter of the vessels
   D. blood cells

6. As peripheral resistance is increased, the blood flow to the peripheral tissue is:
   A. increased
   B. watery
   C. reduced
   D. thin

7. The primary result of aging on the peripheral vessels is the:
   A. vasoconstriction of arteries
   B. vasodilation of veins
   C. increased elasticity of vessel walls
   D. stiffening of vessel walls

8. Aging in the vascular system causes a slowing of the heart rate and a decrease in the stroke volume, resulting in decreased:
   A. cardiac output
   B. tachycardia
   C. peripheral resistance
   D. hypertension

9. The transportation of oxygen is compromised in the aging patient by the decreased:
   A. hematocrit
   B. WBC count
   C. hemoglobin
   D. cardiac enzymes

10. Peripheral vascular disease is a common complication of:
    A. pneumonia
    B. myocardial infarction
    C. diabetes
    D. influenza

11. When documenting the review of the peripheral vascular system, the nurse can best assess the presence of peripheral vascular disease by visualizing changes in the:
    A. integumentary system
    B. nervous system
    C. urinary system
    D. respiratory system

12. If peripheral vascular disease causes limb-threatening ischemia, amputation of a limb may be necessary due to the development of:
    A. cyanosis
    B. gangrene
    C. fractures
    D. hypersensitivity

13. Capillary refill time is assessed in the nail beds to determine the adequacy of peripheral:
    A. edema
    B. infection
    C. movement
    D. perfusion

14. Skin temperature is palpated in patients with PVD to determine the existence of:
    A. infection
    B. bleeding
    C. cyanosis
    D. ischemia

15. The development of paleness in the extremities suggest the presence of peripheral:
    A. hemorrhage
    B. infection
    C. vasoconstriction
    D. vasodilation

16. In the evaluation of edema, when the thumb is depressed in the area for 5 seconds and the depression of the thumb remains in the edematous area, the edema is said to be:
    A. 1+
    B. 2+
    C. 3+
    D. pitting

17. If pain or severe skin color changes occur during exercises with PVD patients, the nurse should:
    A. encourage the exercises to be done gradually
    B. stop the exercises immediately
    C. ambulate the patient to promote venous return
    D. administer muscle relaxants as ordered

18. With a disease process such as PVD, which can result in necrosis and gangrene, any exercise program must be instituted by the:
    A. nurse
    B. patient
    C. physical therapist
    D. physician

19. Emotional stress affects the peripheral vascular system by causing:
    A. vasodilation
    B. vasoconstriction
    C. hypotension
    D. bradycardia

20. It is important for patients with peripheral vascular disease to stop smoking, because smoking causes:
    A. intermittent claudication
    B. skin ulceration
    C. vasoconstriction
    D. vasodilation

21. The primary function of intermittent pneumatic compression devices is to prevent:
    A. infection
    B. hemorrhage
    C. deep vein thrombosis
    D. cyanosis

22. What position should be avoided by patients with peripheral vascular disease?
    A. extended standing
    B. elevation of lower extremities
    C. lowering extremities below the level of the heart
    D. elevation of extremities to nondependent position

23. Which of the following works as a vasodilator that promotes arterial flow to the peripheral tissues?
    A. TED hose
    B. intermittent pneumatic compression
    C. heat
    D. cold

24. Which of the following should be avoided by patients with peripheral vascular disease because the healing process is usually compromised?
    A. walking
    B. going barefoot
    C. wearing TED hose
    D. eating fruit

25. Elevation of the extremity following surgery for patients with PVD aids in the prevention of:
    A. hemorrhage
    B. edema
    C. hypotension
    D. ulceration

26. Disappearance of a peripheral pulse during the postoperative care of patients with PVD alerts the nurse to the development of a:
    A. thrombotic occlusion
    B. massive hemorrhage
    C. severe infection
    D. varicose vein

27. The main adverse action of anticoagulants is:
    A. bleeding
    B. infection
    C. hypertension
    D. oliguria

28. Thrombolytic therapy is employed to:
    A. shorten the clotting time
    B. increase clot formation
    C. prevent the formation of new clots
    D. dissolve an existing clot

29. The use of vasodilators results in increased blood flow by relaxing the vascular smooth muscle and causing:
    A. increased clotting time
    B. decreased elasticity in vessels
    C. decreased resistance in vessels
    D. increased narrowing in vessels

30. A grave risk with a diagnosis of deep vein thrombosis is the development of:
    A. hemorrhage
    B. pneumonia
    C. pulmonary embolus
    D. infection

31. Three precipitating factors (called Virchow's triad) for a thrombus to form include hypercoagulability, damage to the vessel walls, and:
    A. hemorrhage
    B. stasis of the blood
    C. decreased hematocrit
    D. damaged blood cells

32. The primary diagnostic examinations used in the detection of thrombus formation are the plethysmography, Doppler ultrasound and:
    A. venography
    B. ECG
    C. myelography
    D. angioplasty

33. The reason why patients with thrombosis should not be massaged or rubbed is the possible development of:
    A. severe infection
    B. hemorrhage
    C. skin breakdown
    D. pulmonary emboli

34. The placement of antiembolism hose on patients with thrombosis is done to improve circulation and to prevent:
    A. infection
    B. stasis
    C. hemorrhage
    D. ulceration

35. A life-threatening event that requires immediate attention is:
    A. arterial embolism
    B. thrombophlebitis
    C. varicose vein disease
    D. thrombosis

36. The absence of peripheral pulse below the occlusive
    area is a clinical manifestation of:
    A. Raynaud's disease
    B. aneurysms
    C. peripheral arterial occlusive disease
    D. thrombophlebitis

37. During repair of an abdominal aneurysm, the aorta
    is clamped for a period of time. This poses a risk of:
    A. dyspnea
    B. renal failure
    C. pneumonia
    D. incontinence

38. Varicose veins develop dilation due to faulty:
    A. elasticity
    B. smooth muscle
    C. thickness
    D. valves

39. Another name for chronic venous insufficiency is:
    A. varicose veins
    B. postphlebitic syndrome
    C. thrombophlebitis
    D. aortic dissection

40. The initial sign of the development of ulcerations in
    patients with chronic venous insufficiency is:
    A. redness
    B. infection
    C. stasis dermatitis
    D. cyanosis

41. The medical management of lymphangitis necessi-
    tates the administration of:
    A. antimicrobial agents
    B. thrombolytic agents
    C. anticoagulants
    D. analgesics

42. Elastic support hose are utilized for several months
    following an acute attack of lymphangitis to prevent
    the formation of:
    A. infection
    B. hemorrhage
    C. lymphedema
    D. dermatitis

C H A P T E R

33

Hypertension

OBJECTIVES

1. Define hypertension.
2. Explain the physiology of blood pressure regulation.
3. Discuss the risk factors, signs and symptoms, diagnosis, treatment, and complications of hypertension.
4. Identify the nursing considerations when administering selected antihypertensive drugs.
5. List the data to be obtained in the nursing assessment of a person with known or suspected hypertension.
6. Identify the nursing diagnoses for the patient with hypertension.
7. Describe the nursing interventions for the patient with hypertension.

I. Match the definition on the left with the most appropriate term on the right.

___ 1. Sudden drop in systolic blood pressure when changing from a lying or sitting position to a standing position

___ 2. Stationary blood clot

___ 3. Nosebleed

___ 4. Persistent elevation of arterial blood pressure greater than 140/90 mm Hg

___ 5. Fainting

___ 6. Enlargement

___ 7. Excess insoluble fats in the blood

A. Hypertension

B. Syncope

C. Thrombus

D. Hyperlipidemia

E. Orthostatic hypotension

F. Epistaxis

G. Hypertrophy

II. Fill in the blanks.

1. Two good sources of potassium are _____ and _____.

2. The most common cardiovascular problem in the United States today is _____.

3. Hypertension is a persistent elevation of arterial blood pressure greater than_____.

4. Two factors that determine blood pressure are cardiac output and _____

_____.

5. Resistance to blood flow is primarily determined by the diameter of blood vessels and _____

_____.

6. The diameter of blood vessels is regulated largely by the _____.

7. The force in the blood vessels that the left ventricle must overcome to eject blood from the heart is called

   _____.

8. The volume of blood pumped by the heart in one minute is called _____.

9. Stimulation of the sympathetic nervous system causes the release of two hormones: epinephrine and

   _____.

10. Complete the following 2 nursing diagnoses for the patient with hypertension.

    A. Noncompliance related to _____.

    B. High risk for injury related to _____.

11. In finding out whether sexual dysfunction is a side effect of a patient's antihypertensive medication, the nurse may

    ask: _____.

III. Complete the statements on the left with the most appropriate term on the right. Some terms may be used more than once; all terms may not be used.

_____ 1. Epinephrine and norepinephrine constrict blood vessels, increase blood pressure, and _____ the heart rate.

_____ 2. When body position is altered from supine to standing, the diastolic blood pressure normally _____ .

_____ 3. In response to decreased ability of the aorta to distend, pulse pressure _____.

_____ 4. In response to increased peripheral vascular resistance, the systolic pressure _____.

_____ 5. When body position is altered from supine to standing, the systolic blood pressure normally _____.

_____ 6. Epinephrine constricts blood vessels and increases the force of cardiac contraction, causing blood pressure to _____.

_____ 7. When there is a narrowing of the arteries and arterioles, peripheral vascular resistance _____.

A. increase(s)/rise(s)

B. decrease(s)/fall(s)

C. widen(s)

D. narrow(s)

IV. Complete the statements on the left with the most appropriate term on the right. Some terms may be used more than once.

1. An important side effect of alpha-adrenergic receptor blockers is _____.

2. When body position is altered from supine to standing, the systolic blood pressure normally _____.

3. Epinephrine _____ cardiac output.

4. Flushing, dizziness, and headaches are common side effects of _____.

5. The _____ are more susceptible to orthostatic hypotension because their blood vessels respond more slowly to position changes.

6. Elderly patients are at risk for adverse effects of medications because of reduced liver and _____ function.

A. constrict

B. elderly

C. diuretics

D. orthostatic hypotension

E. increased

F. kidney

G. sodium

H. increases

I. calcium channel blockers

J. decreases about 10 mm Hg

K. syncope

7. Norepinephrine stimulates the blood vessels to _____.

8. Increased cardiac output, increased peripheral resistance, and increased blood volume will result in _____ blood pressure.

9. Symptoms of orthostatic hypotension include lightheadedness, dizziness, and _____.

0. Aldosterone stimulates the kidney to reabsorb water and _____.

1. A sudden drop in systolic blood pressure, usually 20 mm Hg, when going from a lying or sitting to a standing position is called _____.

A. constrict

B. elderly

C. diuretics

D. orthostatic hypotension

E. increased

F. kidney

G. sodium

H. increases

I. calcium channel blockers

J. decreases about 10 mm Hg

K. syncope

'. Complete the statements on the left with the most appropriate term on the right.

1. The center for blood pressure regulation in the brain is the _____.

2. If antihypertensive drugs are stopped suddenly, _____ may occur.

3. Symptoms of hypertensive crisis include blurred vision, nausea, restlessness, and _____.

4. The sympathetic nervous system increases the production of epinephrine and _____.

5. Without appropriate treatment for hypertensive crisis, the patient may develop damage to the cardiac and _____ systems.

6. Signs of hypokalemia include confusion, irritability, and _____.

7. The group of antihypertensive drugs that must be used cautiously in patients with asthma, diabetes, and chronic obstructive pulmonary disease is _____.

8. In order to prevent orthostatic hypotension, patients are encouraged to _____.

9. With aging, atherosclerotic changes reduce elasticity of arteries, decrease cardiac output, and _____ peripheral vascular resistance.

10. Three stimulants that may contribute to hypertension include amphetamines, nicotine, and _____.

A. Muscle weakness

B. Rise slowly from a lying or sitting position

C. Beta blockers

D. Norepinephrine

E. Caffeine

F. Rebound hypertension

G. Medulla oblongata

H. Increase

I. Severe headache

J. Renal

VI. Complete the statements on the left with the most appropriate term on the right. Some terms may be used more than once.

1. Nicotine in cigarettes acts as a _____.

2. Hyperlipidemia is a contributing factor for _____.

3. Hyperlipidemia is excess _____ in the blood.

4. Norepinephrine and epinephrine are _____.

5. A serious complication of hypertension in which nocturia and azotemia occur is _____.

6. The long-term effects of hypertension on the eyes include narrow arterioles, retinal hemorrhage, and _____.

7. The long-term effects of hypertension on the heart include coronary artery disease, angina, and _____.

8. Factors that contribute to hypertension include cardiac stimulation, retention of fluid, and _____.

9. The long-term effects of hypertension on the brain include transient ischemic attacks and _____.

A. Vasoconstriction

B. Myocardial infarction

C. Vasoconstrictor(s)

D. Cerebrovascular accidents/ strokes

E. Insoluble fats

F. Renal failure

G. Atherosclerosis

H. Papilledema

VII. Complete the statements on the left with the most appropriate term on the right. Some terms may be used more than once, and some terms may not be used.

1. Patients on diuretics must be monitored for _____ imbalances.

2. People with hypertension are at risk for myocardial infarction and _____.

3. A plan for selecting drugs to treat hypertension, beginning with the administration of a single, relatively safe drug and progressing to combinations of drugs, is called a _____ approach.

4. Optimal blood pressure is generally defined as a diastolic blood pressure of _____ or less.

5. A nonpharmacologic approach to the treatment of hypertension includes weight reduction, smoking cessation, and _____.

6. The first step of a stepped-care approach to the treatment of hypertension recommends starting the patient on a low dose of beta blockers, ACE inhibitors, or _____.

A. Exercise

B. Diuretic(s)

C. Fluid and electrolyte(s)

D. Stepped-care

E. Stroke(s)

F. 120 mm Hg

G. 90 mm Hg

H. Progressive

VIII. Match the description on the left with the correct lifestyle modification on the right. Answers may be used more than once.

____ 1. Reduces water in the body, decreasing the circulating blood volume

____ 2. Decreases blood glucose and cholesterol levels, increasing sense of well-being

____ 3. Eliminates vasoconstriction caused by nicotine

____ 4. Reduce stress and lower blood pressure

____ 5. Improves cardiac efficiency by increasing cardiac output and decreasing peripheral vascular resistance.

____ 6. Reduces blood pressure by reducing the workload of the heart

A. Weight reduction

B. Smoking cessation

C. Sodium reduction

D. Exercise

E. Relaxation therapy; biofeedback

Introductory Nursing Care of Adults

IX. Match the actions of the drugs on the left with the correct classification of drugs on the right. Answers may be used more than once.

_____ 1. Block alpha receptor effects, lowering blood pressure by reducing peripheral resistance

_____ 2. Decrease fluid retention by decreasing the production of aldosterone

_____ 3. Reduce blood pressure by blocking the beta effects of catecholamines

_____ 4. Inhibit impulses from the vasomotor center in the brain, reducing peripheral resistance and lowering blood pressure

_____ 5. Reduce blood volume through promotion of renal excretion of sodium and water

_____ 6. Block the movement of calcium into cardiac and vascular smooth muscle cells, reducing heart rate, decreasing force of cardiac contraction, and dilating peripheral blood vessels

_____ 7. Relax arteriolar smooth muscle

_____ 8. Prevent the conversion of angiotensin I to angiotensin II, a potent vasoconstrictor, decreasing peripheral resistance

A. Central adrenergic blockers

B. Calcium channel blockers

C. Alpha-adrenergic receptor blockers

D. ACE inhibitors

E. Direct vasodilators

F. Beta-adrenergic receptor blockers

G. Diuretics

X. Match the side effects or cautions on the left with the correct classification of drugs on the right. Some classifications may be used more than once, and some side effects may be matched with more than one classification.

_____ 1. Palpitations, dizziness, headache, drowsiness, nausea

_____ 2. Hypoglycemia

_____ 3. Hypovolemia and hypokalemia

_____ 4. Flushing, dizziness, headache

_____ 5. Skin rash; renal failure

_____ 6. Use cautiously with asthma, diabetes, and COPD

_____ 7. Fluid and electrolyte imbalances

A. Beta blocker

B. Calcium channel blocker

C. Alpha-adrenergic receptor blocker

D. Diuretic

E. ACE inhibitors

XI. Match the names of the drugs on the left with the correct classification of drugs on the right.

_____ 1. Prazosin (Minipress)

_____ 2. Hydrochlorothiazide (HCTZ) and spironolactone (Aldactone)

_____ 3. Clonidine (Catapres) and methyldopa (Aldomet)

_____ 4. Propranolol (Inderal)

_____ 5. Hydralazine (Apresoline) diazoxide (Hyperstat IV), and sodium nitroprusside (Nipride)

_____ 6. Captopril (Capoten) and enalapril (Vasotec)

_____ 7. Verapamil (Calan)

A. Calcium channel blockers

B. Beta blockers

C. Direct vasodilators

D. Diuretics

E. Alpha-adrenergic receptor blockers

F. Central adrenergic blockers

G. ACE inhibitors

XII. Choose the most appropriate answer.

1. How many people in the United States have hypertension that requires monitoring and/or treatment?
   A. About 5%
   B. About 10%
   C. About 20%
   D. About 50%

2. The cause of essential hypertension is:
   A. kidney disease
   B. drugs
   C. pregnancy
   D. unknown

XIII. In Figure 33-2 below, label 4 parts of the body (A-D) on which long-term effects of prolonged hypertension occur.

A.

B.

C.

D.

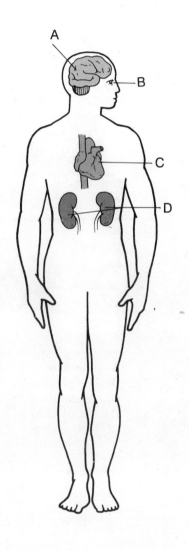

Digestive Tract Disorders

OBJECTIVES

1. List the nursing responsibilities in the care of patients undergoing diagnostic tests and procedures for disorders of the digestive tract.
2. List the data to be included in the nursing assessment of the patient with a digestive disorder.
3. Describe the nursing care of patients with gastrointestinal intubation and decompression, tube feedings, total parenteral nutrition, digestive tract surgery, and drug therapy for digestive disorders.
4. Describe the pathophysiology, signs and symptoms, complications, and medical treatment of selected digestive disorders.
5. Apply the nursing process to develop nursing care plans for patients receiving treatment for digestive disorders.

LEARNING ACTIVITIES

I.   Match the definition on the left with the most appropriate term on the right.

___ 1. Formation of excessive gas in the stomach or intestines	A. Anorexia
	B. Caries
___ 2. Gentle ejection of stomach contents into the mouth without nausea or retching	C. Cathartic
	D. Dyspepsia
___ 3. Agent that softens stool and promotes bowel evacuation	E. Dysphagia
___ 4. Lack of appetite for food	F. Emesis
___ 5. Epigastric discomfort after meals, caused by impaired digestion	G. Eructation
	H. Flatulence
___ 6. Inflammation of the peritoneum	I. Flatus
___ 7. Difficulty swallowing	J. Gingivitis
___ 8. Inflammation of the oral mucosa	K. Laxative
___ 9. Vomiting	L. Peritoneum
___ 10. Gas in the digestive tract that is expelled through the rectum	M. Peritonitis
	N. Regurgitation
___ 11. Expulsion of gas from the stomach through the mouth; belching	O. Stomatitis

I. *Continues*

I. *Continues*

____ 12. Inflammation of the gums

____ 13. Agent that stimulates bowel evacuation; usually rapid in effect and producing a watery stool

____ 14. Membrane that lines the walls of the abdominal and pelvic cavities

____ 15. Destructive process of tooth decay

A. Anorexia

B. Caries

C. Cathartic

D. Dyspepsia

E. Dysphagia

F. Emesis

G. Eructation

H. Flatulence

I. Flatus

J. Gingivitis

K. Laxative

L. Peritoneum

M. Peritonitis

N. Regurgitation

O. Stomatitis

II. Match the definition on the left with the most appropriate term on the right.

____ 1. Pyrosis; burning or tight sensation rising from the lower sternum to the throat

____ 2. Hard white patches on the gums, oral mucosa, or tongue that tend to become malignant

____ 3. Hole or break in a structure

____ 4. Inflammation of the lips

____ 5. Inflammation of the parotid glands

____ 6. Cracking of the lips and corners of the mouth

A. Cheilitis

B. Heartburn

C. Parotitis

D. Cheilosis

E. Leukoplakia

F. Perforation

III. Complete the statements on the left with the most appropriate term on the right. Some terms may be used more than once, and some terms may not be used.

____ 1. Accessory organs of the digestive system include the salivary glands, liver, gallbladder and the _____.

____ 2. The absorption of nutrients takes place in the _____.

____ 3. The place where food digestion begins is the _____.

____ 4. The duodenum, jejunum, and ileum are sections of the _____.

____ 5. Pepsin and hydrochloric acid are _____.

____ 6. The fundus, body, and pylorus are sections of the _____.

A. Mouth

B. Stomach

C. Gastric secretions

D. Pancreas

E. Pyloric sphincter

F. Small intestine

G. Gallbladder

IV. Complete the statements on the left with the most appropriate term on the right. Some terms may be used more than once, and some terms may not be used.

____ 1. Chyme enters the large intestine through the _____.

____ 2. Liver and pancreatic secretions enter the digestive tract in the section of the small intestine known as the _____.

____ 3. The ascending, transverse, and descending colons are sections of the _____.

____ 4. _____ is produced in the liver and stored in the gallbladder.

____ 5. Villi are found in the _____.

A. Stomach

B. Duodenum

C. Bile

D. Maltase

E. Ileocecal valve

F. Large intestine

G. Small intestine

V. Complete the statements on the left with the most appropriate term on the right. Some terms may be used more than once, and some terms may not be used.

____ 1. The head of the bed is elevated during tube feedings in order to prevent _____.

____ 2. An inflammation of the lining of the stomach is called _____.

____ 3. The most serious complication of gastric endoscopy is _____.

____ 4. The best means of diagnosing gastritis is _____.

____ 5. Opiates (such as morphine) are not given to patients with diverticulosis to avoid the common side effect of _____.

____ 6. A complication that occurs when tube feedings of concentrated formula are given rapidly is _____.

____ 7. The most serious complication of acute gastritis is _____.

A. Gastroscopy

B. Hemorrhage

C. Headache

D. Constipation

E. Perforation of the digestive tract

F. Dumping syndrome

G. Diarrhea

H. Aspiration

I. Drowsiness

J. Gastritis

VI.   Complete the statements on the left with the most appropriate term on the right. Some terms may be used more than once, and some terms may not be used.

____ 1. Patients who are vomiting and who are very weak or unable to move are at risk for _____.

____ 2. The gentle ejection of food or fluid without nausea or retching is _____.

____ 3. Drugs that prevent or treat nausea and vomiting are called _____.

____ 4. Two symptoms that are common just before vomiting are increased salivation and _____.

____ 5. The most common side effect of centrally acting antiemetics is _____.

____ 6. A feeling of discomfort sometimes referred to as queasiness is _____.

____ 7. The functions of the digestive tract are digestion, elimination, and _____.

____ 8. Prolonged or severe vomiting can lead to significant losses of fluid and _____.

____ 9. Intravenous fluids may be ordered for patients with vomiting to prevent _____.

____ 10. The breakdown of food into simple nutrient molecules that can be used by the cells is a description of _____.

____ 11. The forceful expulsion of stomach contents through the mouth is _____.

A.   Antimicrobials

B.   Tachycardia

C.   Digestion

D.   Drowsiness

E.   Diarrhea

F.   Nausea

G.   Absorption

H.   Oxygen

I.   Electrolytes

J.   Vomiting

K.   Aspiration

L.   Antiemetics

M.   Osmosis

N.   Regurgitation

O.   Dehydration

VII.   Complete the statements on the left with the most appropriate term on the right. Some terms may be used more than once, and some terms may not be used.

____ 1. Cold sores or fever blisters are caused by a virus called _____.

____ 2. A general term for inflammation of the mouth is _____.

____ 3. Thrush is caused by _____.

____ 4. A bacterial infection of the mouth, sometimes called trench mouth is _____.

____ 5. A yeast-like fungus characterized by bluish white lesions of the mouth is _____.

____ 6. A viral infection in which ulcers and vesicles develop in the mouth and on the lips and that may be treated with antiviral agents is _____.

____ 7. A chronic condition of the mouth characterized by ulcers of the lips and mouth that recur at intervals is _____.

A.   Stomatitis

B.   Pharyngitis

C.   *Candida albicans*

D.   Aphthous stomatitis

E.   *Staphylococcus*

F.   Herpes simplex

G.   Vincent's infection

VIII. Complete the statements on the left with the most appropriate term on the right. Some terms may be used more than once, and some terms may not be used.

___ 1. A substance made up of bacteria, saliva, and cells that sticks to the surface of the teeth is called _____.

___ 2. The presence of hard, white patches in the mouth, which is considered to be a premalignant condition, is _____.

___ 3. A disease that begins with inflammation of the gums and progresses to involve the other structures that support the teeth is called _____.

___ 4. An inflammation of the parotid glands is called _____.

___ 5. Dental decay starts with the development of _____.

___ 6. The primary symptom of esophageal cancer is progressive _____.

___ 7. A destructive process of tooth decay is called _____.

___ 8. A major problem for the patient with esophageal cancer is _____.

A. Leukoplakia

B. Dental caries

C. Pharyngitis

D. Nutrition

E. Candidiasis

F. Periodontal disease

G. Plaque

H. Dysphagia

I. Parotitis

IX. Complete the statements on the left with the most appropriate term on the right. Some terms may be used more than once, and some terms may not be used.

___ 1. Another name for belching, which patients with hiatal hernia may experience, is _____.

___ 2. Acidic gastric fluids can cause inflammation of the esophagus, called _____.

___ 3. The procedure used to assess bowel sounds is _____.

___ 4. Hiatal hernia is thought to be caused by weakness in the _____.

___ 5. The opening in the diaphragm through which the esophagus passes is the esophageal _____.

___ 6. Direct examination of the esophagus with an endoscope is called _____.

___ 7. The procedure used to detect the presence of air, fluid, or masses in tissues is known as ____.

___ 8. The protrusion of the lower esophagus and stomach upward through the diaphragm, into the chest, is _____.

___ 9. A surgical procedure that strengthens the LES by suturing the fundus of the stomach around the esophagus and anchoring it below the diaphragm is _____.

___ 10. Many patients with hiatal hernia report a feeling of burning and tightness rising from the lower sternum to the throat, which is called _____.

A. Hiatus

B. Pyloric sphincter

C. Hiatal hernia

D. Esophagoscopy

E. Gastrectomy

F. Esophagitis

G. Eructation

H. Heartburn

I. Palpation

J. Stomatitis

K. Auscultation

L. Fundoplication

M. Percussion

N. Lower esophageal sphincter

Introductory Nursing Care of Adults

X. Complete the statements on the left with the most appropriate term on the right. Some terms may be used more than once, and some terms may not be used.

___ 1. Two tests that allow the physician to confirm the presence of diverticula are colonoscopy and _____.

___ 2. Ulcerative colitis and Crohn's disease are types of _____.

___ 3. A loss of tissue from the lining of the digestive tract is _____.

___ 4. Regional enteritis is also known as _____.

___ 5. A break in the wall of the stomach or the duodenum that permits digestive fluids to leak into the peritoneal cavity is _____.

___ 6. A common complication of peptic ulcers is _____.

___ 7. Normally, the barrier that protects the digestive tract lining from digestive juices is _____.

___ 8. The most common symptoms of inflammatory bowel disease are bloody diarrhea and _____.

___ 9. A condition characterized by small sac-like pouches in the intestinal wall is called _____.

___ 10. A complication of diverticulitis in which an abnormal opening develops between the colon and the bladder is called _____.

___ 11. Most diverticula are found in the _____.

A. Crohn's disease
B. Hemorrhage
C. Hiatal hernia
D. Sigmoid colon
E. Diverticulosis
F. Barium enema
G. Mucus
H. Perforation
I. Duodenum
J. Fistula
K. MRI
L. Inflammatory bowel disease
M. Abdominal pain
N. Peptic ulcer

XI. Complete the statements on the left with the most appropriate term on the right. Some terms may be used more than once, and some terms may not be used.

___ 1. The stapling of the stomach to create an upper pouch that is anastomosed to the jejunum so that food intake is limited by the reduced stomach capacity is called _____.

___ 2. When a person weighs twice as much as the ideal weight, this is called _____.

___ 3. The removal of adipose tissue from selected sites through a suction cannula used mainly for cosmetic surgery is _____.

___ 4. The primary treatment of obesity is a weight reduction program accompanied by _____.

___ 5. An excessive body fat resulting in increased body weight that is more than 20% higher than the ideal is called _____.

A. Gastrectomy
B. Obesity
C. Gastric bypass
D. Exercise
E. Bulimia
F. Morbid obesity
G. Psychotherapy
H. Liposuction

XII. Complete the statements on the left with the most appropriate term on the right. Some terms may be used more than once, and some terms may not be used.

1. A common symptom of malabsorption is the presence of excessive fat in the stool, which is called _____.

2. A condition in which the large intestine loses the ability to contract effectively enough to propel the fecal mass toward the rectum is _____.

3. The passage of loose, liquid stools with increased frequency is called _____.

4. Increased pressure in the chest and abdominal cavities caused by straining to have a bowel movement is called _____.

5. A term used to describe a condition in which one or more nutrients are not digested or absorbed is _____.

6. Celiac sprue is treated by avoiding products that contain _____.

7. A condition in which a person has hard, dry, infrequent stools that are passed with difficulty is _____.

8. The retention of a large mass of stool in the rectum that the patient is unable to pass is called _____.

9. The diet recommended for acute diarrhea is _____.

10. Two examples of malabsorption are lactase deficiency and _____.

11. Lactase deficiency is treated by eliminating _____.

A. Valsalva maneuver
B. Diarrhea
C. Fecal impaction
D. Gluten
E. High-fiber foods
F. Steatorrhea
G. Anorexia
H. Sprue
I. Constipation
J. Malabsorption
K. Paralytic ileus
L. Milk and milk products
M. Clear liquids
N. Megacolon

XIII. Complete the statements on the left with the most appropriate term on the right. Some terms may be used more than once, and some terms may not be used.

____ 1. The repair of the muscle defect in abdominal hernia by suturing is called _____.

____ 2. For some patients who cannot tolerate the stress of surgical hernia repair, a pad called a _____ is placed over the hernia to provide support for the weak muscles.

____ 3. The bulging portion of the large intestine pushing through the abdominal wall is _____.

____ 4. Factors that cause hernias to appear include heavy lifting and _____.

____ 5. Weak locations where hernias occur include the lower inguinal areas of the abdomen and the _____.

____ 6. Nausea, vomiting, pain, fever, and tachycardia may be signs and symptoms of a hernia complication called _____.

____ 7. Following inguinal hernia repair, a common complication is _____.

____ 8. An irreducible hernia, sometimes called _____, may impair blood flow to the trapped loop of intestine.

A. Umbilicus

B. Hernia

C. Fecal incontinence

D. Scrotal swelling

E. Truss

F. Incarcerated

G. Coughing

H. Gangrene

I. Herniorrhaphy

J. Strangulation

XIV. Complete the statements on the left with the most appropriate term on the right. Some terms may be used more than once, and some terms may not be used.

____ 1. An abnormal opening between the anal and the perianal skin is called _____.

____ 2. The most common symptoms of hemorrhoids are rectal pain and _____.

____ 3. A procedure in which internal hemorrhoids are "tied-off" is called _____.

____ 4. Anorectal abscess is treated with _____.

____ 5. A laceration between the anal canal and the perianal skin is called _____.

____ 6. Small growths in the intestine are called _____.

____ 7. Dilated veins in the rectum are called _____.

____ 8. An infection in the tissue around the rectum is called _____.

____ 9. Signs and symptoms of anorectal abscess include rectal pain, swelling, tenderness, and _____.

A. Polyps

B. Ligation

C. Bluish-white color

D. Anal fissure

E. Redness

F. Itching

G. Anorectal abscess

H. Hemorrhoids

I. Heat therapy

J. Anal fistula

K. Antibiotics

XV. Match the drugs on the left with their actions on the right.

      1. Anticholinergics

      2. H₂ receptor antagonists

      3. Anti-inflammatory agents

      4. Antacids

      5. Sucralfate (Carafate)

      6. Antidiarrheals

      7. Antibiotics

      8. Iron supplements and vitamin B_{12}

A. Prevent(s) or treat(s) infections

B. Neutralize(s) gastric acid

C. Cling(s) to the surface of the ulcer and protect(s) it so that healing can take place

D. Treat(s) anemia

E. Decrease(s) hydrochloric acid production by competing at receptor sites

F. Decrease(s) inflammation

G. Control(s) diarrhea

H. Reduce(s) gastrointestinal motility and secretions

XVI. Match the nursing diagnoses on the left with the appropriate patient conditions on the right.

      1. Self-care deficit: feeding related to paralysis

      2. Altered oral mucous membrane related to trauma, infection

      3. Knowledge deficit of recommended mouth care practices

A. Patient with infections or inflammatory oral conditions

B. Patient with problems of teeth or gums

C. Patient unable to feed himself or herself

XVII. List 2 functions of the large intestine.

1.

2.

XVIII. List age-related changes in the 7 areas of the digestive tract listed below.

1. Gums (gingiva)

2. Teeth

3. Tastebuds

4. Walls of esophagus and stomach

5. Stomach secretions

6. Gastric motor activity

7. Large intestine muscle and mucosa

XIX. Many experts believe constipation is not a normal age-related change. List 6 factors that may cause constipation in the elderly.

1.   4.

2.   5.

3.   6.

XX.   List 1 reason why auscultation is done before palpation.

1.

XXI.   List 8 terms used to describe bowel sounds.

1.   5.

2.   6.

3.   7.

4.   8.

XXII.   List 3 nursing measures following barium enema.

1.

2.

3.

XXIII. List 5 possible signs and symptoms of digestive tract perforation.

1.

2.

3.

4.

5.

XXIV.   List the 3 specimens that are most often tested for occult blood.

1.

2.

3.

XXV.   List 2 reasons why tubes may be inserted into the stomach.

1.

2.

XXVI.   In which position should the patient be for tube feelings?

XXVII. Explain why residual formula should be returned to the patient.

XXVIII. Following tube feedings, the head and chest should be elevated for how long?

XIX. What should the nurse do if the patient who is receiving a tube feeding reports nausea or pain?

XX. List 7 signs and symptoms of dumping syndrome.

1.

2.

3.

4.

5.

6.

7.

XXI. List 2 indications the nurse assesses to determine the return of peristalsis.

1.

2.

XXXII. List 3 complications that may occur if TPN runs in too rapidly.

1.

2.

3.

XXXIII. Explain why an NG tube may be inserted and attached to suction before or during gastric surgery.

XXXIV. List 3 measures the nurse may take for the patient following surgery on the digestive tract.

1.

2.

3.

XXXV. List 2 goals of care for the patient with anorexia.

1.

2.

XXXVI. List 2 nursing diagnoses for patients who are unable to feed themselves due to paralysis.

1.

2.

XXXVII. List 2 criteria for evaluating the success of nursing interventions when patients require help with feeding.

1.

2.

XXXVIII. List 3 nursing diagnoses for patients with infections or inflammatory oral conditions.

1.

2.

3.

XXXIX. List 3 nursing diagnoses for patients with problems of teeth or gums.

1.

2.

3.

XL. List 2 signs which are common just before vomiting.

1.

2.

XLI. List 5 signs of fluid volume deficit.

1.

2.

3.

4.

5.

XLII. List 5 nursing diagnoses for patients who are obese.

1.

2.

3.

4.

5.

XLIII. List 4 signs and symptoms of strangulation in patients with abdominal hernias.

1.

2.

3.

4.

XLIV. Identify the 2 types of malignant tumors that develop in the mouth.

1. Type that occurs on the buccal mucosa, gums, floor of the mouth, tonsils, and tongue:

2. Type that most commonly occurs on the lip:

XLV. Postoperative patients may have stents placed in the esophagus to reduce the risk of regurgitation of stomach contents. List 3 ways the nurse should teach the patient to avoid regurgitation.

1.

2.

3.

XLVI. List 3 interventions to reduce pain in patients with peptic ulcer.

1.

2.

3.

XLVII. List 3 aspects of care which the nurse should teach the patient who experiences dumping syndrome.

1.

2.

3.

XLVIII. List 5 goals of nursing care for patients with diarrhea.

1.

2.

3.

4.

5.

IL. Normal age-related changes in the large intestine do not explain the frequent complaints of constipation by the elderly; list 4 factors that are more likely related to constipation in the elderly.

1.

2.

3

4.

L. Choose the most appropriate answer.

1. The transfer of digested food molecules from the digestive tract into the blood stream is:
   A. digestion
   B. absorption
   C. peristalsis
   D. elimination

2. The removal of solid food wastes from the body is:
   A. elimination
   B. absorption
   C. digestion
   D. metabolism

3. Enzymes that convert complex sugars into simple sugars include:
   A. secretin, bile and insulin
   B. lipase, lactase, and sucrase
   C. pepsin, hydrochloric acid, and chyme
   D. sucrase, lactase, and maltase

4. Normal bowel sounds include:
   A. minimal clicks and gurgles
   B. clicks and gurgles 5–30 times/minute
   C. steady, consistent gurgling sounds
   D. no sounds for 1 full minute

5. If stool specimens are being tested for occult blood, the following should be omitted from the diet for 2-3 days before collecting the specimen:
   A. eggs
   B. cheese
   C. red meat
   D. beets

6. After insertion of a gastric tube, feedings are not started until:
   A. the patient requests food
   B. adequate oxygen levels are achieved on blood gases
   C. placement of tube is certain
   D. oral fluids are tolerated

7. The forceful expulsion of stomach contents is:
   A. regurgitation
   B. vomiting
   C. aspiration
   D. eructation

8. Signs and symptoms of fever, tachycardia, tachypnea, and fluid accumulation in the postoperative care of patients with esophageal cancer are suggestive of:
   A. infection
   B. hemorrhage
   C. cardiac shock
   D. leakage

9. Severe or prolonged vomiting puts the patient at risk for:
   A. fluid volume deficit
   B. altered tissue perfusion
   C. hemorrhage
   D. infection

10. The vomiting patient who is also unconscious or has impaired swallowing is at risk for aspiration and should be placed in what position?
    A. flat in bed
    B. head of bed elevated at least 90 degrees
    C. on the side
    D. head of bed slightly elevated at 30 degrees

11. To prevent nighttime reflux, the sleeping position for patients with hiatal hernia should be:
    A. on the side
    B. head of bed at 90-degree angle
    C. flat
    D. head of bed elevated 6 to 12 inches

12. Sudden, sharp pain starting in the midepigastric region and spreading across the entire abdomen in patients with peptic ulcer may indicate:
    A. infection
    B. perforation
    C. dyspnea
    D. kidney failure

13. If the abdomen becomes rigid and tender and patients draw their knees up to their chest, this may indicate:
    A. peritonitis
    B. perforation
    C. kidney failure
    D. pyloric obstruction

14. The most prominent symptom of pyloric obstruction is persistent:
    A. eructation
    B. heartburn
    C. vomiting
    D. hemorrhage

15. A complication of stomach surgery that occurs because the absence or decreased size of the stomach prevents the normal pacing of chyme moving into the intestine is:
    A. black, tarry stools
    B. dumping syndrome
    C. coffee-ground emesis
    D. obstructed pyloric sphincter

16. When severe constipation is accompanied by trickling of liquid stool, this may suggest:
A. pyloric obstruction
B. fecal impaction
C. intestinal hemorrhage
D. steatorrhea

17. A major complication of appendicitis is:
A. diarrhea
B. constipation
C. fluid volume deficit
D. peritonitis

18. The classic symptom of appendicitis is pain at:
A. McBurney's point
B. the xiphoid process
C. right hypochondriac region
D. inguinal node

19. When appendicitis is suspected, the patient is allowed:
A. clear liquids
B. full liquids
C. nothing by mouth
D. soft foods

20. In addition to fluid volume deficit, patients with peritonitis may go into shock because of:
A. edema
B. convulsions
C. septicemia
D. paralysis

21. Pain is severe for several postoperative days following abdominoperineal resection. At first, the patient will probably be most comfortable in which position?
A. supine
B. sidelying
C. prone
D. Fowler's

22. Following abdominoperinal resection, a procedure that cleans, soothes, and increases circulation to the perineum is:
A. use of a TENS unit
B. Kegel exercises
C. the sitz bath
D. débridement

LI.   In Figure 34–1, label the parts (A–S) of the digestive tract.

A.

B.

C.

D.

E.

F.

G.

H.

I.

J.

K.

L.

M.

N.

O.

P.

Q.

R.

S.

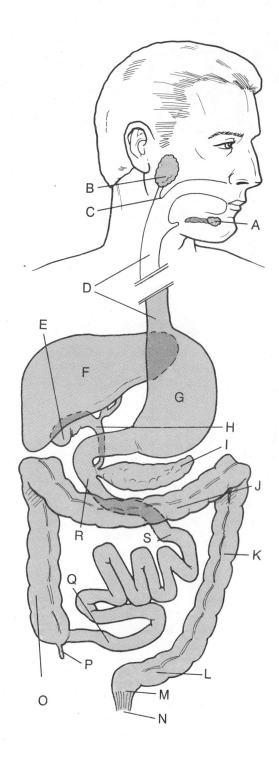

CHAPTER

35

Disorders of the Liver, Gallbladder, and Pancreas

OBJECTIVES

1. Identify nursing assessment data related to the functions of the liver, gallbladder, and pancreas.
2. Identify the nurse's role in tests and procedures performed to diagnose disorders of the liver, gallbladder, and pancreas.
3. Describe the care of the patient who has an esophageal balloon tube in place.
4. Explain the pathology, signs and symptoms, diagnosis, complications, and medical treatment of selected disorders of the liver, gallbladder, and pancreas.
5. Apply the nursing process to develop a nursing care plan for the patient with liver, gallbladder, or pancreatic dysfunction.

LEARNING ACTIVITIES

I.   Match the definition on the left with the most appropriate term on the right

___ 1. Gland that secretes a substance directly into the blood

___ 2. Enlargement of the liver

___ 3. Splitting of glycogen into glucose

___ 4. Presence of gallstones in the gallbladder

___ 5. Inflammation of the liver

___ 6. Obstruction of the common bile duct by a gallstone

___ 7. Golden yellow color of the skin, sclerae, and mucous membranes caused by deposition of bile pigments; associated with liver dysfunction or bile obstruction

___ 8. Ejection of gas from the stomach through the mouth; belching

___ 9. Chronic, progressive liver disease

___ 10. Synthesis of glucose from sources other than carbohydrates

A. Hepatitis
B. Cirrhosis
C. Cholecystectomy
D. Glycogenolysis
E. Cholecystitis
F. Eructation
G. Hepatomegaly
H. Glycogenesis
I. Choledocholithiasis
J. Gluconeogenesis
K. Endocrine gland
L. Ascites
M. Hepatic
N. Cholelithiasis
O. Icterus
P. Jaundice

I. *Continues*

I.   *Continues*

____ 11.   Jaundice; golden yellow skin color caused by deposition of bile

____ 12.   Accumulation of excess fluid in the peritoneal cavity

____ 13.   Removal of the gallbladder

____ 14.   Conversion of glucose from glycogen

____ 15.   Pertaining to the liver

____ 16.   Inflammation of the gallbladder

A.   Hepatitis

B.   Cirrhosis

C.   Cholecystectomy

D.   Glycogenolysis

E.   Cholecystitis

F.   Eructation

G.   Hepatomegaly

H.   Glycogenesis

I.   Choledocholithiasis

J.   Gluconeogenesis

K.   Endocrine gland

L.   Ascites

M.   Hepatic

N.   Cholelithiasis

O.   Icterus

P.   Jaundice

II.   Match the definition on the left with the most appropriate term on the right.

____ 1.   Pathologic changes in the peripheral nervous system

____ 2.   Impaired digestion; epigastric discomfort after meals; heartburn

____ 3.   Removal of ascitic fluid from the peritoneal cavity

____ 4.   Nosebleed

____ 5.   Injection of hardening agents into blood vessels

____ 6.   Inflammation of the pancreas

____ 7.   Inflammation of the biliary ducts

____ 8.   Excess fat in stools

____ 9.   Gland that secretes substances through ducts

____ 10.   Enlarged, tortuous blood or lymphatic vessel

____ 11.   Itching

____ 12.   Enlargement of breast tissue in males

A.   Paracentesis

B.   Steatorrhea

C.   Dyspepsia

D.   Pruritus

E.   Sclerotherapy

F.   Gynecomastia

G.   Varices

H.   Pancreatitis

I.   Neuropathy

J.   Exocrine gland

K.   Epistaxis

L.   Cholangitis

III. Complete the statements on the left with the most appropriate term on the right. Some terms may be used more than once, and some terms may not be used.

____ 1. Bile is produced in the _____.

____ 2. Specialized reticuloendothelial cells in the liver that ingest old red blood cells and bacteria are called _____.

____ 3. When fats pass into the duodenum, the gallbladder and the liver respond by delivering bile to the small intestine through the _____.

____ 4. A golden yellow skin color associated with liver dysfunction or bile obstruction is _____.

____ 5. A product of the normal breakdown of old red blood cells in the liver is _____.

____ 6. The vessel that delivers blood from the aorta to the liver is the _____.

____ 7. The vessel that delivers blood from the intestines to the liver is the _____.

____ 8. Bile produced in the liver passes into the gallbladder for storage through the _____.

____ 9. Bile is stored in the _____.

____ 10. When the sclera turns yellow in patients with liver disease, this condition is called scleral _____.

A. Bilirubin
B. Portal vein
C. Pancreas
D. Kupffer's cells
E. Gallbladder
F. Hepatic artery
G. Pancreatic duct
H. Common bile duct
I. Icterus
J. Liver
K. Cystic duct
L. jaundice

IV. Complete the statements on the left with the most appropriate term on the right. Some terms may be used more than once, and some terms may not be used.

____ 1. A radioactive substance that is injected into a vein is then visualized in a radiograph to reveal tumors and abscesses; this procedure is called _____.

____ 2. The use of sound waves to create an image of the liver, spleen, pancreas, gallbladder, and biliary system that is noninvasive and painless is called _____.

____ 3. A procedure that involves removal of a small specimen of liver tissue for examination is called _____.

____ 4. A primary complication of liver biopsy that occurs because of the liver's rich blood supply and potential for impaired coagulation is _____.

____ 5. A primary complication of liver biopsy that occurs if the lung is accidentally punctured during the biopsy is _____.

A. Liver biopsy
B. Pneumothorax
C. Ultrasonography
D. Hemothorax
E. Liver scan
F. Hemorrhage
G. PET scan

V. Complete the statements on the left with the most appropriate term on the right. Some terms may be used more than once, and some terms may not be used.

____ 1. The second phase of hepatitis, which lasts from 2 to 4 weeks, which is characterized by jaundice and clay-colored stools, is called the _____.

____ 2. Serum hepatitis is transmitted in body fluids and is called _____.

____ 3. When bile channels are compressed due to inflammation in the liver, this results in an elevation in serum bilirubin and is observed as _____.

____ 4. The third phase of hepatitis, in which fatigue, malaise, and liver enlargement last for several months is called the _____.

____ 5. Infectious hepatitis or epidemic hepatitis, which is transmitted by water, food, or contaminated medical equipment is called _____.

____ 6. The first phase of hepatitis, which lasts from 1 to 21 days, when the patient is most infectious is called the _____.

A. Hepatitis B

B. Preicteric phase

C. Angioedema

D. Jaundice

E. Icteric phase

F. Anorexia

G. Posticteric phase

H. Hepatitis A

VI. Complete the statements on the left with the most appropriate term on the right. Some terms may be used more than once, and some terms may not be used.

____ 1. A symptom common in cirrhosis that is characterized by tingling or numbness in the extremities thought to be caused by vitamin B deficiencies is called _____.

____ 2. Cirrhosis that develops as a result of obstruction to bile flow is called _____.

____ 3. Cirrhosis that is caused by nutritional deficiencies or exposure to alcohol is called _____.

____ 4. The accumulation of fluid in the peritoneal cavity that occurs frequently in patients with cirrhosis is called _____.

____ 5. A chronic, progressive disease of the liver that is characterized by degeneration and destruction of liver cells is called _____.

A. Laennec's

B. Peripheral neuropathy

C. Ascites

D. Cirrhosis

E. Postnecrotic cirrhosis

F. Biliary cirrhosis

G. Dyspepsia

VII. Complete the statements on the left with the most appropriate term on the right. Some terms may be used more than once, and some terms may not be used.

____ 1. Two types of drugs used to dissolve gallstones include dissolution agents and _____.

____ 2. A procedure that delivers a series of shock waves through water or a cushion, causing the gallstones to break up, is called _____.

____ 3. In emergency situations, the surgeon may tie off bleeding varices directly; this technique is an example of _____.

____ 4. A newer surgical procedure in which the gallbladder is grasped with forceps, cut free with a laser, and pulled out through a small incision is called _____.

____ 5. A balloon tube, such as the Sengstaken-Blakemore tube, used to apply direct pressure to bleeding veins in the esophagus and stomach is called a _____.

____ 6. The use of endoscopic instruments to incise the sphincter of Oddi and extract stones from the common bile duct is called _____.

____ 7. A procedure in which a solution is injected into the varices or into the veins that supply them, causing them to harden and close, is called _____.

____ 8. The most frequently used treatment for cholelithiasis in which the gallbladder is surgically removed is called _____.

A. Endoscopic cholecystectomy

B. Choleangiography

C. Endoscopic sphincterotomy

D. Lithotripsy

E. Paracentesis

F. Esophageal-gastric balloon tube

G. Anticholinergics

H. Oral bile salts

I. Sclerotherapy

J. Cholecystectomy

K. Surgical treatment of bleeding varices

VIII. Complete the statements on the left with the most appropriate term on the right. Some terms may be used more than once, and some terms may not be used.

____ 1. As an endocrine gland, the pancreas secretes hormones into the blood that regulate the level of _____.

____ 2. The exocrine function of the pancreas is the production of _____ that make up the pancreatic fluid.

____ 3. Through the pancreatic duct, pancreatic fluid is secreted into the _____.

____ 4. The pancreatic enzyme that reduces starch, sucrose, and fructose to glucose, fructose, and galactose is _____.

____ 5. The pancreatic enzyme that acts on emulsified fats to yield fatty acids, glycerides, and glycerol is _____.

____ 6. The beta cells in the pancreas produce and secrete _____.

____ 7. The alpha cells in the pancreas secrete and produce _____.

____ 8. A surgical procedure for cancer of the pancreas involving the removal of the diseased portion of the pancreas, the duodenum, and part of the stomach is called the _____.

A. Duodenum

B. Trypsin

C. Lipase

D. Digestive enzymes

E. Somatostatin

F. Blood glucose

G. Insulin

H. Whipple procedure

I. Stomach

J. Amylase

K. Glucagon

Introductory Nursing Care of Adults

IX. Match the effects of cirrhosis complications on the left with the most appropriate complication of cirrhosis on the right. Some terms may be used more than once, and some may not be used.

___ 1. Results in leaking of lymph fluid and albu-min-rich fluid from the diseased liver

___ 2. Renal failure following diuretic therapy, paracentesis, or GI hemorrhage

___ 3. Caused by excessive ammonia in the blood, resulting in cognitive disturbances

___ 4. May cause fatal hemorrhage

___ 5. Development of collateral vessels

A. Hepatic encephalopathy

B. Esophageal varices

C. Portal hypertension

D. Epistaxis

E. Hepatorenal syndrome

F. Peripheral neuropathy

G. Ascites

X. State the recommended diet for patients with cirrhosis.

XI. List 2 reasons why paracentesis is not used frequently to remove ascitic fluid from the peritoneal cavity.

1.

2.

XII. List 3 reasons why patients with cirrhosis are at risk for impaired skin integrity or skin breakdown.

1.

2.

3.

XIII. When patients with cholethiasis are discharged from the hospital, the nurse should advise them to report the 4 signs of bile duct obstruction which are:

1.

2.

3.

4.

XIV. List 6 functions of the liver.

1.

2.

3.

4.

5.

6.

XV. Choose the most appropriate answer.

1. Stool in the large intestine gets its characteristic brown color from the final breakdown products of:
   A. chyme
   B. pepsin
   C. amylase
   D. bilirubin

2. Patients with liver disease are at increased risk for drug:
   A. incompatibilities
   B. toxicities
   C. idiosyncrasies
   D. synthesis

3. Clay-colored stools are characteristic of:
   A. bile obstruction
   B. pancreatitis
   C. gastritis
   D. Crohn's disease

4. The prescribed diet for patients with hepatitis is usually:
   A. high carbohydrate and vitamins, low protein, low to moderate fat
   B. low carbohydrate, moderate to high protein, high fat
   C. high carbohydrate and vitamins, moderate to high protein, low to moderate fat
   D. low carbohydrate, low protein, low to moderate fat

5. Patients with hepatitis may have impaired skin integrity due to:
   A. jaundice
   B. pruritus or scratching
   C. nausea and vomiting
   D. fluid volume deficit

6. The nurse should explain to patients with hepatitis that rest is necessary to allow the liver to heal by:
   A. producing more white blood cells to fight infection
   B. producing more platelets to assist in clotting
   C. regenerating new cells to replace damaged cells
   D. regenerating new blood vessels to replace damaged ones

7. The nurse should be alert for signs of fluid retention in patients with hepatitis, which include increasing abdominal girth, rising blood pressure and:
   A. dry mucous membranes
   B. tachycardia
   C. edema
   D. concentrated urine

8. Which of the following drugs may be ordered for pruritus, which occurs with hepatitis?
   A. antihistamines
   B. antiemetics
   C. antibiotics
   D. analgesics

9. The patient with hepatitis may be self-conscious about appearance because of:
   A. cyanosis
   B. redness
   C. ulcerations
   D. jaundice

10. People who have had close contact with hepatitis patients should be vaccinated wit:
    A. immune globulin
    B. RhoGam
    C. influenza vaccine
    D. Salk vaccine

11. A frequent problem in cirrhosis for which small, semisolid meals are recommended is:
    A. peripheral neuropathy
    B. jaundice
    C. anorexia
    D. ascites

12. The medical management of ascites aims to promote reabsorption and elimination of the fluid by means of salt restriction and:
    A. antihistamines
    B. analgesics
    C. diuretics
    D. antibiotics

13. Potential complications of peritoneal-venous shunts used to allow ascitic fluid to drain from the abdomen and return to the blood stream are tubing obstruction and:
    A. jaundice
    B. peripheral neuropathy
    C. pruritus
    D. peritonitis

14. The best position for patients with ascites to help them breathe more easily is:
    A. side-lying
    B. prone
    C. supine
    D. elevated head of bed

15. The patient with cirrhosis is at great risk for injury or hemorrhage due to impaired:
    A. coagulation
    B. immunity
    C. skin integrity
    D. breathing patterns

16. Since the esophagus and the trachea are adjacent to each other, upward movement of the esophageal balloon in the patient with cirrhosis may cause:
    A. impaired circulation
    B. airway obstruction
    C. cardiac shock
    D. perforated intestine

17. Bile is essential for the emulsification and digestion of:
    A. carbohydrates
    B. protein
    C. hormones
    D. fats

18. When fats enter the duodenum, the gallbladder contracts and delivers bile to the intestine through the:
    A. hepatic duct
    B. cystic duct
    C. common bile duct
    D. pancreatic duct

19. Bile ducts respond to obstruction (such as gallstones) with spasms in an effort to move the stone: the intense spasmodic pain is called:
    A. hepatic encephalopathy
    B. renal colic
    C. biliary colic
    D. peripheral neuropathy

20. A common symptom of cholecystitis is right upper quadrant pain that radiates to the:
    A. sternum
    B. shoulder
    C. umbilicus
    D. jaw

21. When the cholecystectomy patient first returns from surgery, the drainage from the T tube may be bloody, but it should soon become:
    A. dark amber
    B. clay-colored
    C. bright red
    D. greenish brown

22. What type of diet is recommended for patients with cholecystitis to decrease attacks of biliary colic?
    A. low protein
    B. low fat
    C. low carbohydrate
    D. low salt

23. Patients who have obstructive jaundice due to blockage of the bile ducts often have impaired skin integrity with:
    A. pruritus
    B. infection
    C. hemorrhage
    D. hypersensitivity

24. Patients with obstructed bile flow may have a deficiency of vitamin:
    A. A
    B. C
    C. D
    D. K

25. A complication of endoscopic sphincterotomy is pancreatitis caused by accidental entry of the endoscope into the pancreatic duct; early signs of pancreatitis are:
    A. jaundice and confusion
    B. nausea and vomiting
    C. ascites and hypertension
    D. pain and fever

26. A gland that has both endocrine and exocrine functions is the:
    A. pancreas
    B. adrenal gland
    C. thyroid gland
    D. sebaceous gland

27. Vitamin K is needed for the production of:
    A. bile
    B. calcium
    C. prothrombin
    D. thyroxine

28. Specific blood studies used to assess pancreatic function include serum:
    A. bilirubin
    B. amylase
    C. prothrombin
    D. albumin

29. The most prominent symptom of pancreatitis is:
    A. jaundice
    B. abdominal pain
    C. hypertension
    D. diarrhea

30. To remove the stimulus for secretion of pancreatic fluid in acute pancreatitis, the patient is usually allowed:
    A. nothing by mouth
    B. low fat diet
    C. clear liquid diet
    D. low sodium diet

31. Which drugs do patients with chronic pancreatitis need to take in order to digest food?
   A. analgesics
   B. anticholinergics
   C. antiemetics
   D. pancreatic enzymes

32. Signs of hypocalcemia that may occur in patients with chronic pancreatitis include:
   A. confusion and fatigue
   B. cardiac dysrhythmias
   C. muscle twitching or cramping
   D. easy bruising

33. When patients with pancreatitis are on TPN in order to restrict oral intake and reduce pancreatic fluid secretion, the nurse must monitor for:
   A. hyperkalemia
   B. hypernatremia
   C. hyperchloremia
   D. hyperglycemia

XVI. In Figure 35–10 below, label the anatomic parts (A–J).

A.

B.

C.

D.

E.

F.

G.

H.

I.

J.

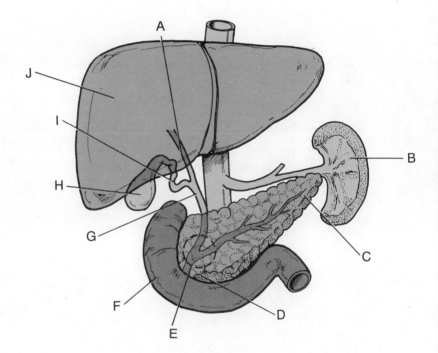

CHAPTER
36

Urologic Disorders

OBJECTIVES

1. List the data to be collected when assessing a patient who has a urologic disorder.
2. Describe the diagnostic tests and procedures for patients with urologic disorders.
3. Explain the nursing responsibilities for patients having tests and procedures to diagnose urologic disorders.
4. Describe the nursing responsibilities for common therapeutic measures employed to treat urologic disorders.
5. Explain the pathophysiology, signs and symptoms, complications, and treatment of disorders of the kidney, ureters, bladder, and urethra.
6. Apply the nursing process to plan care for patients with urologic disorders.

LEARNING ACTIVITIES

I.   Match the definition on the left with the most appropriate term on the right.

___ 1. Concentration, commonly called a stone, formed of mineral salts in hollow organs or their passages

___ 2. Excessive urine volume

___ 3. Decreased urine output

___ 4. Accumulation of nitrogenous compounds in the blood

___ 5. Removal of calculi through an incision in a duct or organ

___ 6. Removal or resection of the urinary bladder or of a cyst

___ 7. Crushing or disintegration of calculi

___ 8. Absence of urine production

___ 9. Blood in the urine

___ 10. Increased production of urine

___ 11. Having a harmful effect on kidney tissue

___ 12. Azotemia; the signs and symptoms typical of chronic renal failure

___ 13. Excessive urination during the night

___ 14. Difficult or painful urination

A. Anuria
B. Azotemia
C. Calculus
D. Cystectomy
E. Diuresis
F. Dysuria
G. Hematuria
H. Lithotomy
I. Lithotripsy
J. Nephrotoxic
K. Nocturia
L. Oliguria
M. Polyuria
N. Uremia

II. Match the definition or description on the left with the most appropriate term on the right. Some terms may be used more than once, and some may not be used.

___ 1. The _____ is the part of the kidney that contains the glomeruli and most of the tubules.

___ 2. The inner portion of the kidney, which contains pyramids, is the _____.

___ 3. The pyramids of the kidney collect urine and drain it into the _____.

___ 4. The calices join to form the _____ of the kidney.

___ 5. The _____ is a tube that transports urine from each kidney pelvis to the bladder.

___ 6. The functional unit of the kidney is the _____.

___ 7. A mass of blood vessels tucked into the Bowman's capsule is the _____.

___ 8. The kidneys lie behind the _____.

___ 9. The outer layer of the kidney, which receives a large blood supply, is the _____.

A. Ureter

B. Calices

C. Bladder

D. Pelvis

E. Peritoneum

F. Medulla

G. Glomerulus

H. Cortex

I. Urethra

J. Nephron

III. Complete the statements on the left with the most appropriate term on the right. Some terms may be used more than once, and some terms may not be used.

___ 1. The upper portion of the bladder is called the _____.

___ 2. The _____ is the muscular sac that stretches to store urine.

___ 3. The bladder rests on the floor of the pelvic cavity behind the _____.

___ 4. The muscular tube that carries urine from the bladder out of the body is called the _____.

___ 5. In the male, the urethra is encircled by a gland called the _____.

___ 6. The _____ nerves stimulate the detrusor muscle and cause the bladder to empty.

___ 7. When 300 to 400 ml of urine collect in the bladder, bladder distention causes the urge to _____.

___ 8. The _____ muscle contracts to empty the bladder.

A. Ureter

B. Prostate

C. Detrusor

D. Peritoneum

E. Parasympathetic

F. Pudendal

G. Bladder

H. Urethra

I. Fundus

J. Micturate

IV. Complete the statements on the left with the most appropriate term on the right. Some terms may be used more than once, and some terms may not be used.

_____ 1. Some nonelectrolyte substances which are reabsorbed by the tubules include uric acid, urea, and _____.

_____ 2. Reabsorption of water by the tubules occurs through the process of _____.

_____ 3. The end product of glomerular filtration and tubular reabsorption is _____.

_____ 4. Aldosterone is secreted by the adrenal glands in response to _____.

_____ 5. Aldosterone causes the reabsorption of water and _____.

_____ 6. Substances secreted by the tubules are called _____.

_____ 7. The amount of water reabsorbed in the kidneys is influenced by antidiuretic hormone and _____.

_____ 8. Urine is moved from the kidney to the bladder by means of _____.

A. Aldosterone
B. Glucose
C. Ions
D. Peristalsis
E. Concentrated urine
F. Urethra
G. Urine
H. Creatinine
I. Osmosis
J. Sodium

V. Complete the statements on the left with the most appropriate term on the right. Some terms may be used more than once, and some terms may not be used.

_____ 1. _____ causes reabsorption of water in the renal tubules, decreasing urine volume.

_____ 2. _____ is released in response to inadequate renal blood flow or low arterial pressure.

_____ 3. The hormone secreted in the kidneys that stimulates the bone marrow to produce red blood cells is _____.

_____ 4. The hormone that is released from the pituitary when stimulated by hypertonic plasma is _____.

_____ 5. Very concentrated plasma is said to be _____.

_____ 6. A common condition that leads to hypertonic plasma is _____.

A. Erythropoietin
B. Angiotensin II
C. Hypertonic
D. Calcium
E. Renin
F. Hypotonic
G. Antidiuretic hormone
H. Dehydration

VI. Complete the statements on the left with the most appropriate term on the right. Some terms may be used more than once, and some terms may not be used.

___ 1. A _____ provides a general outline of the kidneys, revealing their approximate size and contour.

___ 2. Also called an excretory urogram, the _____ permits visualization of the kidneys, ureter, and bladder in order to assess kidney function and structures, ureter size and patency, bladder size and shape and presence of calculi.

___ 3. _____ uses sound waves to detect urinary tract malformations as well as cysts, tumors, and renal calculi.

___ 4. A plain film or a KUB (for kidneys, ureters and bladder) that helps detect tumors, malformations, and calculi is called _____.

___ 5. _____ is the direct visualization of the interior of the urethra, bladder, and ureteral orifices done for diagnostic or treatment purposes.

___ 6. Obtaining a specimen of renal tissue for direct examination to evaluate conditions leading to renal failure is called _____.

___ 7. _____ permits the removal of calculi, tumors, or foreign materials; cauterization of lesions; implantation of radium seeds; insertion of ureteral catheters; and control of bleeding.

___ 8. _____ involves the IV injection of an iodine dye, fluoroscopy and radiography.

___ 9. A study of the renal blood vessels that is used to diagnose renal artery stenosis, aneurysms, vascular tumors, renal cysts, and renal infarctions is the _____.

___ 10. A test which involves the injection of IV radioisotope, followed by radiographs to demonstrate blood flow to each kidney, is called _____.

___ 11. In _____, a lighted tube is inserted through the urethra into the bladder under sterile conditions.

A. Ultrasonography

B. Voiding cystourethrogram

C. Angiogram

D. MRI

E. Cystoscopy

F. Catheterization

G. Renal scan

H. Flat plate

I. Cystometrogram

J. Renal biopsy

K. Intravenous pyelogram

VII. Complete the statements on the left with the most appropriate term on the right. Some
terms may be used more than once, and some terms may not be used.

_____ 1. With normally functioning kidneys, the serum creatinine level is _____.

_____ 2. _____ is a general indicator of the kidneys' ability to excrete urea whose values are
raised by high-protein diets, gastrointestinal
bleeding, dehydration, and some drugs.

_____ 3. A better measurement of kidney functioning
than the BUN because it is elevated only in
kidney disorders is the _____.

_____ 4. With normally functioning kidneys, the urine
creatinine level is _____.

_____ 5. The best test of overall kidney function is
_____.

_____ 6. Two tests that are compared to each other and
which should be opposite each other if kidneys are functioning normally are the creatinine clearance and the _____.

A. Blood urea nitrogen

B. High

C. Serum electrolytes

D. Urine culture

E. Very low

F. Serum creatinine

G. Creatinine clearance

VIII. Complete the statements on the left with the most appropriate term on the right. Some
terms may be used more than once, and some terms may not be used.

_____ 1. A catheter is inserted into the bladder, and
fluid is instilled until the patient reports the
urge to void, to produce a _____.

_____ 2. _____ measures the rate of urine flow
during voiding.

_____ 3. A _____ outlines the contour of the
bladder and shows reflux of urine.

_____ 4. The backward movement of urine from the
bladder into the ureters is called _____.

_____ 5. To produce a _____, a catheter is inserted into the bladder, dye is injected, and
radiographs are taken.

_____ 6. A _____ is used to evaluate bladder tone
in the patient with incontinence or with a
neurogenic bladder.

A. Reflux

B. Urodynamic study

C. Ultrasonography

D. Flat plate

E. Cystometrogram

F. Cystogram

IX. Complete the statements on the left with the most appropriate term on the right. Some terms may be used more than once, and some terms may not be used.

___ 1. _____ is the condition in which calculi are formed in the kidneys and travel through the ureters into the bladder.

___ 2. Three diagnostic tests to confirm the presence and location of calculi in the urinary tract include ultrasound, IVP, and the _____.

___ 3. _____ is inflammation of the renal pelvis.

___ 4. A hereditary disorder in which grape-like cysts replace normal kidney tissue is _____.

___ 5. _____ is the removal of a calculus.

___ 6. The removal of a calculus from the renal pelvis is _____.

___ 7. Inflammation of the urinary bladder is _____.

___ 8. A urinalysis is done in patients with glomerulonephritis to detect red blood cell casts and _____.

___ 9. The formation of calculi in the urinary tract is called _____.

___ 10. The formation of calculi in the kidneys is called _____.

___ 11. The intense, colicky pain of renal calculi may be relieved by narcotic analgesics and _____.

___ 12. Possible complications of lithotripsy include bruising and _____.

___ 13. Inflammation of the capillary loops in the glomeruli is _____.

A. Polycystic kidney disease

B. Anticholinergics

C. Pyelolithotomy

D. Hemorrhage

E. Nephrolithiasis

F. KUB

G. MRI

H. Proteinuria

I. Glomerulonephritis

J. Lithotomy

K. Antispasmodics

L. Urolithiasis

M. Cystitis

N. Platelets

O. Lithiasis

P. Pyelonephritis

X. Complete the statements on the left with the most appropriate term on the right. Some terms may be used more than once, and some terms may not be used.

___ 1. Removal of the kidney is called _____.

___ 2. _____ is a noninvasive procedure to break up calculi.

___ 3. Removal of the bladder is a _____.

___ 4. A procedure to open the bladder is _____.

___ 5. _____ is a surgical procedure that reroutes the flow of urine.

A. Urinary diversion

B. Lithotripsy

C. Cystoscopy

D. Cystectomy

E. Nephrectomy

F. Cystotomy

XI. Complete the statements on the left with the most appropriate term on the right. Some terms may be used more than once, and some terms may not be used.

___ 1. A _____ is a hollow tube placed in the ureter to maintain alignment or to provide a route for urine drainage.

___ 2. A procedure that is sometimes used to measure residual urine is _____.

___ 3. The _____ is threaded through a ureter into the renal pelvis.

___ 4. _____ is the primary cause of nosocomial infections.

___ 5. _____ technique is used to insert a catheter.

___ 6. A _____ is inserted through a flank incision directly into the kidney pelvis when the ureter is completely obstructed.

___ 7. The catheter must be handled gently to avoid trauma to the _____.

___ 8. The introduction of a catheter through the urethra into the bladder for the purpose of removing urine is called _____.

A. Ureteral catheter

B. Urethra

C. Urinary stent

D. Clean

E. Sterile

F. Renal pelvis

G. Catheterization

H. Nephrostomy tube

I. Cystoscopy

XII. Complete the statements on the left with the most appropriate term on the right. Some terms may be used more than once, and some terms may not be used.

___ 1. _____ is removal of a kidney.

___ 2. Following the removal of a kidney, the condition in which peristalsis does not return within 3 to 4 days is called _____.

___ 3. When a calculus obstructs urine flow, the urine may back up into the kidney, causing _____.

___ 4. The placement of a tube in the kidney so that urine may drain through the tube into an external collection device is called.

___ 5. In patients with hydronephrosis, urine is usually strained and examined for _____.

___ 6. Distention of the kidney with urine is called ___.

A. Hydronephrosis

B. Red blood cells

C. Nephrectomy

D. Cystectomy

E. Calculi

F. Paralytic ileus

G. Nephrostomy

XIII. Complete the statements on the left with the most appropriate term on the right. Some terms may be used more than once, and some terms may not be used.

___ 1. Elevated serum potassium is called _____.

___ 2. _____ is an increase in nitrogen waste products in the blood.

___ 3. Elevated blood pressure and edema are signs of _____ .

___ 4. _____ is abnormally low serum calcium.

___ 5. Indications of _____ include headache, lethargy, and delirium.

___ 6. Symptoms of _____ include tetany and irritability.

___ 7. Untreated _____ may result in bradycardia.

___ 8. Fluid restriction and diuretics are used to prevent or treat _____.

A. Insulin resistance

B. Hypercalcemia

C. Azotemia

D. Hyperkalemia

E. Hypocalcemia

F. Metabolic Acidosis

G. Hypokalemia

H. Hypervolemia

XIV. Complete the statements on the left with the most appropriate term on the right. Some terms may be used more than once, and some terms may not be used.

___ 1. With renal failure, cells develop _____, causing blood insulin and glucose levels to rise.

___ 2. Signs of _____ include moist breath sounds, bounding pulse, dependent edema, and dyspnea.

___ 3. Waste product accumulation affects the _____, causing itching and dryness.

___ 4. Hypervolemia, hyperkalemia, and hypocalcemia all affect the _____ system.

___ 5. Patients in chronic renal failure produce less erythropoietin than normal, and those red blood cells that are produced have shorter than normal life spans, resulting in _____.

___ 6. In chronic renal failure, the general _____ is suppressed, including declining antibody production and diminished inflammatory response.

___ 7. _____ effects of chronic renal failure include mental status changes and peripheral neuropathy.

___ 8. Hemodialysis may create _____, which is corrected with the administration of hypertonic glucose.

___ 9. A genetically engineered _____, administered intravenously following hemodialysis or subcutaneously for patients on peritoneal dialysis, improves red bleed cell formation and can reverse anemia.

___ 10. _____ can be caused by the accumulation of calcium phosphate crystals and urea in the skin.

___ 11. _____ may be caused by hyperkalemia or hypocalcemia.

A. Disequilibrium

B. Hemodialysis

C. Immune response

D. Erythropoietin

E. Insulin resistance

F. Neurologic

G. Congestive heart failure

H. Skin

I. Cardiovascular

J. Dysrhythmias

K. Anemia

L. Gastrointestinal

M. Itching

XV. Complete the statements on the left with the most appropriate term on the right. Some terms may be used more than once, and some terms may not be used.

___ 1. _____, which is most often noted around the mouth, is a very late sign in chronic renal failure.

___ 2. Most patients with chronic renal failure retain _____ and water.

___ 3. Emotional and psychological effects of chronic renal failure include depression, emotional lability, and _____.

___ 4. Ovulation and _____ usually cease in females with chronic renal failure.

___ 5. The skeletal changes characteristic of chronic renal failure are known as _____.

___ 6. A diet high in carbohydrates and low in protein is prescribed to reduce the accumulation of _____.

___ 7. _____ is the condition in which calcium is lost from bones and replaced with fibrous tissue.

___ 8. For unknown reasons, patients with chronic renal failure are usually _____.

___ 9. The effects of chronic renal failure on the male reproductive system typically include low sperm counts and _____

A. Anxiety

B. Impotence

C. Osteitis fibrosa

D. Hypothyroid

E. Osteomalacia

F. Sodium

G. Cholesterol

H. Uremic frost

I. Urea

J. Menstruation

K. Renal osteodystrophy

XVI. Match the description of function on the left with the most appropriate function of the urinary system on the right. Some functions may be used more than once, and some may not be used.

___ 1. Maintain fluid balance

___ 2. Elimination of urine

___ 3. Stimulation of red blood cell production

___ 4. Formation of urine

___ 5. Secretion of renin

A. Hormonal

B. Regulatory

C. Excretory

XVII. Complete the statements on the left with the most appropriate term on the right. Some terms may be used more than once, and some terms may not be used.

___ 1. _____ is the passage of molecules through a semipermeable membrane into a special solution.

___ 2. A "_____" is a rippling sensation palpable on the venous side of the cannula or fistula.

___ 3. For temporary peritoneal dialysis, a _____ is used to insert a catheter into the peritoneal cavity through the abdominal wall.

___ 4. Vascular access for hemodialysis may be accomplished by temporary catheter, cannula, graft, or _____.

___ 5. A process by which blood is removed from the body and circulated through an artificial kidney is called _____.

___ 6. The major complication of peritoneal dialysis is _____.

___ 7. Vascular access sites must be assessed for _____.

___ 8. _____ allows a patient to have dialysis performed at night by a machine, giving the patient freedom during the day and reducing the risk of infection.

___ 9. A rushing or roaring noise or "swoosh" heard through a stethoscope with each heartbeat is known as a _____.

___ 10. _____ allows the patient freedom from a machine and the independence to perform dialysis alone.

___ 11. The leading cause of death for hemodialysis patients is _____.

A. Thrill
B. Peritonitis
C. Atherosclerotic cardiovascular disease
D. Nausea
E. Dialysis
F. Bruit
G. Continuous ambulatory peritoneal dialysis
H. Hemodialysis
I. Murmur
J. Fistula
K. Patency
L. Trocar
M. Closed-cycle peritoneal dialysis

XVIII. Match the description on the left with the most appropriate process on the right. Some processes may be used more than once, and some may not be used.

___ 1. Process by which fluids, electrolytes, and some nonelectrolytes are filtered out of the blood

___ 2. Process by which most of the glomerular filtrate is returned to the blood

___ 3. Process involving diffusion and active transport that maintains normal fluid balance

___ 4. The kidney's acid-base regulating mechanism

A. Tubular reabsorption
B. Glomerular filtration
C. Tubular secretion
D. Glomerular secretion

XIX. Match the definition or description on the left with the most appropriate term on the right. Some terms may be used more than once, and some may not be used.

____ 1. Large urine output

____ 2. Low or scanty urine output

____ 3. Absence of urine output

____ 4. Presence of blood in urine

____ 5. Painful urination

____ 6. Involuntary loss of urine

A. Oliguria

B. Incontinence

C. Dysuria

D. Cystitis

E. Hematuria

F. Polyuria

G. Anuria

XX. Match the description on the left with the most appropriate diagnostic test on the right. Some tests may be used more than once, and some may not be used.

____ 1. Examination of voided or catheterized urine specimen for pH, blood, glucose, and protein

____ 2. Clean-catch or midstream urine specimen is collected to determine which antibiotics will be effective against the specific organisms found in the culture

____ 3. Collection of urine for 12 or 24 hours, which is an estimate of the glomerular filtration rate

____ 4. A blood test that is a general indicator of the kidneys' ability to excrete urea

____ 5. A blood test that is indicative of the kidney's ability to excrete wastes

____ 6. A blood test that may show elevated sodium and potassium levels and decreased calcium levels, which indicates renal failure

A. Creatinine clearance

B. Osmolality

C. Serum creatinine

D. Urinalysis

E. Serum electrolytes

F. Blood urea nitrogen (BUN)

G. Urine sensitivity

XXI. Match the description of pain on the left with the location of pain on the right. Some locations may be used more than once, and some may not be used.

____ 1. Dull flank pain

____ 2. Excruciating, abdominal pain that radiates to the groin or perineum

A. Calculus in urethra

B. Calculus in renal pelvis

C. Calculus in ureter

Introductory Nursing Care of Adults
Copyright © 1995 by W.B. Saunders Company. All rights reserved.

XXII. Complete the statements on the left with the most appropriate term on the right. The questions all refer to nursing interventions for patients who have just returned from angiography. Some terms may be used more than once, and some may not be used.

____ 1. Assess for signs of blood loss; look for restlessness, tachycardia, decreasing urine output and _____.

____ 2. The catheter site is assessed for _____ .

____ 3. For the first several hours, a sandbag or ice bag may be ordered for the _____ .

____ 4. Peripheral pulses, color of the extremity, and temperature are frequently monitored on _____ .

____ 5. Complaints from the patient that need to be reported to the physician immediately if they occur, as they may be signs of bleeding, are _____ .

____ 6. For 12 to 24 hours after the procedure, the activity of the patient will probably be _____.

A. the side of the arterial puncture

B. hypotension

C. bleeding or hematoma

D. Insertion site

E. bedrest

F. decreased

G. early ambulation

H. hypertension

I. increased

J. abdominal or flank pain

K. headaches

XXIII. Match the characteristics of acute renal failure on the left with the stage in which they occur on the right. Some stages may be used more than once.

____ 1. Urine output exceeds 400 ml per day and may rise above 4 liters per day

____ 2. Serum electrolytes, BUN, and creatinine return to normal

____ 3. Urine specific gravity becomes fixed at 1.010

____ 4. Primary treatment goal is reversal of failing renal function to prevent further damage

____ 5. Urine output decreased to 400 ml per day or less

____ 6. Lasts 1 to 12 months

____ 7. Lasts up to 14 days

____ 8. Few waste products are excreted despite the production of large quantities of urine

____ 9. Lasts 1 to 3 days

A. Onset stage

B. Oliguric stage

C. Diuretic stage

D. Recovery stage

XXIV. Match the drugs used to treat acute renal failure on the left with the specific condition treated by the drug on the right.

____ 1. Hypertonic glucose and insulin

____ 2. Furosemide (Lasix)

____ 3. Sodium bicarbonate

____ 4. Calcium gluconate

____ 5. Ethacrynic acid (Edecrin)

____ 6. Sodium polystyrene sulfonate (Kayexalate)

A. Oliguria

B. Hyperkalemia

XXV. Match the nursing diagnoses for the patient with chronic renal failure with the most appropriate "related to" statement on the right.

____ 1. Altered nutrition: less than body requirements

____ 2. Constipation

____ 3. Self-care deficit

____ 4. Altered role performance

____ 5. Ineffective individual coping

____ 6. High risk for infection

____ 7. Diarrhea

____ 8. Sensory perceptual alterations

____ 9. High risk for injury

A. Effects of uremia on the nervous system

B. Multiple life changes

C. Inability to fulfill usual roles and responsibilities

D. Impaired immune response, malnutrition, break in skin integrity

E. Anorexia, nausea, vomiting, stomatitis, dietary restrictions

F. Electrolyte imbalances, drug side effects

G. Coagulation disorder, impaired wound healing, bone demineralization, peripheral neuropathy

H. Inactivity, drug side effects, fluid restriction, electrolyte imbalances

I. Lack of knowledge, confusion, anemia, fatigue

XXVI. Fill in the blanks.

1. The removal of a calculus from the ureter is called _____.

2. The term used when the kidneys are unable to maintain fluid and electrolyte or acid-base balance is called

_____.

3. An agent that reduces immune responses is called a(n) _____.

4. The passage of molecules through a semipermeable membrane into a special solution is called

_____.

XXVII. List 2 reasons why women have more bladder infections than men.

1.

2.

XXVIII. List 6 substances other than electrolytes that are found in the glomerular filtrate.

1.   4.

2.   5.

3.   6.

XXIX. List the 7 main components of urine.

1.   5.

2.   6.

3.   7.

4.

XXX. List 6 factors that affect the average daily urine output.

1.   4.

2.   5.

3.   6.

XXXI. Describe the age-related changes in the kidneys that occur with respect to the areas listed below.

1. Function of kidneys:

2. Adaptation of kidneys under stress:

3. Number of nephrons:

4. Renal blood vessels:

5. Renal blood flow:

6. Glomerular filtration:

7. Plasma renin and aldosterone levels:

8. Antidiuretic hormone effect on tubules:

9. Kidney's ability to concentrate and dilute urine:

10. Creatinine clearance:

11. Renal threshold for glucose:

12. Incidence of nocturia:

XXXII. Describe the age-related changes of the bladder that occur with respect to the areas listed below.

1. Bladder muscles:

2. Connective tissue in the bladder:

3. Capacity of bladder:

4. Emptying function of bladder:

5. Prevention of reflux of urine from the bladder into the ureters:

6. Incontinence:

XXXIII. List 2 major causes of female urinary incontinence.

1.

2.

XXXIV. List 4 characteristics of urine that should be recorded.

1.

2.

3.

4.

XXXV. List 8 characteristics of urine that are examined during urinalysis.

1.

2.

3.

4.

5.

6.

7.

8.

XXXVI. Describe what the following colors of urine may indicate in patients with urinary disorders.

1. Straw-colored:

2. Bright red:

3. Tea-colored:

4. Cloudy or smoky appearance:

5. Colorless urine:

XXXVII. List 9 drugs that may increase the blood urea nitrogen.

1.   6.

2.   7.

3.   8.

4.   9.

5.

XXXVIII. Before an IVP, the nurse asks the patient about iodine allergy and informs the radiologist if the patient is allergic to iodine; list 2 effects of dye injection that the nurse should explain to the patient before the procedure.

1.

2.

XXXIX. List 4 symptoms of an allergic reaction to iodine dye.

1.

2.

3.

4.

XL. List 4 signs of blood loss for which the nurse observes when a patient with kidney disease returns from undergoing angiography.

1.

2.

3.

4.

XLI. List 4 signs following renal biopsy that, if observed, must be reported to the physician immediately because they may indicate significant bleeding.

1.

2.

3.

4.

XLII. List 4 common symptoms postcystoscopy patients may experience that can be relieved by warm sitz baths and mild analgesics.

1.

2.

3.

4.

XLIII. List 7 types of drugs that are commonly used following urologic surgery.

1.   5.

2.   6.

3.   7.

4.

XLIV. List 2 reasons why males have fewer UTIs than females.

1.

2.

XLV. List 4 types of drugs used in the medical management of pyelonephritis.

1.   3.

2.   4.

XLVI. Describe the findings that the nurse expects to find in patients with glomerulonephritis related to the following areas.

1. BUN:

2. Serum creatinine:

3. Color of urine:

4. Urine output:

5. Edema:

6. Blood pressure:

7. Glomerular filtration:

8. Blood volume:

9. Red blood cells:

XLVII. List 4 factors that influence the development of renal calculi.

1.

2.

3.

4.

XLVIII. List 5 substances that are known to be toxic to the kidney and may lead to renal failure.

1.

2.

3.

4.

5.

IL. List 5 nursing diagnoses for patients in acute renal failure.

1.

2.

3.

4.

5.

L. List the 3 most common causes of uremia.

1.

2.

3.

LI. Choose the most appropriate answer.

1. Glomerular filtrate and blood plasma are essentially the same except that the filtrate does not have:
   A. water
   B. sodium
   C. potassium
   D. proteins

2. As the blood passes through the glomerulus, which of the following is too large to pass through the semipermeable membrane?
   A. serum sodium
   B. serum potassium
   C. plasma protein
   D. glucose

3. The normal pH of urine is:
   A. 1.0–3.0
   B. 4.0–7.0
   C. 7.5–9.0
   D. 10.0–13.0

4. The body normally excretes how many liters of urine per day?
   A. 0.5 liter
   B. 1 to 2 liters
   C. 5 liters
   D. 7 to 10 liters

5. Two substances that are present in blood but not normally present in urine are:
   A. sodium and chloride
   B. glucose and proteins
   C. calcium and magnesium
   D. potassium and bicarbonates

6. Glomerular damage may be indicated by the presence of which of the following in the urine?
   A. sodium
   B. chloride
   C. proteins
   D. potassium

7. The presence of how much urine usually causes the urge to micturate?
   A. 100–150 ml
   B. 300–400 ml
   C. 500–600 ml
   D. 800–1000 ml

8. Voiding is primarily controlled by:
   A. involuntary reflex
   B. voluntary muscles
   C. peristalsis
   D. tubular secretion

9. A hormone that helps maintain normal serum calcium and phosphate levels is:
   A. antidiuretic hormone
   B. epinephrine
   C. parathormone
   D. aldosterone

10. Blood pressure is regulated through fluid volume maintenance and release of the hormone:
    A. aldosterone
    B. renin
    C. antidiuretic hormone
    D. parathormone

11. A change in blood volume will result in a change in:
    A. body temperature
    B. heart rate
    C. blood pressure
    D. respiratory rate

12. Decreased oxygen in renal blood triggers the secretion of:
    A. aldosterone
    B. antidiuretic hormone
    C. epinephrine
    D. erythropoietin

13. Patients in renal failure have a deficiency of erythropoietin, which causes them to have:
    A. pneumonia
    B. anemia
    C. seizures
    D. hypertension

14. A common problem in males related to the urinary system is:
    A. urethral obstruction
    B. incontinence
    C. relaxed pelvic musculature
    D. lack of testosterone

15. If crystals on the skin are observed during the examination of patients with urinary disorders, this is recorded as:
    A. ashen skin
    B. edema
    C. uremic frost
    D. scaly skin

16. Tissue turgor is evaluated in patients with urinary disorders to detect:
    A. uremic frost
    B. Kussmaul's respirations
    C. infection
    D. dehydration

17. The eyes of patients with urinary disorders are examined for periorbital edema, the presence of which suggests:
    A. dehydration
    B. fluid retention
    C. uremic frost
    D. Kussmaul's respirations

18. If patients with urinary disorders have dyspnea, this may be a sign of:
    A. dehydration
    B. uremic frost
    C. potassium imbalance
    D. fluid overload

19. If patients with urinary disorders have an odor of urine on their breath, this may indicate:
    A. urinary tract infection
    B. kidney failure
    C. cardiac failure
    D. pneumonia

20. Patients with urinary disorders who have potassium imbalances may have:
    A. uremic frost
    B. heart irregularities
    C. hypertension
    D. rapid respirations

21. Swishing sounds caused by the turbulence of blood are called:
    A. bruits
    B. uremic frost
    C. crackles
    D. rhonchi

22. An indication of renal artery stenosis (narrowing) is:
    A. urinary tract infection
    B. crackles
    C. bruits
    D. uremic frost

23. The edema found in renal failure is described as:
    A. dependent
    B. peripheral
    C. pitting
    D. generalized

24. In patients with renal failure, the skin over edematous areas is apt to be described as:
    A. warm and moist
    B. dry and flushed
    C. pink and intact
    D. pale and thick

25. Inspection of the genitalia during the examination of patients with urinary disorders must always be done utilizing:
    A. auscultation
    B. palpation
    C. universal precautions
    D. aseptic technique

26. Normal urine is:
    A. bright red
    B. straw-colored
    C. tea-colored
    D. smoke-colored

27. Urine with a cloudy appearance may be indicative of:
    A. bacterial infection
    B. excessive fluid intake
    C. dehydration
    D. diabetes mellitus

28. Normally, urine is sterile and slightly:
    A. alkaline
    B. acidic
    C. pyuric
    D. hematuric

29. A diagnostic test for the identification of microorganisms present in urine is:
    A. blood urea nitrogen
    B. urinalysis
    C. urine culture
    D. creatinine clearance

30. The best test of overall kidney function, which is an estimate of glomerular filtration rate, is:
    A. blood urea nitrogen
    B. urinalysis
    C. urine culture
    D. creatinine clearance

31. What blood tests need to be within normal limits before a renal biopsy is performed?
    A. electrolytes
    B. BUN
    C. serum creatinine
    D. clotting studies

32. After a renal biopsy, what is the most important assessment to make?
    A. infection
    B. dyspnea
    C. bleeding
    D. fatigue

33. Following cystoscopy, at first the color of the urine will be:
    A. colorless
    B. pink-tinged
    C. tea-colored
    D. orange

34. Following cystoscopy, urine should lighten to its usual color within:
    A. 4 to 6 hours
    B. 8 to 10 hours
    C. 24 to 48 hours
    D. 60 to 72 hours

35. Following cystoscopy, belladonna and opium suppositories may be ordered to reduce:
    A. bladder spasm
    B. hematuria
    C. infection
    D. tachycardia

36. Bladder perforation is rare following cystoscopy, but it may be indicated by severe:
    A. hematuria
    B. abdominal pain
    C. tachycardia
    D. hypotension

37. The major concern with catheterization is the potential for:
    A. hemorrhage
    B. shock
    C. kidney failure
    D. infection

38. To measure residual volume, the patient must be catheterized immediately after voiding; which of the following is an abnormal finding?
    A. 5 ml
    B. 10 ml
    C. 25 ml
    D. 75 ml

39. Following urologic surgery, which of the following outputs should be reported to the physician?
    A. less than 30 ml/hour
    B. less than 50 ml/hour
    C. less than 70 ml/hour
    D. less than 100 ml/hour

40. The most common nosocomial infections are:
    A. skin infections
    B. wound infections
    C. urinary tract infections
    D. blood infections

41. Most urinary tract infections are caused by:
    A. viruses
    B. bacteria
    C. yeasts
    D. fungi

42. Dysuria, frequency, urgency, and bladder spasms are common symptoms of:
    A. pyelonephritis
    B. kidney failure
    C. vaginitis
    D. urethritis

43. The medical treatment for cystitis is:
    A. antibiotics
    B. antihypertensives
    C. antihistamines
    D. diuretics

44. The pain of urethritis may be reduced by:
    A. antiemetics
    B. back massage
    C. sitz baths
    D. bubble baths

45. A common symptom of pyelonephritis is:
    A. polyuria
    B. hypotension
    C. bradycardia
    D. flank pain

46. When forcing fluids on patients with pyelonephritis, the nurse needs to be careful to prevent:
    A. infection
    B. hemorrhage
    C. kidney failure
    D. circulatory overload

47. An elderly patient with pyelonephritis who experiences a suddenly increased fluid volume may develop:
    A. hypotension
    B. congestive heart failure
    C. seizures
    D. thrombophlebitis

48. The most common type of glomerulonephritis follows a respiratory tract infection caused by:
    A. staphylococcus
    B. virus
    C. fungus
    D. streptococcus

49. In addition to antibiotics, acute glomerulonephritis is treated medically with:
    A. diuretics and antihypertensives
    B. antihistamines and antiemetics
    C. anticholinergics and analgesics
    D. narcotics and anticonvulsants

50. In the acute phase of glomerulonephritis, bedrest is ordered to prevent or treat heart failure and severe hypertension that result from:
    A. fluid volume deficit
    B. fluid overload
    C. altered tissue perfusion
    D. respiratory distress

51. A common nursing diagnosis for patients with acute glomerulonephritis is:
    A. fluid volume deficit
    B. fluid volume excess
    C. altered tissue perfusion
    D. high risk for injury

52. A consistent fluid intake of less than 1500 ml per day may contribute to:
    A. renal calculi
    B. hypertension
    C. tachycardia
    D. pneumonia

53. When a person is dehydrated, the kidneys conserve water, causing urine to be:
    A. dilute
    B. cloudy
    C. alkaline
    D. concentrated

54. A diet that can contribute to calculus formation is one which is high in purines and:
    A. sodium
    B. potassium
    C. calcium
    D. fats

55. In order to prevent renal calculi, the nurse should teach patients to have:
    A. a high-calcium diet
    B. a high-purine diet
    C. a high fluid intake
    D. limited physical activity

56. A major nursing concern for patients with renal calculi is:
    A. frequent ambulation
    B. emotional support
    C. range of motion exercises
    D. pain relief

57. The most frequent indication of urologic trauma is:
    A. pyuria
    B. dysuria
    C. oliguria
    D. hematuria

58. The treatment of choice for renal cancer is:
    A. lithotripsy
    B. radical nephrectomy
    C. cystectomy
    D. nephrostomy

59. The location of the flank incision following nephrectomy causes pain with expansion of the:
    A. abdomen
    B. pelvis
    C. cerebrum
    D. thorax

60. When patients following nephrectomy protect the chest by not breathing deeply, this leads to the development of:
    A. hemorrhage
    B. infection
    C. atelectasis
    D. shock

61. The most common malignancy of the urinary tract is:
    A. cancer of the kidney
    B. cervical cancer
    C. bladder cancer
    D. liver cancer

Introductory Nursing Care of Adults

62. The most frequent symptom of bladder cancer is intermittent:
    A. glycosuria
    B. proteinuria
    C. pyuria
    D. hematuria

63. When the bladder is removed completely, urinary diversion is sometimes provided, which allows urine to be excreted through the:
    A. urethra
    B. ileal conduit
    C. ureter
    D. cystoscopy

64. Preoperative care for an ileal or sigmoid conduit includes thorough preparation of the intestinal tract, which includes administration of an antibiotic that is not absorbed from the intestinal tract, called:
    A. Keflex
    B. penicillin
    C. neomycin
    D. tetracycline

65. An effective means of assessing changes in fluid status of patients in acute renal failure is:
    A. monitoring edema
    B. recording intake and output
    C. daily weights
    D. vital signs

66. When 90 to 95% of kidney function is lost, the patient is considered to be in:
    A. acute renal failure
    B. chronic renal failure
    C. renal shock
    D. renal oliguria

67. The most life-threatening effect of renal failure is:
    A. hypernatremia
    B. hyponatremia
    C. hyperkalemia
    D. hypokalemia

68. When a kidney is obtained from a living related donor, the 1-year survival rate for transplantation is about:
    A. 30–33%
    B. 65–70%
    C. 75–80%
    D. 95–97%

69. To control the body's response to foreign tissue, the transplant recipient is given:
    A. analgesics
    B. immunosuppressants
    C. anticholinergics
    D. antihistamines

70. Specific nursing diagnoses related to possibility of organ rejection after renal transplantation may include:
    A. high risk for injury
    B. altered role performance
    C. anxiety
    D. diarrhea

71. Signs of dehydration in the patient who has had a renal transplant may include thready pulse, poor tissue turgor, and:
    A. low blood pressure
    B. high blood pressure
    C. high fever
    D. abnormally low body temperature

LII.   In Figure 36–1 below, label the parts (A–J) of the urinary system.

A.

B.

C.

D.

E.

F.

G.

H.

I.

J.

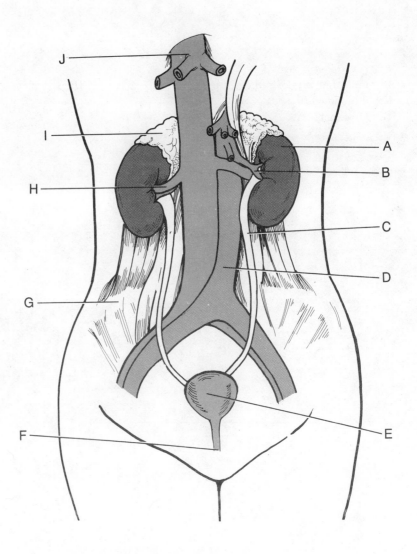

Introductory Nursing Care of Adults

Connective Tissue Disorders

OBJECTIVES

1. Define connective tissue.
2. Describe the function of connective tissue.
3. Describe the characteristics and prevalence of connective tissue diseases.
4. Describe the diagnostic tests and procedures used for assessing diseases of connective tissue.
5. Discuss the drugs indicated for treatment of patients with connective tissue diseases.
6. Describe the pathologic basis for osteoarthritis (degenerative joint disease); rheumatoid arthritis; osteoporosis; gout; systemic lupus erythematosus; progressive systemic sclerosis; polymyositis; periarteritis nodosa; ankylosing spondylitis; polymyalgia rheumatica; Reiter's syndrome; Behçet's syndrome; and Sjögren's syndrome.
7. Identify the data to be collected in the nursing assessment of a patient with a connective tissue disorder.
8. Utilizing the nursing process, formulate a plan of care for a patient whose life has been affected by a connective tissue disease.

LEARNING ACTIVITIES

I. Match the definition on the left with the most appropriate term on the right.

____ 1. Instrument used to measure joint range of motion

____ 2. Around the joint

____ 3. Elevated level of uric acid in the blood

____ 4. Muscle pain

____ 5. Deposit of sodium urate crystals under the skin

____ 6. Protrusions of the distal interphalangeal finger joints; associated with osteoarthritis

____ 7. Enlarged proximal interphalangeal joints of the fingers

____ 8. Pain in a joint

____ 9. Circular, scaly lesions with erythematous raised rim; occurs over scalp, ears, face, and areas exposed to sun

____ 10. Plastic repair of a joint

____ 11. Inflammation of blood vessels

____ 12. Crackling sound or sensation

____ 13. Joint immobility

A. Hyperuricemia

B. Ankylosis

C. Arthralgia

D. Tophus

E. Vasculitis

F. Periarticular

G. Heberden's nodes

H. Crepitus

I. Goniometer

J. Myalgia

K. Discoid lupus

L. Bouchard's nodes

M. Arthroplasty

II. Complete the statements on the left with the most appropriate term on the right. Some terms may be used more than once, and some terms may not be used.

____ 1. Sacs of synovial fluid found in joints that promote smooth articulations of joint structures are _____.

____ 2. The site at which two or more bones are joined is called a _____.

____ 3. Joints that allow no movement at all are called _____.

____ 4. Joints that are slightly movable are _____.

____ 5. Bone, blood, cartilage, ligaments, skin, and tendons are called _____.

____ 6. The hard tissue that makes up most of the skeletal system is _____.

____ 7. Synovial joints are _____.

____ 8. A very smooth membrane, permitting structures to move without friction, is _____.

____ 9. Tough, fibrous cords that bind the joint capsule are called _____.

____ 10. The covering at the end of bones that serves as a shock absorber is _____.

____ 11. Joints that are freely movable are _____.

____ 12. The substance that fills and lubricates the space in the middle of the joint is _____.

A. Ligaments

B. Amphiarthrotic

C. Synovial joints

D. Joint

E. Cartilage

F. Connective tissues

G. Diarthrotic

H. Bone

I. Bursae

J. Synovial fluid

K. Synarthrotic

L. Tendons

M. Synovial membrane

III. Complete the statements on the left with the most appropriate term on the right. Some terms may be used more than once, and some terms may not be used.

____ 1. A liquid type of connective tissue is _____.

____ 2. A specialized fibrous connective tissue that provides firm but flexible support for the embryonic skeleton and part of the adult skeleton is _____.

____ 3. Strong, flexible fibrous bands of connective tissue that connect bones and serve as support for muscles are _____.

____ 4. The largest organ of the body is the _____.

____ 5. The main function of skin is _____.

____ 6. The outermost, nonvascular layer of skin is the _____.

____ 7. The layer of skin composed of bundles of collagen fibers and elastic connective tissue that supports blood vessels, sweat glands, sebaceous glands, and hair follicles is the _____.

____ 8. Dense, fibrous tissues that anchor muscles firmly to bones are _____.

A. Dermis

B. Skin

C. Tendons

D. Cartilage

E. Collagen

F. Epidermis

G. Blood

H. Temperature regulation

I. Ligaments

J. Protection

Introductory Nursing Care of Adults

IV.   Complete the statements on the left with the most appropriate term on the right. Some terms may be used more than once, and some terms may not be used.

____ 1.   A device that is used after joint replacement surgery to move the joints through a set range of motions at a set rate of movements per minute is the _____.

____ 2.   The most common form of arthritis, which is also called degenerative joint disease, is _____.

____ 3.   The surgical treatment of choice for OA is _____.

____ 4.   Joint activities are compromised because the basic structure of the cartilage is altered in _____.

____ 5.   The primary indication for total joint replacement in patients with OA is _____.

____ 6.   A condition that generally affects joints under pressure (such as the spine and knees) is _____.

A.   Total joint replacement

B.   Physical therapy

C.   Continuous passive movement machine

D.   Osteoarthritis

E.   Ankylosing spondylitis

F.   Intractable pain

V.   Complete the statements on the left with the most appropriate term on the right. Some terms may be used more than once, and some terms may not be used.

____ 1.   The synovium thickens and fluid accumulates in the joint space of patients with _____.

____ 2.   A loss of joint mobility which occurs in RA is called _____.

____ 3.   Morning stiffness lasting more than 1 hour is a common symptom of _____.

____ 4.   If blood vessels are affected by RA, they become inflamed, a condition called _____.

____ 5.   Subcutaneous nodules over bony prominences, which are often present in RA, are called _____.

____ 6.   Aa chronic, progressive inflammatory disease is _____.

A.   Rheumatoid arthritis

B.   Osteoarthritis

C.   Rheumatoid nodules

D.   Systemic lupus erythematosus

E.   Vasculitis

F.   Polymyositis

G.   Ankylosis

VI. Complete the statements on the left with the most appropriate term on the right. Some terms may be used more than once, and some terms may not be used.

___ 1. A disease characterized by dry mouth, dry eyes, and dry vagina is called _____.

___ 2. An uncommonly seen disease that consists of enlarged liver and spleen and neutropenia is called _____.

___ 3. A disease marked by rheumatoid nodules in the lungs that occurs most often in coal miners and asbestos workers is called _____.

___ 4. A condition in which there is loss of bone mass, making the patient susceptible to fractures, is _____.

___ 5. Common sites of fractures due to osteoporosis are the wrist, vertebrae, and _____.

___ 6. Bone mass can be measured using a technique called _____.

___ 7. A systemic disease characterized by the deposition of urate crystals in the joints and other body tissues is _____.

___ 8. An excessive rate of uric acid production or decreased uric acid excretion by the kidneys results in _____.

___ 9. The joint commonly affected by gout is that of the _____.

___ 10. Deposits of sodium urate crystals under the skin that are seen in patients with gout are called _____.

___ 11. A diet low in _____ is recommended for patients with gout.

A. Caplan's syndrome
B. Absorptiometry
C. Great toe
D. Felty's syndrome
E. Periarteritis nodosa
F. Hyperuricemia
G. Purines
H. Hip
I. Systemic lupus erythematosus
J. Tophi
K. Sjögren's syndrome
L. Doppler ultrasound
M. Osteoporosis
N. Gout
O. Ankle
P. Milk and milk products

VII. Complete the statements on the left with the most appropriate term on the right. Some terms may be used more than once, and some terms may not be used.

____ 1. Decreased elasticity, stenosis, and occlusion of vessels are manifestations of _____.

____ 2. _____ is an inflammatory disease that primarily affects the vertebral column, causing spinal deformities.

____ 3. The management of Raynaud's phenomenon is aimed at elimination of anything that causes _____.

____ 4. A butterfly-shaped rash over the nose and cheeks is a common symptom of _____.

____ 5. Scleroderma may be brought into remission with high doses of immunosuppressants or _____.

____ 6. _____ is a condition characterized by inflammation and damage to blood vessels that is present in nearly all connective tissue diseases.

____ 7. A chronic, inflammatory disease of unknown cause, which is classified as an autoimmune disease, is _____.

____ 8. The primary symptom of polymyositis is _____.

____ 9. _____ is a disease that is a form of systemic necrotizing vasculitis.

____ 10. A chronic, multisystem disease that draws its name from the characteristic hardening of the skin is _____.

____ 11. Patients with scleroderma who have esophageal involvement may be given drugs to neutralize _____.

____ 12. A relatively rare inflammatory disease that primarily affects the skeletal muscle is _____.

____ 13. The antigout agent that inhibits the synthesis of uric acid is _____.

____ 14. _____ is the antigout agent that increases urinary excretion of uric acid.

A. Periarteritis nodosa

B. Furosemide (Lasix)

C. Muscle weakness

D. Probenecid (Benemid)

E. Systemic lupus

F. Polymyositis

G. Vasculitis

H. Steroids

I. Sjögren's syndrome

J. Progressive systemic sclerosis (scleroderma)

K. Ankylosing spondylitis

L. Antihypertensives

M. Gastric acid

N. Vasospasm

O. Allopurinol (Xyloprim)

P. Shoulder pain

VIII. Match the purpose or description on the left with the most diagnostic test on the right. Some tests may be used more than once, and some may not be used.

____ 1. Results of this test are elevated in any inflammatory process, especially RA.

____ 2. Detection of blood dyscrasias; differentiation of anemias, leukemia; decreased in RA and SLE.

____ 3. Increased in infection, tissue necrosis, and inflammation; sometimes decreased in SLE.

____ 4. Determines the presence of antibodies; present in about 80% of persons with RA.

____ 5. Assesses renal function; elevated in SLE, scleroderma, and polyarteritis.

____ 6. Positive reading in active inflammation. Often positive for RA and SLE.

____ 7. Measures presence of antibodies that react with a variety of nuclear antibodies; positive in SLE, RA, scleroderma, Raynaud's disease, Sjögren's syndrome.

A. C-reactive protein

B. Rheumatoid factor (RF)

C. Erythrocyte sedimentation rate (ESR)

D. White blood cell count (WBC)

E. Antinuclear antibodies (ANA)

F. Red blood cell count (RBC)

G. Platelet count

H. Creatinine

IX. Match the purpose or description on the left with the most appropriate radiologic test on the right. Some tests may be used more than once, and some may not be used.

____ 1. Intravenous radioactive material that is taken up by bone is injected for visualization of entire skeletal system. Procedure detects malignancies, osteoporosis, osteomyelitis, and some fractures.

____ 2. Determines density, texture, and alignments of bone; assesses soft tissue involvement.

____ 3. Scans the soft tissues and bones by use of both x-rays and computers. Determines presence of tumors or some spinal fractures.

____ 4. Examines soft tissue joint structures. Performed most commonly on shoulder or knee when a traumatic injury is suspected and determines presence of bone chips, torn ligaments or other loose bodies.

____ 5. Contrast medium injected directly into vertebral disk being examined.

____ 6. Visualization of soft tissue produced by sound waves.

____ 7. A noninvasive procedure that makes use of magnetic energy sources to view soft tissue.

A. Ultrasound

B. Magnetic resonance imaging (MRI)

C. Radiographs

D. Diskogram

E. Bone scan

F. PET scan

G. Computed tomography (CT) scan

H. Arthrogram

X. Match the purpose or description on the left with the most appropriate test on the right. Some tests may be used more than once, and some may not be used.

___ 1. Needle aspiration of synovial fluid from within joint cavity or to remove excess fluid. Local anesthesia is used. Procedure is useful in diagnosis of joint inflammation.

___ 2. Confirms inflammatory connective tissue diseases such as SLE or scleroderma.

___ 3. A surgical procedure performed in the operating room. Visualization of joint cavity and structure. Used as treatment to remove loose bodies and as diagnostic test by collecting fluid for biopsy.

___ 4. Procedure consists of microscopic examination of skeletal muscle obtained by surgical incision. Tissue reveals features of inflammatory reaction as in polymyositis.

A. Arthroscopy

B. Organ biopsy

C. Muscle biopsy

D. Skin biopsy

E. Joint aspiration

XI. List 4 functions of bones.

1.

2.

3.

4.

XII. List 2 functions of joints.

1.

2.

XIII. List 6 age-related joint changes.

1.

2.

3.

4.

5.

6.

XIV. List the results of age-related joint changes in the 3 areas below.

1. Mobility and movement:

2. Musculoskeletal injury:

3. Bone surfaces:

XV. List the changes that occur to the following 3 structures in patients with osteoarthritis.

1. Articular cartilage:

2. Underlying and adjacent bone:

3. Surrounding synovium:

XVI. List 6 signs and symptoms other than pain about which osteoarthritis patients may complain.

1.

2.

3.

4.

5.

6.

XVII. Impaired physical mobility can significantly interfere with the patient's ability to carry out usual activities in the home or work setting; list 10 modifications of daily activities and joint protection measures that the nurse should teach patients with osteoarthritis.

1.

2.

3.

4.

5.

6.

7.

8.

9.

10.

XVIII. Following joint replacement, the patient is taught to recognize signs and symptoms of dislocation; list 3 signs and symptoms of dislocation to teach the patient that should be reported to the physician if they are observed.

1.

3.

3.

XIX. When mobility is severely impaired following hip replacement surgery, list 4 complications for which the patient is at risk.

1.

2.

3.

4.

XX. List 5 signs and symptoms of deep vein thrombosis for which the nurse should observe in patients following joint replacement surgery.

1.   4.

2.   5.

3.

XXI. List 4 observations of the surgical wound that the nurse makes in order to assess the risk of infection after joint replacement surgery.

1.   3.

2.   4.

XXII. List risk factors for osteoporosis related to the 5 areas below.

1. Physical characteristics:

2. Surgical history:

3. Dietary factors:

4. Substance use/abuse:

5. Activity:

XXIII. List 5 characteristics of gout.

1.   4.

2.   5.

3.

XXIV. List 6 factors to assess in patients with gout.

1.   4.

2.   5.

3.   6.

XXV. List 4 signs and symptoms that patients with gout should be advised to report to the physician promptly because they may indicate kidney stones.

1.   3.

2.   4.

XXVI. List the 2 overall goals of treatment for gout.

1.

2.

XXVII. Choose the most appropriate answer.

1. The extracellular compartments and components of the body that provide the body's structure and support are called:
   A. thrombocytes
   B. connective tissues
   C. cytoplasm
   D. mitochondria

2. The only bone in the human body that does not articulate with at least one other bone is the:
   A. humerus
   B. hyoid
   C. mandible
   D. femur

3. What type of joints are found in the skull?
   A. synarthrotic
   B. diarthrotic
   C. amphiarthrotic
   D. synovial

4. The shoulder joint is:
   A. synarthrotic
   B. amphiarthrotic
   C. immovable
   D. diarthrotic

5. Important changes in the connective tissue of the body that occur with aging include loss of bone strength and:
   A. nutrients
   B. mass
   C. vitamins
   D. minerals

6. Which layer of the skin becomes thinner with age owing to decreased collagen?
   A. epidermis
   B. subcutaneous
   C. dermis
   D. epithelium

7. Which of the following connective tissue components remains unchanged with aging?
   A. joint capsule
   B. dermis
   C. bone
   D. blood volume

8. During the physical examination of persons with connective tissue disorders, what is assessed by asking the patient to move each extremity through the normal range of motion?
   A. joint pain and range of motion
   B. fever and tachycardia
   C. weight loss and nutritional deficiencies
   D. tachypnea and bone function

9. When assessing patients for joint pain and range of motion, the nurse watches for signs of pain and listens for the crackling sound called:
   A. bursitis
   B. grinding
   C. crepitus
   D. scraping

10. Besides a complete blood count, the routine blood studies for evaluation of musculoskeletal disorders should include the:
    A. prothrombin time
    B. BUN
    C. electrolytes
    D. erythrocyte sedimentation rate

11. Anti-inflammatory drugs used for musculoskeletal disorders include NSAIDs and:
    A. prednisone
    B. morphine
    C. furosemide
    D. digoxin

12. Following joint replacement surgery, a CPM machine may be used to prevent formation of scar tissue and promote:
    A. phagocytosis
    B. clotting
    C. flexibility
    D. circulation

13. Often the pain in osteoarthritis (OA) can be controlled with:
    A. beta blockers
    B. salicylates
    C. anticholinergics
    D. narcotics

14. Symptoms of salicylate toxicity in the elderly may be atypical; instead of the common symptoms of gastrointestinal complaints or ototoxicity, the older person may exhibit:
    A. drowsiness
    B. confusion
    C. malaise
    D. hypotension

15. A nursing diagnosis that patients with OA may have related to pain and limited range of motion is:
    A. knowledge deficit
    B. altered self-esteem
    C. altered tissue perfusion
    D. impaired physical mobility

16. Bathroom grab bars, a seat in the shower, and a raised toilet seat may promote independence and safety for the patient with poor:
A. shoulder mobility
B. ankle mobility
C. upper arm mobility
D. hip mobility

17. A nursing diagnosis following total joint replacement that is related to improper alignment, dislocated prosthesis, and/or weakness is:
A. altered peripheral tissue perfusion
B. high risk for injury
C. high risk for infection
D. knowledge deficit

18. Uncontrolled pain may make the patient reluctant to participate in rehabilitation measures following total joint replacement surgery; an intervention to improve patient participation is:
A. assess nerve and circulatory status before exercises
B. check vital signs at least every 4 hours
C. assist patient in and out of bed
D. administer analgesics 30 minutes to 1 hour before exercises

19. Prosthetic joints can become dislocated if they are not maintained in proper alignment; after hip replacement, the affected leg must be kept in a position of:
A. abduction
B. adduction
C. slight elevation
D. supination

20. Body areas distal to the operative joint are monitored for circulatory adequacy by assessing warmth, color, and:
A. peripheral pulses
B. ulceration
C. skin necrosis
D. wound drainage

21. Pillows and pads should not be placed under the legs of patients with joint replacements in order to reduce the risk of:
A. ulceration
B. gangrene
C. deep vein thrombosis
D. infection

22. A positive Homans's signs in patients who have had joint replacement surgery is indicative of:
A. wound infection
B. deep vein thrombosis
C. septicemia
D. cardiac shock

23. After joint replacement, the patient has altered tissue perfusion and is at risk for:
A. headache
B. hemorrhage
C. seizures
D. pneumonia

24. If a patient shows signs of cerebral blood vessel occlusion, headache, confusion, or loss of consciousness, the patient may have:
A. deep vein thrombosis
B. hemorrhage
C. fat embolus
D. neuropathy

25. Pressure caused by edema or constrictive dressings following joint replacement surgery can cause nerve damage, which may be manifested as:
A. paresthesia
B. infection
C. positive Homans's sign
D. hemorrhage

26. If the nurse suspects that a dressing is too tight and is causing nerve damage, the nurse monitors sensations:
A. at the wound site
B. proximal to the joint
C. distal to the joint
D. within the joint

27. A nursing intervention related to the patient's high risk for infection is that the nurse will:
A. place the call light in easy reach
B. instruct patient to keep legs slightly abducted
C. use strict sterile technique for dressing changes
D. assess nerve and circulatory status

28. Drugs that are administered to patients who have had joint replacements who are at risk for infection are:
A. antihistamines
B. antimicrobials
C. antiemetics
D. anticoagulants

29. A measure to control morning pain and stiffness in patients with RA is to:
A. take a warm shower
B. increase intake of fluids
C. eat foods low in purines
D. use aseptic technique

30. A factor that slows bone loss and improves strength, balance, and reaction time (reducing the risk of falls and fractures) is:
A. vitamin C
B. increased fluid intake
C. regular exercise
D. protein

31. Patients with gout may have altered urinary elimination related to:
    A. dehydration
    B. restricted fluid intake
    C. kidney stones
    D. edema

32. To prevent the complication of kidney stones in patients with gout, the patient is advised to:
    A. protect affected joints from trauma
    B. keep walking pathways lighted and free of obstacles
    C. obtain assistance with activities of daily living
    D. drink at least 8 glasses of fluid daily

33. The effects of SLE on specific body tissues include damage to the kidneys, heart, lungs, central nervous system, and:
    A. sternum
    B. mouth
    C. eyes
    D. joints

34. Polymyalgia rheumatica, Reiter's syndrome, Behçet's syndrome, and Sjögren's syndrome all involve:
    A. urinary tract disorders
    B. connective tissue disorders
    C. central nervous system disorders
    D. cardiac disorders

35. A patient with scleroderma may be unable to tolerate anything touching the affected skin during acute episodes of:
    A. SLE
    B. Raynaud's phenomenon
    C. syncope
    D. esophageal reflux

XXVIII. In Figure 37–1 below, label the major structures (A–H) of the normal synovial joint.

(Figure from Ignatavicius, D. D., & Bayne, M. V. [1991]. *Medical-surgical nursing: A nursing process approach* [p. 720]. Philadelphia: W. B. Saunders.)

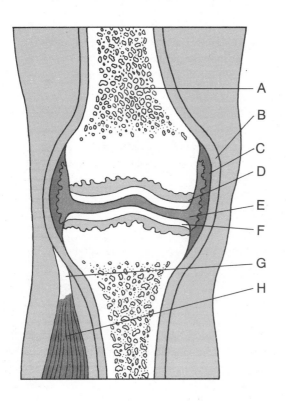

A.

B.

C.

D.

E.

F.

G.

H.

38

Fractures

OBJECTIVES

1. Identify the various types of fractures.
2. Describe the five stages of the healing process.
3. Discuss the major complications of a fracture, including infection, fat embolism, and compartment syndrome.
4. Compare the types of medical treatment for fractures, particularly reduction and fixation.
5. Describe common therapeutic measures for fractures, including casts, traction, crutches, walkers, and canes.
6. Discuss the nursing care of a patient with a fracture.
7. Describe specific types of fractures, specifically hip fracture, Colles' fracture, and pelvic fracture.

LEARNING ACTIVITIES

I. Match the definition on the left with the most appropriate term on the right.

____ 1. Condition in which fat globules are released from the marrow of the broken bone into the blood stream, migrate to the lungs, and cause pulmonary hypertension

____ 2. Fracture in which the broken bone does not break through the skin

____ 3. Fracture in which the fragments of the broken bone break through the skin

____ 4. Serious complication of a fracture caused by internal or external pressure to the affected area, resulting in decreased blood flow, pain, and tissue damage

____ 5. Failure of a fracture to heal

____ 6. Fracture in which the break extends across the entire bone, dividing it into two separate pieces

____ 7. Procedure done during the open reduction surgical procedure to attach the fragments of the broken bone together when reduction alone is not feasible

____ 8. Process of bringing the ends of the broken bone into proper alignment

A. Compartment syndrome

B. Open reduction

C. Fixation

D. Closed or simple fracture

E. Delayed union

F. Incomplete fracture

G. Fracture

H. Nonunion

I. Bone remodeling

J. Closed reduction or manipulation

K. Fat embolism

L. Complete fracture

M. Stress fracture

N. Open or compound fracture

O. Reduction

I. *Continues*

I. *Continues*

___ 9. Fracture in which the bone breaks only part way across, leaving some portion of the bone intact

___ 10. Non surgical realignment of the bones to their previous anatomic position using traction, angulation, or rotation, or a combination of these

___ 11. Surgical procedure in which an incision is made at the fracture site, usually on patients with open (compound) or comminuted fractures, to cleanse the area of fragments and debris

___ 12. Fracture caused by either sudden force or prolonged stress

___ 13. Process in which immature bone cells are gradually replaced by mature bone cells

___ 14. Fracture healing does not occur in the normally expected time

___ 15. Break or disruption in the continuity of a bone

A. Compartment syndrome
B. Open reduction
C. Fixation
D. Closed or simple fracture
E. Delayed union
F. Incomplete fracture
G. Fracture
H. Nonunion
I. Bone remodeling
J. Closed reduction or manipulation
K. Fat embolism
L. Complete fracture
M. Stress fracture
N. Open or compound fracture
O. Reduction

II. Complete the statements on the left with the most appropriate term on the right. Some terms may be used more than once, and some terms may not be used.

___ 1. Pins in the bone are attached to an external frame in _____.

___ 2. The first sign of a fat embolism is _____.

___ 3. _____ can cause irreversible muscle damage within 4 to 6 hours following fractures.

___ 4. A primary symptom of compartment syndrome is _____.

___ 5. The use of rods, pins, nails, screws, or metal plates to align bone fragments and keep them in place for healing is _____.

___ 6. A condition in which fat globules are released from the marrow of the broken bone is called _____.

___ 7. A fracture that occurs because of a pathologic condition in the bone, such as a tumor or disease process that causes a spontaneous break, is called _____.

___ 8. The goal of treatment for compartment syndrome is to relieve _____.

___ 9. Infections associated with fractures result from indwelling hardware used to repair the broken bone or from _____.

___ 10. In deep, grossly contaminated fracture wounds, _____ is likely to develop.

___ 11. _____ is infection of the bone.

A. Internal fixation
B. Petechiae
C. Pathologic fracture
D. Respiratory distress
E. Pressure
F. Stress fracture
G. Pain
H. Gangrene
I. External fixation
J. Osteomyelitis
K. Fat embolism
L. Compartment syndrome
M. Wound contamination

III. Complete the statements on the left with the most appropriate term on the right. Some terms may be used more than once, and some terms may not be used.

___ 1. A cast used for breaks in the shoulder, arm, wrist, and hand is called a(n) _____.

___ 2. A cast used for breaks in the upper and lower leg, ankle, and foot is called a(n) _____.

___ 3. A(n) _____ encircles the trunk.

___ 4. A(n) _____ encases the trunk plus one or two extremities.

A. Body cast

B. Upper extremity cast

C. Leg cylinder cast

D. Spica cast

E. Lower extremity cast

IV. Complete the statements on the left with the most appropriate term on the right. Some terms may be used more than once, and some terms may not be used.

___ 1. A pulling force on a fractured extremity to proved alignment of the broken bone fragments is _____.

___ 2. Traction applied directly to a bone is called _____.

___ 3. Traction applied directly to the skin is called _____.

___ 4. A type of traction used for immobilization of fractures of the cervical vertebrae is called _____.

___ 5. A type of traction used for hip and knee contractures, muscle spasms, and alignment of hip fractures is called _____.

___ 6. Crutchfield's traction and halo vest are examples of _____.

___ 7. A type of traction in which tongs are inserted into either side of the skull is called _____.

___ 8. Buck's traction with a Velcro boot is an example of _____.

A. Plastic traction

B. Skin traction

C. Buck's traction

D. Contracture traction

E. Traction

F. Vest traction

G. Crutchfield's traction

H. Skeletal traction

V. Match the definition or description on the left with the most appropriate stage of healing on the right. Some stages may be used more than once, and some may not be used.

____ 1. Granulation tissue forms a collar around each end of the broken bone, gradually becoming firm

____ 2. Within 2 to 3 weeks after the break, a permanent bone callus forms; ends of the broken bone begin to "knit"

____ 3. Formation of a clot between the 2 broken ends of the bones in 48 to 72 hours

____ 4. The distance between bone fragments closes and immature bone cells are replaced by mature bone cells

____ 5. Formation of a temporary splint by the end of the first week; granulation tissue turns into formation of cartilage, osteoblasts, calcium, and phosphorus

A. Collar formation

B. Consolidation and remodeling

C. Callus formation

D. Cellular proliferation

E. Ossification

F. Hematoma formation

VI. Match the signs and symptoms of fracture on the right with the most appropriate cause on the left. Some causes may be used more than once, and some may not be used.

____ 1. Strong muscle pull may cause bone fragments to override

____ 2. Edema may appear rapidly from localization of serous fluid at the fracture site and extravasation of blood into adjacent tissues

____ 3. Caused by subcutaneous bleeding

____ 4. Involuntary muscle contraction near the fracture

____ 5. Occurs over fracture site due to underlying injuries

____ 6. Severe at the time of injury; following injury this symptom may result from muscle spasm or damage to adjacent structures

____ 7. Results from nerve damage

____ 8. Grating sensations or sounds felt or heard if the injured part is moved; results from broken bone ends rubbing together

____ 9. Results from blood loss or other injuries

A. Muscle spasm

B. Crepitus

C. Pain

D. Hypovolemic shock

E. Swelling

F. Impaired sensation (numbness)

G. Abnormal mobility

H. Bruising (ecchymosis)

I. Fever

J. Deformity

K. Tenderness

VII.   Match the proper positioning on the left with the fracture location on the right.

1. Before medical treatment, keep supine and immobilize neck; after treatment, turn with head well supported

A.   Pelvis

B.   Forearm/foreleg

____   2.   Avoid high sitting positions; logroll

C.   Cervical spine

____   3.   When fracture is stable or after fixation, turn to side opposite fracture

D.   Lumbar spine

E.   Shoulder/humerus

____   4.   Elevate head of bed to comfort; turn to side opposite fracture

____   5.   Elevate distal portion of extremity higher than heart

VIII.   List 5 risk factors for hip fractures.

1.

2.

3.

4.

5.

IX.   List 3 factors that affect healing.

1.

2.

3.

X.   List 4 causes of delayed union or nonunion.

1.

2.

3.

4.

XI.   List 3 goals of medical treatment for a fracture.

1.

2.

3.

XII.   List 4 complications of body or spica casts.

1.

2.

3.

4.

XIII. Concerning patient teaching for patients with casts, list 5 circumstances that patients should *avoid*.

1.

2.

3.

4.

5.

XIV. Choose the most appropriate answer.

1. In adults, the bones most commonly fractured are:
   A. femurs
   B. ribs
   C. pelvic bones
   D. wrists

2. In young and middle-aged adults, the most common fractures are fractures of the :
   A. femur
   B. ribs
   C. wrist
   D. pelvis

3. The most common fractures in the elderly are fractures of the wrist and:
   A. femur
   B. ribs
   C. hip
   D. shoulder

4. Which of the following is a characteristic of fat embolism following a fracture?
   A. bradycardia
   B. decreased respirations
   C. oliguria
   D. petechiae

5. The most common diagnostic test used first to reveal bone disruption, deformity, or malignancy following a fracture is:
   A. myelogram
   B. standard x-ray films
   C. ultrasonography
   D. bone scan

6. The use of rods, pins, nails, screws, or metal plates to align bone fragments is called:
   A. external fixation
   B. closed reduction
   C. internal fixation
   D. mechanical reduction

7. Which of the following is used for external fixation of extensive fractures and fractures of the extremities?
   A. casts
   B. rods
   C. pins
   D. metal plates

8. A condition in which a patient in a body cast may have feelings of claustrophobia is called:
   A. compartment syndrome
   B. cardiac shock
   C. cast syndrome
   D. fat embolus

9. After a fracture of the lower extremity, crutches are used to assist with ambulation and to increase:
   A. pain relief
   B. deep breathing
   C. mobility
   D. circulation

10. Crutch use requires good:
    A. lower extremity function
    B. cardiac function
    C. lung expansion
    D. upper body strength

11. When walking with crutches, the patient's weight should be put on the:
    A. top of the crutches
    B. hand grips
    C. lower extremities
    D. shoulders

12. The type of gait pattern used with bilateral lower extremity prostheses is called:
    A. four-point
    B. swing-to
    C. swing-through
    D. two-point

13. When climbing stairs, which body part goes up the step first while the body is supported by the crutches?
    A. unaffected leg
    B. affected leg
    C. upper extremities
    D. spine

14. Which gait is used with a walker?
    A. two-point
    B. four-point
    C. modified swing-to
    D. modified swing-through

15. Canes should be held close to the body on the:
    A. left side
    B. right side
    C. affected side
    D. unaffected side

16. When the nurse is assessing the patient with a fracture, the affected extremity is compared with the:
    A. proximal body parts
    B. distal body parts
    C. unaffected extremity
    D. normal skeleton

17. In order to assess circulation and sensation in the affected and unaffected extremity, the nurse should perform neurovascular checks in the areas:
    A. distal to the wound
    B. proximal to the wound
    C. surrounding the wound
    D. inside the wound

18. A good indication of circulation to the extremity in patients with a fracture is:
    A. size of wound
    B. edema
    C. skin color
    D. infection

19. If pallor is observed in the extremity of patients with fractures, this may be an indication of:
    A. infection
    B. poor circulation
    C. hemorrhage
    D. skin breakdown

20. The primary method of pain relief for patients with fractures is:
    A. application of cold to the affected part
    B. application of heat to the affected part
    C. wrapping the affected part with a blanket
    D. immobilization of the affected part

21. An appropriate intervention for patients with fractures who have impaired physical mobility is:
    A. strict aseptic technique
    B. monitor for fever
    C. isolation precautions
    D. gait training

22. An appropriate intervention for patients with fractures who have altered tissue perfusion is:
    A. strict aseptic technique
    B. gait training
    C. elevate affected part above the head
    D. rest periods to preserve strength

23. Patients with fractures are at high risk for impaired skin integrity; treatment measures such as casts or traction to immobilize parts may result in:
    A. pressure sores
    B. petechiae
    C. palmar erythema
    D. paralysis

24. For older patients with hip fractures, the treatment of choice is:
    A. immobilization
    B. antibiotic therapy
    C. surgical repair
    D. traction

25. Colles' fracture is a break in the distal:
    A. humerus
    B. tibia
    C. radius
    D. fibula

26. Colles' fractures frequently occur in older adults when they use their hands to:
    A. sew or knit
    B. break a fall
    C. write letters
    D. reach for objects above their heads

27. Interventions for Colles' fractures are aimed at relieving pain and preventing edema; for the first few days, the extremity should be:
    A. below the heart
    B. exercised
    C. elevated
    D. flat

28. Patients with Colles' fractures are encouraged to move their fingers and thumb to promote circulation and reduce:
    A. temperature
    B. swelling
    C. infection
    D. dyspnea

29. Patients with Colles' fractures are encouraged to move their shoulder to prevent:
    A. infection
    B. circulation
    C. cyanosis
    D. stiffness

30. The most common cause of pelvic fractures in young adults is:
    A. head injury
    B. motor vehicle accidents
    C. falls
    D. myocardial infarction

31. The main cause of pelvic fractures in older adults is:
    A. motor vehicle accidents
    B. head injury
    C. falls
    D. heart attacks

32. The nurse needs to observe the patient with a pelvic fracture closely for signs of:
    A. internal injury
    B. convulsions
    C. tachycardia
    D. dyspnea

33. Which of the following is restricted in patients with pelvic fractures until healing is complete?
    A. using trapeze in bed
    B. range of motion exercises
    C. cough and deep breathing exercises
    D. weight bearing

XV. In Figure 38–1 below, label each type of fracture (A–H) from the following list: closed, nondisplaced; comminuted (fragmented); displaced; greenstick; impacted; oblique; open (compound); spiral. (Figure from Ignatavicius, D. D., & Bayne, M. V. [1991]. *Medical-surgical nursing: A nursing process approach* [p. 781]. Philadelphia: W. B. Saunders.)

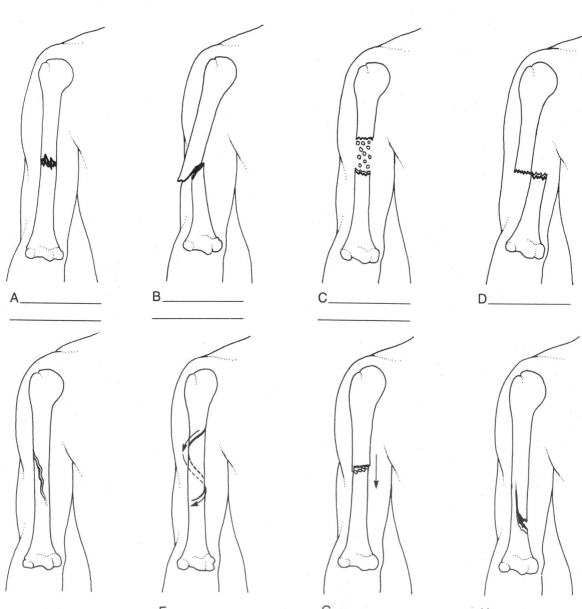

A_____
_____

B_____
_____

C_____

D_____

E_____

F_____

G_____

H_____

CHAPTER

39

Amputations

OBJECTIVES

1. Identify clinical indications for amputations.
2. Describe different types of amputations.
3. Discuss medical and surgical management of the amputation patient.
4. Identify appropriate nursing interventions during the preoperative and postoperative phases of care.
5. Use the nursing process to develop a plan of care for the amputation patient.

LEARNING ACTIVITIES

I.   Match the definition on the left with the most appropriate term on the right.

____ 1. Type of amputation in which a limb or portion of a limb is severed from the body and the wound is left open; a type of open amputation

____ 2. Amputation that is done over the course of several surgeries; usually done to control the spread of infection or necrosis

____ 3. Amputation in which a limb or part of a limb is removed and surgically closed

____ 4. Individual who has undergone an amputation

____ 5. Necrosis or death of tissue, usually due to a deficient or absent blood supply; may result from inflammatory processes, injury, arteriosclerosis, frostbite, or diabetes mellitus

____ 6. Deformity of absence of a limb or limbs occurring during fetal development in the uterus

____ 7. Illusion, following an amputation of a limb, that the limb still exists

____ 8. Amputation that is left open; usually done in cases of infection or necrosis

A.   Phantom limb

B.   Amputee

C.   Guillotine amputation

D.   Staged amputation

E.   Gangrene

F.   Open amputation

G.   Replantation

H.   Closed amputation

I.   Congenital amputation

J.   Stump

K.   Amputation

Continues

I.   *Continued*

___   9.   Refers to the distal portion of an amputated limb

___   10.   Removal of a limb, part of a limb, or an organ; may be done by surgical means or in an accident

___   11.   Surgical reattachment of an organ to its original site; reimplantation

A.   Phantom limb

B.   Amputee

C.   Guillotine amputation

D.   Staged amputation

E.   Gangrene

F.   Open amputation

G.   Replantation

H.   Closed amputation

I.   Congenital amputation

J.   Stump

K.   Amputation

II.   List 6 common types of accidents leading to amputation.

1.

2.

3.

4.

5.

6.

III.   Vascular diseases can lead to the need for amputation. List 3 examples of diseases leading to impaired circulation that may lead to the need for an amputation.

1.

2.

3.

IV.   Explain why vascular diseases may lead to the need for an amputation.

V.   Surgical management of the patient is aimed at performing an amputation at the lowest level that will still accomplish what 2 goals?

1.

2.

VI.   Two types of amputations are closed amputations and open amputations. List one reason for performing each.

1. Closed:

2. Open:

VII. List 8 complications associated with amputations.

1.   5.

2.   6.

3.   7.

4.   8.

VIII. In extremities with a diminished supply of blood, capillary refill should be reported to the physician if it takes how long?

IX. List (A) 3 nursing diagnoses, (B) 3 nursing goals, (C) 3 interventions, and (D) 3 criteria for evaluating care for the preoperative amputation patient.

A. <u>Nursing Diagnoses</u>   B. <u>Nursing Goals</u>

  1.   1.

  2.   2.

  3.   3.

C. <u>Nursing Interventions</u>   D. <u>Criteria for Evaluation</u>

  1.   1.

  2.   2.

  3.   3.

X. Priorities for the postoperative amputee patient are based on three distinct needs. List these 3 needs.

1.

2.

3.

XI. Explain why upper body training for a patient with a lower extremity amputation is important.

XII. List the 4 most common postoperative problems for patients with amputations.

1.   3.

2.   4.

XIII. List 2 causes of postoperative pain in the patient following amputation.

1.

2.

XIV. How many days must the nurse wait postoperatively to massage the stump to promote circulation?

XV. Related to impaired physical mobility that occurs in the postoperative amputation patient, an important goal is to prevent contractures. Contractures are most common in what 3 areas of the body?

1.

2.

3.

XVI. Patient instruction for stump care is extremely important. Describe teaching for each of the 8 topics listed below.

1. Stump:

2. Prosthetic socket and stump sock:

3. Shoes:

4. Lotions, ointments, and powders:

5. Prosthesis, if redness or irritation develops on the stump:

6. Size of stump:

7. Care of prosthesis:

8. Problems with prosthesis:

XVII. Explain why amputations above the wrist do not lend themselves as readily to replantation as do amputations of the hand and fingers.

XVIII. What is one essential aspect of nursing care after replantation, in addition to monitoring vital signs, intake and output, and level of consciousness?

XIX. List 5 areas of baseline documentation related to circulatory status that must be completed upon the patient's arrival to the unit following replantation surgery.

1.

2.

3.

4.

5.

XX. List findings in the 4 areas below that are signs of (A) arterial occlusion and (B) venous congestion following replantation.

	Arterial occlusion	Venous congestion
1. Color	A.	B.
2. Capillary refill	A.	B.
3. Appearance	A.	B.
4. Temperature	A.	B.

XXI. Explain why elevation of the limb is important following replantation.

XXII. Why are the following interventions recommended postoperatively following replantation?
Abstain from cigarette smoking 7–10 days postoperatively; abstain from caffeine for 7–10 days postoperatively; maintain room temperature at 80°F degrees; discourage tight or restrictive gowns.

XXIII. In the postoperative replantation patient, why is the limb not elevated above the level of the heart?

XXIV. The nurse should provide the postoperative replantation patient an opportunity to discuss thoughts and feelings about the replantation, disfigurement, and loss of function. List 3 ways the nurse can assist with this.

1.

2.

3.

XXV. Complete the statements on the left with the most appropriate term on the right. Some terms may be used more than once, and some terms may not be used.

____ 1. The removal of the lower leg at the middle of the shin is called a _____.

____ 2. Removal of part or all of a limb during a serious accident is called _____.

____ 3. Three conditions that lead to the need for an amputation include trauma, disease, and _____.

____ 4. An amputation through the joint is called _____.

A. Tumors

B. Open amputation

C. Traumatic amputation

D. Disarticulation

E. Below-knee amputation

XXVI. Match the indications on the left with the name of the appropriate diagnostic test relating to amputation on the right.

_____ 1. Record heat present to measure amount of blood flow to certain part of body

_____ 2. Amount of oxygen present at skin surface

_____ 3. Infection

_____ 4. Nature of tumor

_____ 5. Volume of blood flow to extremity

_____ 6. Pulses in extremities

_____ 7. Compromised circulation

A. Biopsy

B. Pulse volume recording (plethysmography)

C. Transcutaneous Doppler recordings (ultrasound)

D. WBC

E. Transcutaneous PO_2

F. Vascular studies (angiography)

G. Thermography

XXVII. Match postoperative nursing diagnoses of amputation patients on the left with the related conditions on the right.

_____ 1. Ineffective individual coping

_____ 2. Acute pain

_____ 3. Self-care deficit

_____ 4. Knowledge deficit

_____ 5. High risk for infection

_____ 6. Decreased cardiac output

_____ 7. Impaired skin integrity

_____ 8. Body image disturbance

_____ 9. Anxiety/fear

_____ 10. Activity intolerance

_____ 11. Impaired physical mobility

_____ 12. High risk for injury

_____ 13. Sensory-perceptual alteration

A. Blood loss

B. Surgical incision, scar formation on a severed nerve

C. Surgical wound

D. Loss of a body part

E. Postoperative procedures and therapy

F. Inability to carry out ADLs

G. Perceived threat of disability

H. Inadequate support system

I. Incision, decreased mobility, advanced age

J. Phantom limb

K. Loss of limb, weakness

L. Loss of limb

M. Prolonged bedrest, weakness

XXVIII. Match the postoperative goals on the right with the nursing diagnoses on the left.

____ 1. High risk for injury

____ 2. Ineffective individual coping

____ 3. Body image disturbance

____ 4. Impaired physical mobility

____ 5. Activity intolerance

____ 6. High risk for infection

____ 7. Impaired skin integrity

____ 8. Decreased cardiac output

____ 9. Knowledge deficit

____ 10. Self-care deficit

____ 11. Anxiety/fear

____ 12. Sensory-perceptual alteration

____ 13. Acute pain

A. Acceptance of altered body image

B. Well-healed wound

C. Reduced anxiety

D. Normal blood volume

E. Patient knowledge of procedures and therapies

F. Patient understanding of phantom limb sensation

G. Freedom from falls/injuries

H. Reduced pain

I. Absence of infection

J. Restored mobility

K. Adjustment to amputation

L. Performance of ADLs without fatigue

M. Patient self-care

XXIX. For each of the postoperative nursing diagnoses on the left, match the appropriate nursing intervention on the right.

____ 1. High risk for injury

____ 2. Decreased cardiac output

____ 3. Body image disturbance

____ 4. Impaired skin integrity

____ 5. Impaired physical mobility

____ 6. High risk for infection

____ 7. Pain

____ 8. Phantom limb sensation

A. Active and passive range of motion exercises; use of overbed trapeze, if indicated; prosthesis fitting

B. Check temperature; watch for foul or unpleasant odor from stump; check lab work (WBC)

C. Encourage patient to do exercises as ordered; keep environment free of clutter

D. Whirlpool, massage, or TENS stimulation of ordered

E. Check vital signs; observe for excessive bleeding

F. Administer analgesics as ordered

G. Wrap bandage smoothly; inspect stump for irritation and edema; elevate stump.

H. Encourage patient to talk about changes and effects of amputation

XXX. Match the evaluation criteria on the right with the nursing goals on the left relating to the postoperative patient.

____ 1. Acceptance of altered body image	A. Patient statement of reduced anxiety and calm demeanor
____ 2. Absence of infection	
____ 3. Adjustment to amputation	B. Patient statement of relief of phantom limb sensation
____ 4. Reduced pain	C. Normal pulse and blood pressure
____ 5. Well-healed wound	D. Absence of fever, purulent drainage, redness
____ 6. Normal blood volume	E. Patient statement of pain relief; relaxed expression
____ 7. Patient knowledge of procedures and therapies	F. Patient caring for stump without distress
____ 8. Freedom from falls	G. Patient demonstration of stump care and rehabilitation exercises
____ 9. Patient understanding of phantom limb sensation	H. Well-healed incision
	I. Freedom from injury

XXXI. Match the interventions on the right with characteristics of the elderly on the left.

____ 1. Elderly may have one or more chronic health problems.	A. Emphasize high-calorie and high-protein diet
____ 2. Elderly are sometimes easily distracted.	B. Remind them that phantom sensations are not unusual or bizarre
____ 3. Elderly may have decreased appetites and poor nutritional status.	C. Skip unnecessary details when teaching; make sure patients with glasses or hearing aids have them in place
____ 4. Elderly may feel foolish in describing phantom sensations.	D. Provide prosthesis with extra padding and support to patients for diabetes; recognize that poor vision and decreased sensation may keep the older person from recognizing complications

XXXII. Match the goal on the left with evaluation criteria on the right for postoperative replantation patients.

____ 1. Adjustment to appearance and function	A. Patient verbalization of microvascular precautions
____ 2. Adequate circulation in replanted limb	B. Patient statements reflecting acceptance of altered appearance or function
____ 3. Knowledge of therapeutic measures	C. Patient statement of pain relief
____ 4. Pain relief	D. Presence of warmth, normal skin color, and arterial pulses in replanted limb

XXXIII.   Choose the most appropriate answer.

1. The post-operative drainage from an amputation site should gradually:
   A. increase in amount and become lighter
   B. increase in amount and become darker
   C. decrease in amount and become lighter
   D. decrease in amount and become darker

2. The purpose of giving heparin to a postoperative replantation patient is to reduce the risk of:
   A. thrombosis
   B. edema
   C. infection
   D. hypersensitivity

3. A complication of amputation that is due to inadequate hemostasis and that involves bleeding into the tissue is called:
   A. necrosis
   B. hemorrhage
   C. gangrene
   D. contracture

4. A complication of amputation that is manifested by redness, warmth, swelling, and exudate formation at the stump site due to invasion of tissues by pathogens is called:
   A. contracture
   B. infection
   C. edema
   D. necrosis

5. Which of the following may be prevented by frequent position changes and range of motion exercises?
   A. infection
   B. hemorrhage
   C. necrosis
   D. contractures

6. Which of the following is an opening of the suture line (due to early removal of sutures or falling) that requires reclosure?
   A. gangrene
   B. necrosis
   C. wound dehiscence
   D. contracture

CHAPTER
40

Thyroid and Parathyroid Disorders

OBJECTIVES

1. Identify nursing assessment data related to the functions of the thyroid and parathyroid glands.
2. Describe tests and procedures used to diagnose disorders of the thyroid and parathyroid glands and identify nursing responsibilities relevant for each.
3. Describe the pathophysiology, signs and symptoms, complications, and treatment of hyperthyroidism, hypothyroidism, hyperparathyroidism, and hypoparathyroidism.
4. Develop nursing care plans for patients with disorders of the thyroid or parathyroid glands, including assessment, nursing diagnoses, goals, interventions, and evaluation criteria.

LEARNING ACTIVITIES

I.   Match the definition on the left with the most appropriate term on the right.

____ 1.   Facial edema that develops with severe, long-term hypothyroidism; sometimes used as a synonym for hypothyroidism

____ 2.   Carpopedal spasm following compression of the nerves in the upper arm; a sign of hypocalcemia

____ 3.   Enlargement of the thyroid gland, causing the neck to appear swollen

____ 4.   Steady muscle contraction; caused by hypocalcemia

____ 5.   Small mass of tissue that can be palpated

____ 6.   Spasmodic closure of the larynx

____ 7.   Permanent mental and physical retardation caused by congenital deficiency of thyroid hormones

____ 8.   Excessive metabolic stimulation caused by elevated thyroid hormone level

____ 9.   Spasm of the facial muscles when the facial nerve is tapped; indicative of hypocalcemia

____ 10. Inflammation of the parotid (salivary) gland

____ 11. Inflammation of the thyroid gland

____ 12. Substance that suppresses thyroid function

____ 13. Protrusion of the eyeballs associated with hyperthyroidism

A.   Goiter

B.   Goitrogen

C.   Exophthalmos

D.   Myxedema

E.   Nodule

F.   Cretinism

G.   Parotiditis

H.   Trousseau's sign

I.   Chvostek's sign

J.   Tetany

K.   Laryngospasm

L.   Thyroiditis

M.   Thyrotoxicosis

Introductory Nursing Care of Adults
Copyright © 1995 by W.B. Saunders Company. All rights reserved.

II. For each sign or symptom on the left, indicate whether it is characteristic of (A) hyperthyroidism or (B) hypothyroidism.

___ 1. Heat intolerance

___ 2. Apathy

___ 3. Increased appetite

___ 4. Tachycardia

___ 5. Cold intolerance

___ 6. Weight loss

___ 7. Anorexia

___ 8. Bradycardia

___ 9. Nervousness and restlessness

___ 10. Weight gain

A. Hyperthyroidism

B. Hypothyroidism

III. Fill in the blanks.

1. An important nursing diagnosis for the patient with exophthalmos is _____

_____.

2. Three actions of PTH include (1) increasing the absorption of calcium from the intestines, (2) transferring calcium from the bones to the blood, and (3) signalling the kidneys to _____.

3. Causes of hyperparathyroidism include adenomas, vitamin D deficiencies, elevated serum phosphate, and

_____.

4. High levels of PTH cause calcium to shift from the bones into the _____.

5. If hypercalcemia is untreated, _____ of the bones may occur.

6. Hypoparathyroidism is an uncommon condition. When it does occur, it is usually due to accidental removal of or damage to _____.

7. For patients with hyperthyroidism, _____ should be reported immediately.

IV. List 2 things that should be placed at the bedside before the thyroidectomy patient returns from surgery.

1.

2.

V. List 2 reasons why respiratory distress can result following thyroidectomy.

1.

2.

VI. Following thyroidectomy surgery, where should the nurse check for bleeding?

VII. After total thyroidectomy, how long will patients take thyroid hormones?

VIII. If thyroid enlargement is mild and thyroid hormone production is normal, what treatment is required?

IX. List 1 reason why thyroidectomy surgery may be followed with radioactive iodine treatment.

1.

X. When assessing the patient who has a parathyroid disorder, list 2 body systems on which the nurse should focus.

1.

2.

XI. List 1 reason why an electrocardiogram may be ordered for patients with parathyroid disorders.

1.

XII. Under what conditions will demineralization be apparent on radiographs of patients with parathyroid disorder?

XIII. List (A) 7 nursing diagnoses and (B) 7 criteria for the evaluation of nursing care for the hyperthyroid patient.

1.   1.

2.   2.

3.   3.

4.   4.

5.   5.

6.   6.

7.   7.

XIV. List 6 nursing diagnoses for patients undergoing thyroidectomies.

1.

2.

3.

4.

5.

6.

XV.   List 8 nursing diagnoses for patients with hyperparathyroidism.

1.

2.

3.

4.

5.

6.

7.

8.

XVI.   Complete the sentences on the left with (A) increases or (B) decreases on the right.

___   1.   When thyroid hormones are elevated, the pulse rate _____.

___   2.   Excess thyroxine _____ the body's metabolic rate.

___   3.   High levels of PTH _____ retention of calcium.

___   4.   When thyroid hormones are elevated, blood pressure _____.

___   5.   High levels of PTH _____ loss of phosphates by the kidneys.

A.   Increase(s)

B.   Decrease(s)

XVII.   Complete the statements on the left with the most appropriate term on the right. Some terms may be used more than once, and some terms may not be used.

___   1.   The thyroid gland is located in the lower portion of the _____.

___   2.   The function of the thyroid gland is to regulate _____.

___   3.   When the metabolic rate falls, the hypothalamus stimulates the pituitary gland to secrete _____.

___   4.   Another name for the thyroid hormone is _____.

___   5.   The mineral that is required by the thyroid gland to manufacture hormones is _____.

___   6.   An abnormally increased production of thyroid hormones results in _____.

___   7.   The substance that is secreted when serum calcium levels are very high in order to limit the shift of calcium from the bones into the blood is _____.

A.   Iodine

B.   TSH

C.   PTU

D.   Thyroxine

E.   Hypothyroidism

F.   Neck

G.   Calcitonin

H.   Face

I.   Hyperthyroidism

J.   Metabolism

XVIII. Complete the statements on the left with the most appropriate term on the right. Some terms may be used more than once, and some terms may not be used.

____ 1. The most common forms of hyperthyroidism are Graves' disease and _____.

____ 2. If untreated, hyperthyroidism may lead to _____.

____ 3. Symptoms of thyrotoxicosis include tachycardia, heart failure, and _____.

____ 4. Drugs that block the synthesis, release, or activity of thyroid hormones are _____.

____ 5. The two classes of drugs commonly used as antithyroid drugs are thioamides and _____.

____ 6. When a patient is on drugs that interfere with thyroxine secretion, the nurse should monitor for edema, weight gain, and _____.

____ 7. Examples of thioamides are methimazole (Tapazole) and _____.

____ 8. One main disadvantage of the thioamides is that they can cause _____.

A. Antithyroids

B. Cold intolerance

C. Agranulocytosis

D. Heat intolerance

E. Hyperthermia

F. Iodides

G. Propylthiouracil (PTU)

H. Multinodular goiter

I. Hypothermia

J. Thyrotoxicosis

XIX. Complete the statements on the left with the most appropriate term on the right. Some terms may be used more than once, and some may not be used.

____ 1. For patients receiving thioamides _____ should be reported to the physician immediately.

____ 2. The production of thyroid hormones is inhibited by _____.

____ 3. The most popular forms of iodides used to treat hyperthyroidism are saturated solution of potassium and _____.

____ 4. Side effects of iodine solutions are gastric upset and _____.

____ 5. Grave's disease is often treated with the surgical procedure called _____.

____ 6. The escape of thyroid hormones into the blood stream during thyroidectomy may cause _____.

____ 7. Due to a high metabolic rate, hyperthyroid patients usually have _____.

____ 8. Hyperthyroid patients need diets high in calories, minerals, and _____.

A. Cold intolerance

B. Vitamins

C. Signs of heart failure

D. Iodides

E. Thyroid storm

F. Lugol's solution

G. Total thyroidectomy

H. Heat intolerance

I. Protein

J. Signs of infection

K. Teeth discoloration

L. Subtotal thyroidectomy

XX. Complete the statements on the left with the most appropriate term on the right. Some terms may be used more than once, and some terms may not be used.

____ 1. A condition in which deposits of fat and fluid behind the eyeballs make them bulge forward is called _____.

____ 2. A complication of patients undergoing thyroidectomies that can be prevented by preoperative treatment with antithyroid drugs is _____.

____ 3. Signs and symptoms of poor oxygenation due to airway obstruction that may occur after thyroidectomy include restlessness, increased pulse, and _____.

____ 4. Signs of laryngeal nerve damage include inability to speak and _____.

____ 5. A complication of thyroidectomies includes injury to parathyroid glands, which results in _____.

____ 6. The most serious side effect of hypocalcemia is _____.

____ 7. Tetany is treated with _____.

____ 8. Signs of severe hyperthyroidism include fever, confusion, and _____.

____ 9. Symptoms of infection that should be reported after thyroidectomy include fever, wound swelling, and _____.

____ 10. The result of inadequate secretion of thyroid hormones is called _____.

A. Hyperthyroidism
B. Dyspnea
C. Laryngospasm
D. Bradycardia
E. Tetany
F. Hypothyroidism
G. Calcium salts
H. Foul discharge
I. Hoarseness
J. Exophthalmos
K. Tachycardia
L. Thyroid crisis
M. Tetany

XXI. Complete the statements on the left with the most appropriate term on the right. Some terms may be used more than once, and some may not be used.

____ 1. If not treated early, hypothyroidism during infancy causes _____.

____ 2. Facial edema that develops with long-term hypothyroidism is _____.

____ 3. Foods and drugs that suppress thyroid hormone production are called _____.

____ 4. Symptoms of hypothyroidism include decreased metabolic rate, pulse, and _____.

____ 5. Signs of hypothyroidism include lethargy, irritability, and _____.

____ 6. Thyroid enlargement with normal thyroid hormone production is called _____.

____ 7. Four small glands located on the back of the thyroid gland are called _____.

A. Weight gain
B. Thyroid glands
C. Myxedema
D. Intolerance to cold
E. Weight loss
F. Parathyroid glands
G. Goitrogens
H. Intolerance to heat
I. Simple goiter
J. Cretinism

XXII. Complete the statements on the left with the most appropriate term on the right. Some terms may be used more than once, and some terms may not be used.

___ 1. The parathyroid hormone (parathormone, PTH) plays a critical role in regulating _____.

___ 2. The most notable effect of hyperparathyroidism is _____.

___ 3. The term used to describe enlargement of the thyroid gland is _____.

___ 4. People who have kidney transplants after being on dialysis for a long time may experience _____.

___ 5. When the serum calcium level falls, what is secreted? _____.

___ 6. Generally, calcium retention by the kidney is balanced by the loss of _____.

___ 7. A spasm of the facial muscle when the face is tapped over the facial nerve is _____.

___ 8. A carpopedal spasm that occurs when a blood pressure cuff is inflated beyond that patient's systolic blood pressure and left in place for several minutes is _____.

___ 9. An element that is an important component of strong bones, and that plays a vital role in the functions of nerve and tissue cells, is _____.

___ 10. The secretion of excess PTH is called _____.

A. Trousseau's sign

B. Goiter

C. Phosphates

D. Hypoparathyroidism

E. Chvostek's sign

F. Calcium

G. PTH

H. Hyperparathyroidism

I. TSH

J. Hypercalcemia

K. Sodium

XXIII. Complete the statements on the left with the most appropriate term on the right. Some terms may be used more than once, and some terms may not be used.

___ 1. Medical treatment for patients with hyper-parathyroidism includes high fluid intake, sodium and phosphorus replacements, and restricted _____ intake.

___ 2. In treating hyperparathyroidism, furosemide (Lasix) is given to promote the excretion of _____ in the urine.

___ 3. In treating hyperparathyroidism, propranolol (Inderal) is given to reduce the secretion of _____.

___ 4. Because hypercalcemia can cause urinary calculi and serious kidney damage, patients with hyperparathyroidism should have their _____ closely monitored.

A. Sodium

B. Intake and output

C. Hypercalcemia

D. Calcium

E. Oxygenation

F. Sharp flank pain

G. TSH

H. Hypocalcemia

I. PTH

J. Tetany

K. Dyspnea

XXIII. *Continues*

Introductory Nursing Care of Adults

XXIII. *Continues*

____ 5. In treating hyperparathyroidism, plicamycin and calcitonin are given to inhibit the release of _____ from bones.

____ 6. Findings consistent with urinary calculi that should be reported to the physicians are decreased urine output, hematuria, and _____.

____ 7. Treatment for hyperparathyroidism includes high fluid intake and a diet low in _____.

____ 8. Two potential complications specific to parathyroidectomy are airway obstruction and _____.

____ 9. In parathyroidectomy patients, increasing pulse and respiratory rates, accompanied by restlessness, suggest inadequate _____.

____ 10. Due to the postoperative decrease in parathyroid hormones, the nurse should be alert for _____.

A. Sodium

B. Intake and output

C. Hypercalcemia

D. Calcium

E. Oxygenation

F. Sharp flank pain

G. TSH

H. Hypocalcemia

I. PTH

J. Tetany

K. Dyspnea

XXIV. Complete the statements on the left with the most appropriate term on the right. Some terms may be used more than once, and some terms may not be used.

____ 1. Tetany is a symptom of _____.

____ 2. An early symptom of tetany is _____.

____ 3. Later symptoms of tetany include laryngospasm and _____.

____ 4. Tetany is treated with _____.

____ 5. In order to assess bleeding of the patient after parathyroidectomy, the nurse should assess the dressing and the _____.

____ 6. Hypoparathyroidism is a deficiency of _____.

____ 7. In patients with hypoparathyroidism, a medication that may be ordered with meals to reduce the absorption of phosphates in the intestines is _____.

____ 8. Lowering serum phosphate levels tends to raise the levels of _____.

____ 9. A deficiency of PTH is called _____.

____ 10. Acute hypoparathyroidism is sometimes treated with _____.

____ 11. On a long-term basis, the patient with chronic hypoparathyroidism is treated with calcium salts and _____.

A. Front of the patient's neck

B. Calcium

C. Sodium

D. Aluminum hydroxide

E. Tingling sensations

F. Back of the patient's neck

G. PTH

H. Vitamin D

I. Calcium supplements

J. Hypoparathyroidism

K. Muscle spasms and cramps

L. Hypercalcemia

M. Hypocalcemia

XXV. Choose the most appropriate answer.

1. What is secreted when serum calcium levels are high to limit the shift of calcium from the bones into the blood?
   A. calcitonin
   B. thyroxine
   C. thymine
   D. phosphorus

2. Hyperthyroid patients often experience sleep disturbances and:
   A. sedation
   B. bradycardia
   C. restlessness
   D. hypotension

41

Diabetes Mellitus and Hypoglycemia

OBJECTIVES

1. Describe the role of insulin in the body.
2. Explain the pathophysiology of diabetes mellitus and hypoglycemia.
3. Describe the signs and symptoms of diabetes mellitus and hypoglycemia.
4. Demonstrate knowledge of tests and procedures used to diagnose diabetes mellitus and hypoglycemia.
5. Verbalize treatment of diabetes mellitus and hypoglycemia.
6. Explain the difference between insulin-dependent diabetes mellitus and non–insulin–dependent diabetes mellitus.
7. Differentiate between insulin shock and diabetic ketoacidosis.
8. Describe the treatment of a patient experiencing insulin shock and diabetic ketoacidosis.
9. Describe the complications of diabetes mellitus.
10. Develop a care plan for a patient diagnosed with diabetes mellitus or hypoglycemia.
11. Develop a care plan for a patient diagnosed with ketoacidosis.

LEARNING ACTIVITIES

I.   Match the definition on the left with the most appropriate term on the right.

____ 1. Decreased subcutaneous fat mass

____ 2. Metabolic acidosis related to accumulated ketone bodies in the blood

____ 3. Normal blood glucose level

____ 4. Abnormally low level of glucose in the blood

____ 5. Pertaining to the large blood vessels

____ 6. Products of fatty acid metabolism

____ 7. Presence of glucose in the urine

____ 8. Internally produced or caused by internal factors

____ 9. Kidney disease

____ 10. Disease of the retina of the eye

____ 11. Pertaining to the small blood vessels (i.e., arterioles, capillaries, and venules)

A.   Endogenous
B.   Euglycemia
C.   Glycosuria
D.   Hypoglycemia
E.   Ketoacidosis
F.   Ketone bodies
G.   Lipoatrophy
H.   Lipohypertrophy
I.   Macrovascular
J.   Microvascular
K.   Nephropathy
L.   Neuropathy
M.   Polydipsia
N.   Polyphagia
O.   Polyuria
P.   Retinopathy

I.   *Continues*

I. *Continued*

___ 12. Excessive urine output

___ 13. Pathologic changes in the peripheral nervous system

___ 14. Excessive thirst

___ 15. Increased subcutaneous fat mass

___ 16. Excessive food ingestion

A. Endogenous
B. Euglycemia
C. Glycosuria
D. Hypoglycemia
E. Ketoacidosis
F. Ketone bodies
G. Lipoatrophy
H. Lipohypertrophy
I. Macrovascular
J. Microvascular
K. Nephropathy
L. Neuropathy
M. Polydipsia
N. Polyphagia
O. Polyuria
P. Retinopathy

II. Match the definition on the left with the most appropriate term on the right.

___ 1. Loss of muscle tone

___ 2. Rebound response to excess insulin, causing hyperglycemia

___ 3. Small, involuntary muscle contraction

___ 4. Externally produced or caused by external factors

___ 5. Electronic device used to measure blood glucose

A. Somogyi effect
B. Fasciculation
C. Amyopathy (amyotonia)
D. Glucometer
E. Exogenous

II. Complete the statements on the left with the most appropriate term on the right. Some terms may be used more than once, and some terms may not be used.

____ 1. A diminished or inadequate amount of insulin to meet daily requirements characterizes _____.

____ 2. The more severe form of diabetes mellitus is _____.

____ 3. Insulin is released in the body in response to the ingestion of _____.

____ 4. The absence of endogenous insulin characterizes _____.

____ 5. Because the cells of the body are not able to use carbohydrates without insulin, the body uses fat stores for heat and energy, and so the patient experiences _____.

____ 6. Tissue breakdown and burning of lean body mass send hunger signals to the hypothalamus, and so the patient experiences _____.

____ 7. The hormone that stimulates the active transport of glucose into the cells of muscle and adipose tissue is _____.

A. Weight loss

B. Insulin

C. IDDM

D. NIDDM

E. Glycogen

F. Polydipsia

G. Carbohydrates

H. Polyphagia

V. Complete the statements on the left with the most appropriate term on the right. Some terms may be used more than once, and some terms may not be used.

____ 1. Insulin promotes fatty acid synthesis and the conversion of fatty acids into fat, which is stored as _____.

____ 2. A collection of symptoms characterized by the body's inability to utilize glucose is _____.

____ 3. When insulin is absent, the increased osmolality of blood stimulates the thirst centers in an effort to dilute the glucose, and so the patient experiences _____.

____ 4. Insulin promotes the conversion of glucose to _____, which is stored in the liver.

____ 5. Lack of insulin permits fat stores to break down and increases the amount of _____ stored in the liver.

____ 6. The kidneys, in an effort to reduce the glucose concentration, increase urine output, and so the patient experiences _____.

____ 7. _____ regulates the rate at which carbohydrates are consumed by the body for energy.

____ 8. A hormone produced by the beta cells in the islets of Langerhans located in the pancreas is _____.

A. Polydipsia

B. Triglycerides

C. Polyphagia

D. Glycogen

E. Insulin

F. Adipose tissue

G. Glucose

H. Diabetes mellitus

I. Polyuria

V. Complete the statements on the left with the most appropriate term on the right. Some terms may be used more than once, and some terms may not be used.

____ 1. Characteristics of diabetic retinopathy include a thickened basement membrane due to leakage of the blood vessels and increased _____.

____ 2. With diabetic retinopathy, the vitreous becomes cloudy and vision is lost due to _____.

____ 3. A symptom of eye problems for patients with diabetes is the presence of spots, which are called _____.

____ 4. Persons with diabetes account for a large percentage of patients with renal disease, which is called _____.

____ 5. In patients with diabetes, the kidneys have an increased workload due to _____.

____ 6. Elevated pressure in the *renal* vessels, over a period of years, destroys the kidney's _____ ability.

____ 7. Elevated insulin levels circulating in the blood of patients with diabetes contribute to the premature development of _____.

A. Floaters

B. Neuropathy

C. Polyuria

D. Hemorrhage

E. Atherosclerosis

F. Capillary permeability

G. Filtering

H. Nephropathy

VI. Complete the statements on the left with the most appropriate term on the right. Some terms may be used more than once, and some terms may not be used.

____ 1. A loss of muscle tone that causes pain in the muscles of the pelvic girdle and thighs is called diabetic _____.

____ 2. Signs and symptoms of peripheral vascular disease that may be seen in patients with diabetes include diminished pedal pulses and _____.

____ 3. Neuropathy is related to the body's poor control of _____.

____ 4. Urinary retention with overflow (in the absence of prostatic obstruction) is a symptom of _____.

____ 5. Pain in the calf, back, or buttocks while walking is a sign of _____.

____ 6. Tingling, numbness, burning, or sharp pains that are usually worse in the legs or arms are complaints of patients with _____.

A. Glucose

B. Neuropathy

C. Glycogen

D. Amyopathy

E. Nephropathy

F. Atonic bladder

G. Claudication

VII. Complete the statements on the left with the most appropriate term on the right. Some terms may be used more than once, and some terms may not be used.

____ 1. Treatment of ketoacidosis is aimed at correction of the 3 main problems, which are acidosis, dehydration, and _____.

____ 2. The patient with ketoacidosis may have lost a large volume of fluid as the result of vomiting, diarrhea, hyperventilation, and _____.

____ 3. Replacement of potassium is vital in patients with ketoacidosis because hypokalemia can lead to severe _____.

____ 4. A life-threatening emergency caused by lack of insulin or inadequate amounts of insulin is called diabetic _____.

____ 5. Air hunger, seen in patients with ketoacidosis, is observed as _____.

____ 6. The movement of potassium from the extracellular compartment into the cells is enhanced by _____.

____ 7. Ketoacidosis results in disorders in the metabolism of carbohydrates, fats, and _____.

____ 8. The electrolyte of primary concern in ketoacidosis is _____.

A.   Glucose

B.   Ketoacidosis

C.   Insulin

D.   Electrolyte imbalance

E.   Potassium

F.   Cardiac dysrhythmias

G.   Kussmaul's respirations

H.   Proteins

I.   Sodium

J.   Polyuria

VIII. Complete the statements on the left with the most appropriate term on the right. Some terms may be used more than once, and some terms may not be used.

____ 1. _____ occurs when insulin is absent or insufficient, causing ketone bodies to accumulate as the result of the breakdown of fats for energy.

____ 2. The treatment for diabetic patients with acidosis is the IV infusion of _____.

____ 3. _____ occurs when a patient becomes comatose from extremely high glucose levels but has no evidence of elevated ketones.

____ 4. _____ causes increased osmolality, affects the sensorium, and causes the patient to lapse into a coma.

____ 5. A patient's persistent hyperglycemia causes osmotic diuresis, resulting in the loss of _____.

____ 6. Three conditions that patients in hyperosmolar nonketotic coma experience are hyperglycemia, dehydration, and _____.

A.   Hyperosmolar nonketotic coma

B.   Acidosis

C.   Glycogen

D.   Hyperglycemia

E.   Hypernatremia

F.   Insulin

G.   Fluid and electrolytes

IX. Complete the statements on the left with the most appropriate term on the right. Some terms may be used more than once, and some terms may not be used.

___	1.	The goal of managing diabetes is to help the patient remain _____.
___	2.	The American Diabetes Association recommends that 12 to 20% of the total daily calories should come from _____.
___	3.	Two elevated blood levels that occur often in patients with NIDDM, increasing the risk of cardiovascular disease, are serum cholesterol and _____.
___	4.	_____ has a potential glucose-lowering effect due to the slower rate of glucose absorption from the gastrointestinal tract.
___	5.	_____ is a very effective nonpharmacologic treatment in NIDDM patients that can dramatically decrease serum glucose.
___	6.	Much of the morbidity and mortality in NIDDM patients occurs because of increased _____.
___	7.	If IDDM or NIDDM patients have a serum glucose level of 300 mg/dl or greater, they should avoid _____.
___	8.	The utilization of too much glucose during exercise coupled with an excess of insulin in the blood stream causes _____.
___	9.	All IDDM patients need _____.
___	10.	When diet and exercise fail to control diabetes in patients with NIDDM, the physician may prescribe _____.

A.   Hypoglycemia

B.   Protein

C.   Exercise

D.   Hyperglycemia

E.   Carbohydrate

F.   Insulin

G.   Triglycerides

H.   Oral hypoglycemic agents

I.   Atherosclerosis

J.   Euglycemic

K.   Fiber

X. Complete the statements on the left with the most appropriate term on the right. Some terms may be used more than once, and some terms may not be used.

___	1.	The major complication of insulin therapy is _____.
___	2.	If a person injects too much insulin, does not eat enough, or exercises too vigorously, the serum _____ level may suddenly drop.
___	3.	The IDDM patient should always carry or keep _____ close at hand.
___	4.	In order to prevent rebound hypoglycemia, the patient should be given some form of _____.
___	5.	When a patient goes into insulin shock, the patient will be given _____.

A.   Somogyi effect

B.   Hypoglycemia

C.   IV dextrose

D.   Hyperglycemia

E.   Glucagon

F.   Growth hormone

G.   Glycogen

H.   Carbohydrate

I.   Glucose

J.   Epinephrine

___ 6. The _____ is a rebound response that occurs in the presence of too much insulin.

___ 7. The low serum glucose induced by too much insulin triggers the release of _____.

___ 8. The combination of low blood glucose and epinephrine stimulates the pituitary to release adrenocorticotropic hormone and _____.

A. Somogyi effect

B. Hypoglycemia

C. IV dextrose

D. Hyperglycemia

E. Glucagon

F. Growth hormone

G. Glycogen

H. Carbohydrate

I. Glucose

J. Epinephrine

XI. Indicate for each action or condition on the left whether insulin (A) increases or (B) decreases it.

___ 1. Rate of metabolism of carbohydrates

___ 2. Conversion of glucose to glycogen

___ 3. Conversion of glycogen to glucose

___ 4. Fatty acid synthesis and conversion of fatty acids into fat

___ 5. Breakdown of adipose tissue

___ 6. Rate of glucose utilization

___ 7. Mobilization of fat

___ 8. Conversion of fats to glucose

___ 9. Protein synthesis in tissue

___ 10. Conversion of protein into glucose

A. Increases

B. Decreases

XII. Match the causes of neuropathic ulcers on the left with the type of injury on the right.

___ 1. Caused by rough shoe linings or incorrectly shaving calluses or cutting toenails.

___ 2. Caused by hot-water bottle or sitting too close to a fire or radiator

___ 3. Caused from substances such as salicylic acid, found in many corn plasters

A. Chemical irritation

B. Mechanical irritation

C. Burns

XIII.   List 4 organs of the body that do not depend on insulin for the transport of glucose into them.

1.

2.

3.

4.

XIV.   List 6 groups of people who are at risk for diabetes.

1.

2.

3.

4.

5.

6.

XV.   List 3 signs and symptoms of kidney failure that the nurse would observe in patients with diabetes.

1.

2.

3.

XVI.   List 2 causes of foot problems in the diabetic.

1.

2.

XVII.   Explain why the diabetic patient may have an ulcer or necrotic area in the foot and be unaware of the problem.

XVIII.   Complete the table below, listing the changes that occur when the foot's nerve supply is impaired and when the foot's blood supply is impaired.

	Impaired nerve supply	Impaired blood supply
Color:	1. _____	2. _____
Pulses:	3. _____	4. _____
Sensation:	5. _____	6. _____

XIX. List 3 long-term complications of diabetes that can be controlled with intensive treatment of IDDM.

1.

2.

3.

XX. List 11 signs and symptoms of ketoacidosis.

1.   7.

2.   8.

3.   9.

4.   10.

5.   11.

6.

XXI. List 4 situations that put the diabetic patient at risk for ketoacidosis.

1.

2.

3.

4.

XXII. List 2 reasons why it is better to run the IV bottle containing potassium by the piggyback method at a prescribed rate, which will be slower than the hydration rate.

1.

2.

XXIII. Explain why patients receiving total parenteral nutrition or dialysis are apt to have hyperosmolar nonketotic coma.

XXIV. List the criteria needed in each category below for patients to be diagnosed as diabetics. (A patient is considered to have DM if he or she meets one or more of the criteria)

1. Fasting glucose level:

2. Random glucose level:

3. 4 classic symptoms of DM:

4. Glucose tolerance test:

XXV. List the 6 food groups that make up the exchange list for diabetics

1.   4.

2.   5.

3.   6.

XXVI. Indicate the 5 types of food exchanges and the amounts of each exchange that may be included in a taco made with hamburger meat, browned and drained well, with grated skim milk cheese, lettuce, and a diced tomato.

1.   4.

2.   5.

3.

XXVII. List 4 areas of injection sites for insulin.

1.   3.

2.   4.

XXVIII. List 2 advantages and 4 disadvantages of an insulin pump.

1.   1.

2.   2.

                                     3.

                                     4.

XXIX. List 3 actions of oral hypoglycemic drugs (sulfonylureas).

1.

2.

3.

XXX. Indicate how the following factors can cause serum glucose levels to drop.

1. Insulin

2. Food

3. Exercise

XXXI. List 10 initial signs and symptoms of hypoglycemia.

1.   6.

2.   7.

3.   8.

4.   9.

5.   10.

XXXII.   List 4 outside factors that act on the body to produce exogenous hypoglycemia.

1.

2.

3.

4.

XXXIII.   Choose the most appropriate answer.

1. Which of the following inhibits the conversion of glycogen to glucose?
   A. fatty acids
   B. insulin
   C. triglycerides
   D. ketones

2. The priority need for diabetic patients with dehydration is replacement of fluids so that the kidneys can:
   A. get rid of excess glucose
   B. lower the body temperature
   C. lower the blood pressure
   D. increase the blood alkalinity

3. The diagnosis of diabetes is based on serum:
   A. amylase levels
   B. red blood cell count
   C. hemoglobin
   D. glucose levels

4. Normal fasting serum glucose levels are between:
   A. 30 and 50 mg/dl
   B. 80 and 120 mg/dl
   C. 200 and 300 mg/dl
   D. 900 and 1000 mg/dl

5. The American Diabetes Association recommends that 55 to 60% of the total daily calories should come from:
   A. protein
   B. fat
   C. carbohydrates
   D. dairy products

6. The insulin with the lowest concentration is:
   A. U-40
   B. U-80
   C. U-100
   D. U-500

7. The type of insulin that has the least immunogenic effect and that does not need as high a dose to be effective is:
   A. animal
   B. human
   C. beef
   D. pork

8. The prescription for insulin including times, types, and amounts, is written to mimic the action of a normal:
   A. stomach
   B. liver
   C. gallbladder
   D. pancreas

9. Regular insulin should be given:
   A. at bedtime
   B. before meals
   C. during meals
   D. after meals

10. To prevent bubbles, the bottle of insulin for injection should be:
    A. heated
    B. cooled
    C. rolled
    D. shaken

11. Which injection site has the fastest rate of absorption for insulin?
    A. upper arm
    B. upper buttocks
    C. abdomen
    D. thighs

12. The 2 oral hypoglycemic agents that are recommended for elderly patients are glipizide (Glucotrol) and:
    A. chlorpropamide (Diabinese)
    B. glyburide (DiaBeta, Micronase)
    C. tolbutamide (Orinase)
    D. acetohexamide (Dymelor)

13. When mixing regular and longer-acting insulins, which should be drawn into the syringe first?
    A. regular insulin
    B. protamine zinc insulin
    C. ultralente insulin
    D. lente insulin

14. A reason for avoiding long-acting oral hypoglycemic agents in the elderly is that decreased renal function in the elderly makes them more prone to:
    A. hyponatremia
    B. hypernatremia
    C. hypoglycemia
    D. hyperglycemia

15. Which is a side effect of oral agents used in the treatment of diabetes mellitus?
    A. hyperglycemia
    B. hypoglycemia
    C. hyperkalemia
    D. hypokalemia

16. Patients who require insulin injections need to self-monitor levels of:
    A. serum cholesterol
    B. red blood cells
    C. amylase
    D. blood glucose

17. Late signs of hypoglycemia include:
    A. palpitations and dyspnea
    B. oliguria and hypotension
    C. peripheral edema and tachypnea
    D. confusion and unconsciousness

18. To detect possible changes in the eyes associated with DM, the nurse inquires whether the patient has had floaters, blurred vision, or:
    A. hemorrhage
    B. infection
    C. diplopia
    D. conjunctivitis

19. During the physical assessment of the diabetic patient, the nurse inspects the feet carefully for lesions, discoloration, and:
    A. edema
    B. ability to dorsiflex
    C. ability to evert
    D. dehydration

20. A nursing diagnosis for patients with diabetes is chronic pain related to:
    A. abnormal blood glucose levels
    B. adverse effects of drugs
    C. neuropathy
    D. alterations in urine output

21. Patients with diabetes may have sensory-perceptual alterations related to:
    A. dietary restrictions
    B. anxiety and fear
    C. imbalance between food intake and activity expenditure
    D. neurologic and circulatory changes

22. Alterations in tactile sensations in diabetic patients may result in:
    A. burns or frostbite
    B. floaters or diplopia
    C. altered urine output or oliguria
    D. abnormal blood glucose levels

23. Altered thought processes in diabetic patients, including confusion, anger, and decreased level of consciousness, may be due to:
    A. neuropathy
    B. nephropathy
    C. ketoacidosis
    D. hyperglycemia

24. Hypoglycemia is defined as a syndrome that develops when the blood glucose level falls to less than:
    A. 10 to 15 mg/dl
    B. 45 to 50 mg/dl
    C. 80 to 120 mg/dl
    D. 200 to 300 mg/dl

25. Endogenous hypoglycemia occurs when internal factors cause an excessive secretion of insulin or an increase in the metabolism of:
    A. protein
    B. fats
    C. calcium
    D. glucose

26. When blood glucose levels fall rapidly, the four substances that are secreted by the body in an attempt to increase glucose levels are cortisol, glucagon, growth hormone, and:
    A. antidiuretic hormone
    B. epinephrine
    C. aldosterone
    D. thyroxine

27. Early signs of hypoglycemia include:
    A. bradycardia and edema
    B. oliguria and constipation
    C. infection and red skin
    D. weakness and hunger

28. A diagnostic test used to evaluate hypoglycemia is:
    A. fasting blood glucose
    B. serum amylase
    C. prothrombin time
    D. hemoglobin

29. Patients with hypoglycemia are at high risk for injury related to:
    A. oliguria and constipation
    B. bradycardia and edema
    C. dizziness and weakness
    D. retinopathy and hypertension

30. Diabetes mellitus is a condition characterized by insulin deficiency that impairs:
    A. circulation
    B. respiration
    C. metabolism
    D. elimination

31. Hyperosmolar nonketotic coma is loss of consciousness due to extremely high serum:
    A. sodium
    B. glucose
    C. calcium
    D. potassium

42

Adrenal and Pituitary Disorders

OBJECTIVES

1. Identify nursing assessment data relevant to the function of the adrenal and pituitary glands.
2. Describe the tests and procedures used to diagnose disorders of the adrenal and pituitary glands and identify nursing considerations relevant for each.
3. Describe the pathophysiology and medical treatment of adrenocortical insufficiency, excess adrenocortical hormones, hypopituitarism, diabetes insipidus, and pituitary tumors.
4. Develop a nursing care plan for patients with selected disorders of the adrenal and pituitary glands.

LEARNING ACTIVITIES

I. Match the definition on the left with the most appropriate term on the right.

____ 1. Ductless gland that produces an internal secretion discharged into the lymph or blood stream and circulated to all parts of the body. Hormones, the active substances of these glands, cause an effect on certain organs or tissues

____ 2. Disease resulting from a deficiency of adrenocorticotropic hormone caused by destruction or dysfunction of the adrenal glands. Characterized by increased pigmentation of the skin and mucous membranes, weakness, fatigue, hypotension, nausea, weight loss, and hypoglycemia.

____ 3. Disease caused by inadequate secretion of antidiuretic hormone by the posterior portion of the pituitary; symptoms include excessive urination, thirst, and dehydration

____ 4. Disease of middle-aged adults resulting from overproduction of growth hormone by the anterior pituitary. Characterized by enlargement of the facial bones, nose, lips, and jaw. Also associated with decreased libido, moodiness, fatigue, muscle pains, sweating, and headache

____ 5. Type of hormone secreted by the adrenal cortex and involved in the regulation of fluid and electrolyte levels in the body

A.   Acromegaly

B.   Addison's disease

C.   Adrenaline

D.   Androgens

E.   Catecholamines

F.   Cushing's disease

G.   Cushing's syndrome

H.   Diabetes insipidus

I.   Endocrine gland

J.   Estrogens

K.   Gigantism

L.   Glucocorticoid

M.   Hypophysectomy

N.   Mineralocorticoid

O.   Syndrome of inappropriate antidiuretic hormone

I.   *Continues*

I. *Continues*

___ 6. Disorder caused by excess antidiuretic hormone production; symptoms include decreased urination, edema, and fluid overload

___ 7. Disorder resulting from excessive glucocorticoids in the body as a result of tumor or hypersecretion of the pituitary. May also be caused by prolonged administration of large doses of exogenous steroids. Symptoms include fat deposits in the neck and abdomen, fatigue, weakness, edema, excess hair growth, glucose intolerances, skin discoloration, and mood swings

___ 8. Class of adrenocortical hormones that affect protein and carbohydrate metabolism and help protect the body against stress

___ 9. Chemical (dopamine, epinephrine, norepinephrine) released at sympathetic nerve endings in response to stress

___ 10. Hormones produced by the ovaries, adrenal glands, and fetoplacental unit in females that are responsible for the development and maturation of females

___ 11. Disease caused by excessive growth hormone in children and young adolescents resulting in excessive proportional growth

___ 12. Disease caused by the hypersecretion of glucocorticoids due to excessive release of adrenocorticotropic hormone by the pituitary

___ 13. Hormones produced by the adrenal cortex, the testes, and the ovaries that stimulate the development of male characteristics

___ 14. Surgical removal of all or part of the pituitary gland

___ 15. Epinephrine; a powerful vasoactive substance produced by the medulla or adrenal gland in times of stress or danger, allowing the body to react by fighting or fleeing

A. Acromegaly

B. Addison's disease

C. Adrenaline

D. Androgens

E. Catecholamines

F. Cushing's disease

G. Cushing's syndrome

H. Diabetes insipidus

I. Endocrine gland

J. Estrogens

K. Gigantism

L. Glucocorticoid

M. Hypophysectomy

N. Mineralocorticoid

O. Syndrome of inappropriate antidiuretic hormone

II.   Match the definition on the left with the most appropriate term on the right.

___ 1.   Posterior portion of the pituitary gland

___ 2.   Organ or structure that secretes substances used in other areas of the body

___ 3.   Continuous adjustment of the body to maintain a relatively constant interval environment

___ 4.   Abnormal growth of tissue or tumor formation of the epithelial layer of a gland

___ 5.   Hormone released by the posterior portion of the pituitary gland that causes the reabsorp-tion of water in the distal tubules and collecting ducts of the kidney

___ 6.   Anterior lobe of the pituitary gland

A.   Homeostasis

B.   Antidiuretic hormone

C.   Gland

D.   Adenohypophysis

E.   Neurohypophysis

F.   Adenoma

III.   Complete the statements on the left with the most appropriate term on the right. Some terms may be used more than once, and some terms may not be used.

___ 1.   The first symptom of a problem in hyperpituitarism is often _____.

___ 2.   Radiographic films of the skull of persons with hyperpituitarism may show a large sella turcica and increased _____.

___ 3.   A hormone is a substance composed of amines, peptides, or _____.

___ 4.   A disease that occurs in early childhood or puberty in which the diaphysis of the long bones grows to great lengths stimulated by excess GH is _____.

___ 5.   A disease that appears when adults are in their 30s and 40s in which bones increase in thickness and width after the epiphyseal closure is _____.

___ 6.   The pituitary gland is also called the _____.

___ 7.   The pituitary gland is connected to the _____.

___ 8.   For patients diagnosed with pituitary tumors, the treatment of choice is _____.

A.   Gigantism

B.   Hypothalamus

C.   Cushing's syndrome

D.   Hypophysectomy

E.   Bone density

F.   Parathyroid gland

G.   Acromegaly

H.   Visual deficit

I.   Hypophysis

J.   Steroids

IV. Complete the statements on the left with the most appropriate term on the right. Some terms may be used more than once, and some terms may not be used.

____ 1. When inadequate secretion of GH occurs during preadolescence, a condition that results is called _____.

____ 2. If growth has been completed and some pathologic process impairs the function of the pituitary, _____ can occur.

____ 3. A condition of shock and hypotension during the postpartum period that can lead to infarction of the pituitary gland is _____.

____ 4. When panhypopituitarism exists, a syndrome in which muscle and organ wasting and disruptions of digestion and metabolism occur is _____.

____ 5. A lack of thyroid hormone that occurs in hypopituitarism produces a state referred to as _____.

A. Sheehan's syndrome

B. Dwarfism

C. Addison's disease

D. Myxedema

E. Panhypopituitarism

F. Simmonds' cachexia

V. Complete the statements on the left with the most appropriate term on the right. Some terms may be used more than once, and some terms may not be used.

____ 1. A way to monitor fluid volume deficit in patients with diabetes insipidus is to complete daily _____.

____ 2. Another name for ADH is _____.

____ 3. A hormone that functions by allowing the renal tubules of the nephron to reabsorb water is _____.

____ 4. When urine output is excessive as it is in diabetes insipidus, an essential intervention is adequate _____.

____ 5. Increased ADH results in increased intravascular volume and decreased urine _____.

____ 6. Related to self-care deficit in patients with diabetes insipidus, extreme fatigue or _____ can interfere with the patient's ability to participate in activities of daily living.

____ 7. Ulcerations of mucous membranes, chest tightness, and upper respiratory infections are risks to patients with DI related to the prolonged use of _____.

____ 8. _____ is related to a deficit in production and synthesis of ADH.

____ 9. Disorders of the posterior pituitary are directly related to deficient or excess _____.

____ 10. Increased ADH release causes increased water _____.

____ 11. Patients with diabetes insipidus are sometimes taught to measure specific gravity at home with _____.

A. Muscle weakness

B. Hydration

C. Antihistamines

D. Weights

E. Diabetes insipidus

F. ADH

G. Thyroid hormone

H. Vasopressin

I. Hydrometers

J. Nasal sprays

K. Glucose monitors

L. Output

M. Retention

Introductory Nursing Care of Adults

VI. Complete the statements on the left with the most appropriate term on the right. Some terms may be used more than once, and some terms may not be used.

____ 1. A syndrome characterized by a water imbalance related to an increase in ADH secretion is called _____.

____ 2. Kidneys retain fluid due to the elevation of _____.

____ 3. Plasma volume expands when ADH is elevated in SIADH, causing an increased ____.

____ 4. When ADH is elevated, the patient develops water intoxication and the body sodium is diluted, resulting in _____.

____ 5. Weight gain without edema is one of the main symptoms of _____.

____ 6. The treatment for SIADH promotes the elimination of _____.

____ 7. In patients with SIADH, fluids are restricted and patients are given _____.

____ 8. Patients with SIADH have fluid volume excess related to excess secretion of _____.

A. Blood pressure
B. Potassium
C. Excess water
D. SIADH
E. Hyponatremia
F. Heart rate
G. ADH
H. Diabetes insipidus
I. Sodium chloride

VII. Complete the statements on the left with the most appropriate term on the right. Some terms may be used more than once, and some terms may not be used.

____ 1. The adrenal glands are located on the superior portion of each kidney in the _____.

____ 2. Norepinephrine and epinephrine act as _____.

____ 3. Epinephrine and norepinephrine help the body adapt to _____, as characterized by the "fight or flight" response.

____ 4. Ten percent of the adrenal gland is composed of the adrenal _____ .

____ 5. The _____ are a pair of small, highly vascularized, triangular-shaped organs.

____ 6. The outer portion of the adrenal gland is called the _____.

____ 7. Norepinephrine and epinephrine are released into the circulation and transported to target organs, where they exert their effects by binding to _____.

____ 8. Stimulation of the sympathetic nervous system causes the adrenal medulla to secrete two _____.

____ 9. The inner portion of the adrenal gland is called the _____.

____ 10. A major function of the catecholamines is the maintenance of _____.

A. Stress
B. Thoracic cavity
C. Adrenal glands
D. Neurotransmitters
E. Homeostasis
F. Catecholamines
G. Medulla
H. Cerebrum
I. Cortex
J. Retroperitoneal cavity
K. Ganglia
L. Adrenergic receptors

VIII. Complete the statements on the left with the most appropriate term on the right. Some terms may be used more than once, and some terms may not be used.

____ 1. The hormones synthesized and secreted by the adrenal cortex are known as _____.

____ 2. The most abundant mineralocorticoid is _____.

____ 3. Mineralocorticoids play a key role in maintaining an adequate _____.

____ 4. Aldosterone promotes the reabsorption of _____.

____ 5. Angiotensin II stimulates the secretion of aldosterone, which preserves or increases extracellular fluid volume, subsequently increasing _____.

____ 6. The most abundant and potent glucocorticoid is _____.

____ 7. Ninety percent of the adrenal gland is composed of the adrenal _____ .

____ 8. Aldosterone promotes the excretion of _____.

____ 9. The secretion of aldosterone is regulated by serum levels of potassium, the renin-angiotensin mechanism, and _____.

____ 10. A substance whose release is stimulated by a decrease in extracellular fluid volume that acts on plasma proteins to release angiotensin is _____.

____ 11. The hormones produced by the adrenal cortex include androgens or estrogens, glucocorticoids, and _____.

A. Blood pressure

B. Catecholamines

C. Steroids

D. Renin

E. Sodium

F. Cortex

G. Aldosterone

H. Mineralocorticoids

I. Heart rate

J. Potassium

K. Extracellular fluid volume

L. Cortisol

M. ACTH

IX. Complete the statements on the left with the most appropriate term on the right. Some terms may be used more than once, and some terms may not be used.

____ 1. Addison's disease results in the loss of aldosterone and _____.

____ 2. A test that is necessary for a definitive diagnosis of hypoadrenalism, such as Addison's disease, is _____.

____ 3. The mainstay of treatment of patients with Addison's disease is replacement therapy with mineralocorticoids and _____.

____ 4. Potassium excretion is decreased when cortisol is not secreted, resulting in _____.

____ 5. Secondary adrenal insufficiency is a result of dysfunction of the hypothalamus or the _____.

____ 6. Decreased levels of aldosterone alter the clearance of potassium, water, and _____.

____ 7. When sodium and water excretion accelerates, problems such as hyponatremia and _____ can result.

____ 8. Acute adrenal crisis is also called _____.

____ 9. Impaired secretion of cortisol results in decreased liver and muscle glycogen and decreased _____.

____ 10. Secondary adrenal insufficiency leads to decreased production of cortisol and _____.

____ 11. Primary adrenal insufficiency is also called _____.

____ 12. Decreased supplies of available glucose, which occurs as a result of impaired secretion of cortisol, is called _____.

____ 13. Patients with either primary or secondary adrenal insufficiency are at risk for episodes of _____.

____ 14. A condition that occurs because hyperkalemia promotes hydrogen ion retention is _____.

A. Hypovolemia

B. Pituitary

C. Addison's disease

D. Gluconeogenesis

E. Norepinephrine

F. Glucocorticoids

G. Tachycardia

H. ACTH stimulation test

I. SIADH

J. Hypoglycemia

K. Hyperkalemia

L. Metabolic acidosis

M. Sodium

N. Androgen

O. Cortisol

P. Addisonian crisis

Q. Androgens

X. Complete the statements on the left with the most appropriate term on the right. Some terms may be used more than once, and some terms may not be used.

____ 1. Prolonged administration of high doses of corticosteroids may cause Cushing's syndrome; this is an example of an _____ cause.

____ 2. An initial screening for Cushing's syndrome is the overnight _____ test.

____ 3. In the immediate postoperative period of adrenalectomy patients, _____ may be needed to maintain blood pressure.

____ 4. The most common cause of Cushing's syndrome is long-term exogenous _____ use.

____ 5. Corticotropin-secreting pituitary tumors may cause Cushing's syndrome; this is an example of an _____ cause.

____ 6. Patients with a pheochromocytoma exhibit episodes of hypertension, hypermetabolism, and _____.

____ 7. Excessive production of ACTH because of a pituitary tumor is called _____.

____ 8. Hypersecretion of the adrenal cortex may result in the production of excess amounts of _____.

____ 9. The prevention of infections in adrenalectomy patients is maintained through observance of _____.

____ 10. A tumor of the adrenal medulla that causes secretion of excessive catecholamines is a _____.

____ 11. The condition that results from excessive cortisol is called _____.

____ 12. Patients who take drugs that suppress adrenal function are at risk of acute _____.

A. Cushing's disease

B. SIADH

C. Exogenous

D. Pheochromocytoma

E. Steroid

F. Cushing's syndrome

G. Hyperglycemia

H. Corticosteroids

I. Diabetes insipidus

J. Dexamethasone

K. Endogenous

L. Adrenal crisis

M. Vasopressors

N. Asepsis

XI. Match the definition or description on the left with the most appropriate term on the right. Some terms may be used more than once, and some may not be used.

_____ 1. Stimulates the growth and development of bone, muscles, or organs

_____ 2. Controls ovulation or egg release in the female and testosterone production in the male

_____ 3. Controls the release of glucocorticoids and adrenal androgens

_____ 4. Stimulates the development of the eggs in the ovary of the female and sperm production in the male

_____ 5. Another name for the somatotrophic hormone

_____ 6. Stimulates breast milk production in the female

_____ 7. Promotes pigmentation

_____ 8. Another name for the lactogenic hormone

_____ 9. Causes the reabsorption of water from the renal tubules of the kidney

_____ 10. Causes contractions of the uterus in labor and the release of breast milk

_____ 11. Another name for vasopressin

_____ 12. Controls the secretory activities of the thyroid gland

A. Luteinizing hormone

B. Thyroid-stimulating hormone

C. Oxytocin

D. Melanocyte-stimulating hormone

E. Growth hormone

F. Norepinephrine

G. Antidiuretic hormone

H. Adrenocorticotropic hormone

I. Prolactin

J. Follicle-stimulating hormone

XII. Match the purpose of the diagnostic test on the left with the test on the right.

_____ 1. Commonly performed test that identifies whether adequate levels of hormones are present using radioactively tagged hormones; based on antigen-antibody displacement reactions

_____ 2. An accurate test for levels of hormones in the blood, utilizing enzyme-labeled hormones

_____ 3. Serial blood glucose levels are measured to detect hyperpituitarism, since glucose will suppress GH levels via a negative feedback process

_____ 4. A test that stimulates the release of ADH to detect diabetes insipidus

A. Glucose tolerance test

B. Hypertonic saline test

C. Enzyme-linked immunosorbent assay

D. Radioimmunoassay

XIII. Match the definition or description on the left with the most appropriate term on the right. Some terms may be used more than once, and some may not be used.

____ 1. A pathologic state caused by excess production of an anterior pituitary hormone

____ 2. One of the hormones most likely to be produced in excess with hyperpituitarism

____ 3. A condition caused by over-production of GH

____ 4. The most common factor in hyperpituitarism

A. Pituitary adenoma

B. Hyperpituitarism

C. Growth hormone

D. Gigantism

E. ACTH

XIV. Match the characteristics on the left with the term describing diabetes insipidus on the right. Some terms may be used more than once, and some may not be used.

____ 1. Inherited defect in which the renal tubules of the kidney do not respond to ADH, resulting in inadequate water reabsorption by the kidneys

____ 2. Caused by a defect in the posterior pituitary gland related to familial or idiopathic causes

____ 3. The result of hypothalamic tumors, head trauma, infection, surgical procedures (hypophysectomy), or metastatic tumors originating in the lung or breast

____ 4. Caused by lithium or demeclomycin, which affect the kidney by inhibiting its response to ADH

____ 5. ADH hormone deficiency results in the excretion of large volumes of very dilute urine

A. Polyuria

B. Secondary DI

C. Nephrogenic DI

D. Primary DI

E. Oliguria

F. Drug-related DI

XV. Complete the statements on the left with the most appropriate term on the right. Some terms may be used more than once, and some terms may not be used.

____ 1. Increased plasma osmolarity stimulates the osmoreceptors, which in turn relay information to the cerebral cortex, causing the persons to experience _____.

____ 2. Massive dehydration leads to severe _____ imbalances.

____ 3. With ADH deficiency, massive dehydration occurs, which leads to decreased intravascular volume, circulatory collapse, and _____.

____ 4. Electrolyte imbalances contribute to circulatory collapse by causing arrhythmias and impaired contractility of the _____.

____ 5. Massive diuresis results in increased plasma _____.

A. Thirst

B. Skeletal muscles

C. Heart

D. Electrolytes

E. Osmolarity

F. Hypotension

XVI. Match the descriptions on the left with the physiologic actions of glucocorticoids on the right. Some terms may be used more than once, and some terms may not be used.

___ 1. Increase hepatic gluconeogenesis and inhibit peripheral glucose use

___ 2. Release glycerol and free fatty acids

___ 3. Migration of inflammatory cells to sites of injury

A. Increased lypolysis

B. Increased protein catabolism

C. Maintenance of glucose levels

D. Increased anti-inflammatory effects

XVII. Indicate whether the following laboratory study results would be expected to (A) increase or (B) decrease in patients with Addison's disease.

___ 1. Serum cortisol level

___ 2. Fasting glucose

___ 3. Sodium

___ 4. Potassium

___ 5. Blood urea nitrogen

A. Increase

B. Decrease

XVIII. Match the nursing diagnoses for persons with Cushing's syndrome on the left with the most appropriate "related to" statements on the right.

___ 1. High risk for infection

___ 2. Altered thought processes

___ 3. High risk for impaired skin integrity

___ 4. High risk for injury (fracture)

___ 5. Body image disturbance

A. Changes in skin and connective tissue and edema

B. Changes in physical appearance and function

C. Fluid and electrolyte imbalance

D. Osteoporosis

E. High serum cortisol levels

XIX. Match the interventions on the left with the nursing diagnoses for patients with Cushing's syndrome on the right. Some nursing diagnoses may be used more than once, and some may not be used.

___ 1. Avoid exposure to infections

___ 2. Report minor signs, such as low-grade fever, sore throat, or aches to the physician

___ 3. Seek a psychiatric referral if mood swings continue to be a problem

___ 4. Assist patient to change positions at least every 2 hours

___ 5. Protect from falls or trauma

___ 6. Discuss bruises, abnormal fat distribution, and hirsutism with the patient if they cause embarrassment

___ 7. Teach the patient about the importance of continuing drug therapy under medical supervision

A. High risk for injury

B. High risk for impaired skin integrity

C. Sexual dysfunction

D. Body image disturbance

E. High risk for infection

F. Knowledge deficit

G. Altered thought processes

XX. List 6 functions of hormones.

1.

2.

3.

4.

5.

6.

XXI. Indicate age-related changes in the healthy older person regarding pituitary function.

1. Pituitary function:

2. ADH secretion:

3. Ability to concentrate urine:

XXII. List 5 conditions that may result from pituitary adenomas that secrete hormones.

1.

2.

3.

4.

5.

XIII. List 2 functions of GH.

1.

2.

XXIV. Monitoring the postoperative hypophysectomy patient for signs and symptoms of infection is important; list 4 signs and symptoms that may be indications of meningitis.

1.

2.

3.

4.

XXV. List 2 medications that will be given as hormone replacement therapy following a complete hypophysectomy.

1.

2.

XXVI. The postoperative hypophysectomy patient is instructed to avoid any activities that can cause a Valsalva maneuver; list 4 activities that may create enough intracranial pressure to disrupt the surgical site and cause CSF leakage.

1.

2.

3.

4.

XXVII. List 5 causes of panhypopituitarism.

1.

2.

3.

4.

5.

XXVIII. List 4 signs and symptoms of dwarfism.

1.

2.

3.

4.

XXIX. List 3 signs of decreased gonadotropins (when gonads become atrophied) which occur in both males and females.

1.

2.

3.

XXX. List 6 topics which should be addressed in the teaching plan of a patient with hypopituitarism.

1.

2.

3.

4.

5.

6.

XXXI. List 3 common signs and symptoms of diabetes insipidus.

1.

2.

3.

XXXII. List 10 possible signs and symptoms of dehydration.

1.   6.

2.   7.

3.   8.

4.   9.

5.   10.

XXXIII. List 4 signs that patients with DI should be taught to report to physicians if they occur, because they may indicate the need for additional treatment.

1.   3.

2.   4.

XXXIV. List 6 factors that may cause or contribute to the development of SIADH.

1.   4.

2.   5.

3.   6.

XXXV. List 8 main symptoms of SIADH that reflect the effects of hyponatremia and water retention.

1.   5.

2.   6.

3.   7.

4.   8.

XXXVI. List 3 measures the nurse can take to help enforce fluid restrictions in patients with SIADH, which may be as little as 500 ml per 24 hours.

1.

2.

3.

XXXVII. List 3 functions of glucocorticoids.

1.

2.

3.

XXXVIII. List 5 symptoms of adrenal dysfunction that may cause a patient to seek medical attention.

1.

2.

3.

4.

5.

XXXIX. List 8 manifestations of an addisonian crisis related to the areas listed.

1. Blood pressure:

2. Heart rate:

3. Fluid balance:

4. Mental status:

5. Sodium level:

6. Potassium level:

7. Calcium level:

8. Glucose level:

XL. List 4 symptoms of hypoglycemia that patients with Addison's disease should report to the physician if they occur.

1.   3.

2.   4.

XLI. List 6 components of a teaching plan for patients with Addison's disease.

1.   4.

2.   5.

3.   6.

XLII. List 5 hallmark findings that lead to a diagnosis of Cushing's syndrome.

1.

2.

3.

4.

5.

XLIII. Choose the most appropriate answer.

1. In the healthy older person, there may be increased secretion of ADH, which may lead to:
   A. edema
   B. dyspnea
   C. hypertension
   D. dehydration

2. The production of excess GH may lead to the development of:
   A. atherosclerosis and hyperglycemia
   B. edema and congestive heart failure
   C. dyspnea and pneumonia
   D. oliguria and kidney failure

3. Growth hormone antagonizes insulin and interferes with its effects, thus leading to:
   A. hyperkalemia
   B. hypokalemia
   C. hyperglycemia
   D. hypoglycemia

4. Because growth hormone mobilizes stored fat for energy, levels of free fatty acids are elevated in the blood stream, leading to the development of:
   A. pneumonia
   B. kidney failure
   C. hypotension
   D. atherosclerosis

5. Visual problems occur in hyperpituitarism due to pressure on the:
   A. occipital lobe
   B. optic nerves
   C. frontal lobe
   D. occulomotor nerves

6. Patients with gigantism and acromegaly initially present with increased strength, progressing rapidly to complaints of:
   A. hypotension and syncope
   B. weakness and fatigue
   C. edema and dry skin
   D. dehydration and bradycardia

7. Some patients with gigantism and acromegaly experience elevated levels of prolactin, which may present as:
   A. distorted facial features
   B. abdominal distention
   C. peripheral neuropathies
   D. galactorrhea

8. Radiation is sometimes used to treat GH adenomas, but overall response is slow and complications occur, such as hypopituitarism and:
   A. auditory defects
   B. hypertension
   C. visual defects
   D. fractures

9. One drug commonly prescribed for patients with hyperpituitarism is:
   A. bromocriptine (Parlodel)
   B. furosemide (Lasix)
   C. levothyroxine (Synthroid)
   D. digoxin

10. A common nursing diagnosis for patients with hyperpituitarism is:
    A. altered tissue perfusion
    B. altered skin integrity
    C. high risk for infection
    D. body image disturbance

11. Bromocriptine (Parlodel) inhibits the release of prolactin and GH by activating:
    A. antidiuretic hormone
    B. thyroid gland
    C. adrenal gland
    D. dopamine receptors

12. Following hypophysectomy, the nurse asks the patient to place the chin to the chest to assess for nuchal rigidity, which is associated with:
    A. bone density
    B. meningeal irritation
    C. cerebral edema
    D. impaired circulation

13. Changes in assessment findings following hypophysectomy that may reflect edema due to the manipulation of tissues or bleeding intracranially include:
    A. unequal pupil size
    B. decreasing alertness
    C. decreasing blood pressure
    D. rising body temperature

14. Strict documentation of intake and output and measurement of specific gravity are important because postoperative hypophysectomy patients are at risk for:
    A. congestive heart failure
    B. kidney failure
    C. pneumonia
    D. diabetes insipidus

15. Because CSF leaks sometimes occur in postoperative hypophysectomy patients, the nurse should check:
    A. intake and output
    B. pupil reactivity
    C. nasal packing
    D. vital signs

16. A bedside test can be done with a chemical strip to detect whether drainage is CSF, since CSF has a high content of:
    A. glucose
    B. protein
    C. white blood cells
    D. red blood cells

17. Decreased pigmentation of the skin results in:
    A. edema
    B. pallor
    C. pruritus
    D. erythema

18. The patient who has a complete hypophysectomy requires hormone replacements:
    A. preoperatively
    B. during the postoperative recovery period
    C. for 6 months to 1 year
    D. for a lifetime

19. In myxedema, insufficient thyroid hormone is available for normal metabolism and:
    A. visual acuity
    B. muscle tone
    C. heat production
    D. bone growth

20. If there is a lack of melanocyte-stimulating hormone, the skin exhibits decreased:
    A. sensory perception
    B. immunity
    C. pigmentation
    D. thermoregulation

21. Deficiency of thyroid-stimulating hormones necessitates thyroid replacement with a drug such as:
    A. ocreotide acetate (Sandostatin)
    B. bromocriptine (Parlodel)
    C. levothyroxine (Synthroid)
    D. vasopressin (Pitressin)

22. To produce or maintain libido, secondary sexual characteristics, and well-being, males with hypopituitarism should receive:
    A. testosterone
    B. estrogen
    C. Synthroid
    D. Parlodel

23. For patients with hypopituitarism, which hormone replacement is necessary in children but not in adults?
    A. thyroid hormone
    B. estrogen
    C. testosterone
    D. growth hormone

24. Drug-related diabetes insipidus is often caused by:
    A. bromocriptine (Parlodel)
    B. lithium carbonate (Eskalith)
    C. levothyroxine (Synthroid)
    D. digitalis

25. A 24-hour urine output of greater than 4 liters of fluid suggests a diagnosis of:
    A. hypertension
    B. kidney infection
    C. congestive heart failure
    D. diabetes insipidus

26. With diabetes insipidus, the specific gravity is extremely low, and the urine is:
    A. concentrated
    B. red
    C. pyuric
    D. dilute

27. In order to maintain adequate blood volume in patients with DI, two measures that are required include intravenous fluid volume replacement and:
    A. diuretics
    B. vasopressors
    C. anticholinergics
    D. antihistamines

28. A common nursing diagnosis for patients with diabetes insipidus is fluid volume deficit related to:
    A. altered tissue perfusion
    B. fatigue and weakness
    C. high risk for infection
    D. excessive urine output

29. The level of consciousness deteriorates and the patient may have seizures or lapse into a coma when water intoxication affects the:
    A. respiratory system
    B. urinary system
    C. cardiovascular system
    D. central nervous system

30. A nursing diagnosis for patients with SIADH is high risk for injury related to:
    A. acute adrenal insufficiency
    B. impaired physiologic response to stress
    C. water intoxication
    D. decreased ADH secretion

31. To prevent progressive cerebral edema in patients with SIADH, patients are placed in what position in bed?
    A. flat
    B. semi-Fowler's
    C. full Fowler's
    D. side-lying

32. The primary function of adrenal androgens is:
    A. metabolism
    B. masculinization
    C. feminization
    D. diuresis

33. In postmenopausal women, the primary source of endogenous estrogen is the:
    A. hypothalamus
    B. thyroid gland
    C. adrenal cortex
    D. ovarian follicle

34. A common skin finding in patients with adrenal dysfunction is:
    A. protruding bones
    B. erythema
    C. bronze pigmentation
    D. pruritus

35. Age-related changes of adrenal function are that the adrenal function:
    A. decreases in epinephrine
    B. remains adequate
    C. becomes hyperactive
    D. increases in metabolism

36. The response to sodium restriction and to position changes is less efficient in the elderly due to declines in the secretion of plasma renin and:
    A. thyroxine
    B. aldosterone
    C. estrogen
    D. androgens

37. Signs and symptoms of hyperkalemia that should be reported to the physician by patients with Addison's disease include:
    A. dyspnea and coughing
    B. oliguria and flank pain
    C. constipation and fatty stools
    D. weakness and paresthesia

38. A characteristic of acute addisonian crisis that must be treated immediately is sudden profound weakness with:
    A. intense headache
    B. dyspnea
    C. postural hypotension
    D. tachycardia

39. Patients with Addison's disease are weighed daily to monitor:
    A. fluid balance
    B. edema
    C. dietary intake
    D. hypertension

40. What substance may be used liberally in the diet of patients with Addison's disease?
    A. carbohydrates
    B. salt
    C. saturated fats
    D. caffeine

41. The majority of patients with Cushing's syndrome are at high risk for infection due to:
    A. fluid and electrolyte balance
    B. altered skin tissue
    C. high serum cortisol levels
    D. osteoporosis

42. Hyperpituitarism leads to:
    A. Addison's disease
    B. adrenal crisis
    C. personality changes
    D. gigantism

XLIV. In the following figure, label the organs of the endocrine system (A–F).

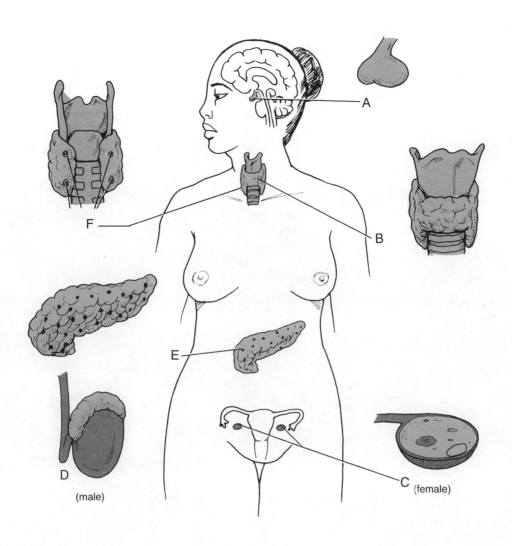

A.   D.

B.   E.

C.   F.

CHAPTER

43

Female Reproductive Disorders

OBJECTIVES

1. List data to be collected when assessing the female reproductive system.
2. Describe the nursing interventions for women who are having diagnostic tests and procedures for reproductive system disorders.
3. Identify the nursing interventions associated with douche, cauterization, heat therapy, and topical medications used to treat disorders of the female reproductive system.
4. Explain the pathophysiology, signs and symptoms, complications, diagnostic procedures, and medical or surgical treatment for selected disorders of the female reproductive system.
5. Apply the nursing process to plan care for the patient with common disorders of the female reproductive system.
6. Describe the nursing interventions for the patient who is menopausal.

LEARNING ACTIVITIES

I. Match the definition on the left with the most appropriate term on the right.

____ 1. Surgical excision of a fallopian tube and ovary
____ 2. Difficult or painful sexual intercourse in women
____ 3. Bending backward of an entire organ
____ 4. A condition in which endometrial tissue is located abnormally outside the uterus
____ 5. Inflammation of breast tissue
____ 6. Inflammation of the vulva
____ 7. Herniation of the urinary bladder into the vagina
____ 8. Bleeding or spotting between menstrual periods
____ 9. Surgical removal of the uterus
____ 10. Abnormal cells
____ 11. Cessation of menstruation
____ 12. Herniation of part of the rectum into the vagina
____ 13. Age at which the first menstrual period occurs
____ 14. Inflammation of the vagina
____ 15. Painful menstruation
____ 16. Menstrual periods characterized by profuse or prolonged bleeding

A. Cystocele
B. Menopause
C. Vaginitis
D. Endometriosis
E. Menorrhagia
F. Metrorrhagia
G. Rectocele
H. Dyspareunia
I. Hysterectomy
J. Vulvitis
K. Mastitis
L. Menarche
M. Salpingo-oophorectomy
N. Dysmenorrhea
O. Dysplasia
P. Retroversion

Introductory Nursing Care of Adults

II. Match the definition on the left with the most appropriate term on the right.

____ 1. An operation that narrows the vagina by suturing the vaginal wall

____ 2. Bending forward of an entire organ

____ 3. Number of pregnancies that terminated after 20 weeks of gestation

____ 4. Bending backward of the upper portion of an organ

____ 5. Inflammation of the cervix

____ 6. State of being unable to reproduce

____ 7. A device inserted into the vagina to support the uterus

____ 8. Total number of pregnancies

____ 9. The inability to conceive and produce viable offspring

____ 10. Bending forward of the top of an organ

A. Anteversion
B. Infertility
C. Parity
D. Pessary
E. Sterility
F. Anteflexion
G. Colporrhaphy
H. Gravidity
I. Retroflexion
J. Cervicitis

III. Complete the statements on the left with the most appropriate term on the right. Some terms may be used more than once, and some terms may not be used.

____ 1. The _____ is a pad of fatty tissue that covers and protects the symphysis pubis.

____ 2. Extensions of fatty tissue that cover and protect inner vulvar structures and that extend from the mons pubis to the perineum are the _____.

____ 3. Another name for the vaginal opening is the _____.

____ 4. A canal that extends from the vulva to the uterus is the _____.

____ 5. The external genitalia are called the _____.

____ 6. The pelvic floor area between the posterior labia minora and the anus is the _____.

____ 7. The two ovaries, two fallopian tubes, the uterus, and the vagina make up the _____.

____ 8. The hood over the clitoris is called the _____.

____ 9. The _____ is a small female structure that corresponds to the male penis and that is composed of erectile tissue with sensory nerve endings.

____ 10. Thin folds of smooth skin that form a hood over the clitoris and extend to the posterior edge of the vagina are called _____.

A. Vagina
B. Labia minora
C. Prepuce
D. Perineum
E. Introitus
F. Frenulum
G. Mons pubis
H. Hymen
I. Internal genitalia
J. Clitoris
K. Labia majora
L. Vulva

IV. Complete the statements on the left with the most appropriate term on the right. Some terms may be used more than once, and some terms may not be used.

___ 1. The site of fertilization, where the sperm and ovum unite, is the _____.

___ 2. The female structure that corresponds to the male testis is the _____.

___ 3. Paired mammary glands located on the chest wall are called _____.

___ 4. The _____ is a firm, muscular organ that is pear shaped and hollow.

___ 5. The neck of the uterus is the _____.

___ 6. The upper segment of the uterus, which is the site of insertions of the fallopian tubes, is called the _____.

___ 7. The tubular structure that receives an ovum from an ovary is called the _____.

___ 8. Glandular and ductal tissue, fibrous tissue, and fat make up the inner structure of _____.

___ 9. Pigmented structures located at the midline of each breast are called _____.

A. Uterus

B. Fundus

C. Vagina

D. Breasts

E. Cervix

F. Endometrium

G. Fallopian tube

H. Introitus

I. Nipples

J. Ovary

V. Complete the statements on the left with the most appropriate term on the right. Some terms may be used more than once, and some terms may not be used.

___ 1. A type of invasive surgery procedure in which a large amount of cervical tissue is removed to treat cancer is called the _____.

___ 2. An invasive surgical procedure that provides direct visualization of the female pelvic cavity is called _____.

___ 3. The test for which specimens are collected routinely to detect cervical cancer and dysplasia is called the _____.

___ 4. The procedure that is commonly done before cervical biopsies is _____.

___ 5. A type of biopsy done in physician's offices or outpatient clinics to diagnose cervical cancer is called _____.

___ 6. Specimens for cultures and smears may be collected to identify suspected _____.

___ 7. The procedure that is done to identify ectopic pregnancy or pelvic masses is _____.

___ 8. A test performed to diagnose uterine cancer is the _____.

___ 9. A procedure in which an instrument is used to inspect the cervix under magnification and to identify abnormal and potentially cancerous tissue is _____.

A. Multiple punch biopsy

B. Papnicolaou (Pap) smear

C. Dilation and curettage

D. Infections

E. Cone biopsy

F. Aspiration biopsy

G. Endometrial biopsy

H. Culdoscopy

I. Breast biopsy

J. Colposcopy

VI. Complete the statements on the left with the most appropriate term on the right. Some terms may be used more than once, and some terms may not be used.

____ 1. A test that patients can be taught to perform by themselves that helps detect abnormalities such as puckering or lumps is _____.

____ 2. An invasive surgical procedure in which an instrument is used to visualize abdominal organs is _____.

____ 3. A procedure that can be performed in a doctor's office or outpatient clinic to aid in the diagnosis when uterine cancer is suspected is _____.

____ 4. A radiologic test used for breast cancer screening is _____.

____ 5. The only method of diagnosing breast cancer is _____.

____ 6. An invasive surgical procedure in which an instrument is used to perform minor surgery such as a tubal ligation is _____.

____ 7. The procedure in which the entire area of uterine lining is scraped is endometrial _____.

____ 8. A procedure in which the instrument is inserted through a small abdominal buttonhole incision is _____.

A. Breast biopsy

B. Dilation and curettage

C. Papanicolaou (Pap) smear

D. Laparotomy

E. Breast self-examination

F. Mammography

G. Curettage

H. Laparoscopy

VII. Complete the statements on the left with the most appropriate term on the right. Some terms may be used more than once, and some terms may not be used.

____ 1. When the body of the uterus bends backward on itself, this is called _____.

____ 2. A forward tilt of the uterus at a sharp angle to the vagina is called _____.

____ 3. When the uterus bends forward on itself, this is called _____.

____ 4. A backward tilt of the uterus with the cervix pointed downward toward the anterior vaginal wall is called _____.

A. Antiflexion

B. Introversion

C. Retroversion

D. Retroflexion

E. Extraversion

F. Anteversion

VIII. Complete the statements on the left with the most appropriate term on the right. Some terms may be used more than once, and some terms may not be used.

___ 1. Mastectomy patients are at high risk for injury related to _____.

___ 2. The removal of the tumor with a margin of surrounding healthy tissue but preserving most of the breast is called _____.

___ 3. A low-incidence cancer of the nipple and areola is _____.

___ 4. The implantation of a tissue expander followed by injections of normal saline is called _____.

___ 5. The removal of all breast tissue, overlying skin, axillary lymph nodes, and underlying pectoral muscles is called _____.

___ 6. If breast cancer cells removed during surgery need estrogen for cell replication, they are said to be _____.

A. Paget's disease
B. ER negative
C. Radical mastectomy
D. Lumpectomy
E. Silicone implant
F. ER positive
G. Lymphedema
H. Reconstruction

IX. Complete the statements on the left with the most appropriate term on the right. Some terms may be used more than once, and some terms may not be used.

___ 1. If a woman has conceived at least one time but is not able to conceive again, this type of infertility is referred to as _____.

___ 2. If the woman has never conceived, this type of infertility is referred to as _____.

___ 3. The ability to conceive but inability to deliver a live infant is called _____.

___ 4. If the woman has conceived at least one time but is not able to deliver a viable infant, this type of infertility is referred to as _____.

___ 5. If the man has never impregnated a woman, this type of infertility is referred to as _____.

___ 6. The inability to conceive within 1 year of regular unprotected sexual intercourse is called _____.

A. Primary
B. Secondary
C. Tertiary
D. Quaternary
E. Infertility
F. Anorgasmia

X. Match the description on the left with the most appropriate days of a typical menstrual cycle on the right.

___ 1. Preparation of the uterine lining for implantation of the fertilized ovum

___ 2. Maturation of an ovarian follicle

___ 3. Unfertilized ovum does not implant; corpus luteum degenerates; necrosis of uterine lining

___ 4. Production of estrogen by the maturing follicle

___ 5. Production of progesterone

___ 6. Menstruation

A. Days 6–14

B. Days 1–14

C. Days 1–5

D. Days 6–26

E. Days 15–26

F. Days 27–28

XI. Match the terms on the left with the most appropriate numerical ranges on the right. These terms refer to the variations within normal menstrual periods. Some ranges may be used more than once, and some may not be used.

___1. Length of cycle (days)

___2. Duration of menstruation (days)

___3. Amount of blood loss (ml)

A. 2–8

B. 10–14

C. 21–40

D. 40–100

E. 150–200

XII. Match the description on the left with the most appropriate term on the right. Some terms may be used more than once, and some may not be used.

___ 1. Often seen with diabetes

___ 2. A sexually transmitted disease that is the primary cause of ectopic pregnancy and infertility

___ 3. Includes profuse, frothy, and yellow-gray discharge

___ 4. A source of non-STD associated pelvic inflammatory disease along with contamination during gynecologic surgery, childbirth, and abortion

___ 5. Includes cottage cheese-like appearance of discharge

___ 6. Protozoal infection

___ 7. Condition that includes scarring and adhesions

___ 8. Fungal infection

___ 9. Infection often caused by disruption of the normal vaginal flora

___10. The sexually transmitted disease that causes most pelvic inflammatory disease

A. *Trichomonas vaginalis*

B. Endometriosis

C. Chlamydia

D. Gonorrhea

E. *Candida albicans*

F. Multiple sexual partners

G. Pelvic examinations

XIII. Match the definition or description on the left with the most appropriate term on the right. Some terms may be used more than once, and some may not be used.

____ 1. Level of prolapse if the cervix protrudes from the vaginal opening

____ 2. A vaginal disorder caused by weakness of supportive structures between the vagina and bladder

____ 3. Level of prolapse if the vagina is inverted and both the cervix and the body of the uterus protrude from the vaginal opening

____ 4. Method used to diagnose first-degree uterine prolapse

____ 5. Nonsurgical treatment of uterine prolapse that is aimed at elevating the uterus

____ 6. A vaginal disorder caused by weakness of supportive structures between the vagina and rectum

____ 7. A condition in which the uterus descends into the vagina from its usual position in the pelvis

____ 8. Method used to diagnose second- and third-degree uterine prolapse

____ 9. Level of prolapse if the cervix is above the vaginal opening

A. Pessary

B. Third degree

C. Visual inspection

D. First degree

E. Rectocele

F. Uterine prolapse

G. Second degree

H. Fourth degree

I. Cystocele

J. Laparoscopy

K. Pelvic examination

XIV. Match the "related to" statements on the left with the nursing diagnoses for patients with cystocele and rectocele on the right.

____ 1. Pelvic muscle weakness

____ 2. Collection of feces in herniated bowel

____ 3. Painful intercourse

____ 4. Incomplete bladder emptying

A. Sexual dysfunction

B. Stress incontinence

C. High risk for infection

D. Constipation

XV. Match the nursing diagnoses for patients with cystocele and rectocele on the left with the nursing goals on the right.

____ 1. Stress incontinence

____ 2. Constipation

____ 3. Sexual dysfunction

____ 4. High risk for infection

A. Absence of urinary tract infections

B. Normal bowel elimination

C. Urinary continence

D. Satisfying sexual practices

XVI. Match each nursing diagnosis for patients with cystocele and rectocele with the most appropriate nursing interventions on the left. Some interventions may be used more than once.

1. Initial application of cold to reduce pain and swelling

2. Teach the patient pelvic floor exercises

3. Emphasize to patient the need for maintaining soft stool consistency and regular bowel elimination

4. Subsequent application of heat via sitz baths and heat lamps

5. Instruct the patient to report signs of urinary frequency, burning, or foul odor, which may indicate UTI

6. Emphasize including plenty of fluids, wide variety of high-fiber foods such as fruits, vegetables, and grains in the diet

___ A. Stress incontinence

___ B. Constipation

___ C. High risk for infection

___ D. Pain

XVII. Match the "related to" statements on the left with the most appropriate nursing diagnoses for the patient with infertility on the right. Some diagnoses may be used more than once, and some may not be used.

___ 1. Unmet expectations of conception

___ 2. Feeling of failure related to inability to conceive

___ 3. Loss of spontaneity

___ 4. Feelings of loss

___ 5. Structured efforts to conceive

A. Situational low self-esteem

B. Anxiety and fear

C. Altered sexuality patterns

D. Ineffective individual coping

XVIII. Match the preoperative and postoperative nursing diagnoses on the left for a patient with a hysterectomy with possible interventions on the right.

_____ 1. Knowledge deficit related to information or misinterpretation of effects of ERT

_____ 2. High risk for fluid volume deficit related to postoperative bleeding

_____ 3. Urinary retention related to surgical manipulation, local tissue edema, temporary sensory or motor impairment

_____ 4. Self-esteem disturbance related to perceived potential changes in femininity, effect on sexual relationship

_____ 5. Altered tissue perfusion related to reduction of cellular components necessary for delivery of oxygen, hypovolemia, reduction of blood flow, intraoperative trauma

_____ 6. Colonic constipation related to weakening of abdominal musculature, abdominal pain, decreased physical activity, dietary changes, environmental changes

A. Assist patient to bathroom or commode; use bedpan only if absolutely necessary

B. Instruct and assist with foot and leg exercises while confined to bed; encourage and assist with ambulation when allowed

C. Explain that positions for sexual intercourse should avoid pressure on the abdominal incision for as long as incisional tenderness persists

D. Check mucous membranes for moisture; offer frequent mouthwashes during nothing by mouth status

E. Encourage early and frequent ambulation

F. Explain that estrogen may increase fluid retention, which may make one "feel fat"

XIX. Match the use/action on the left with the most appropriate drug used to treat disorders of the female reproductive system on the right.

_____ 1. Enhances bone formation; depresses beta-lipoprotein and cholesterol plasma levels; used to replace natural hormones after menopause, treat advanced breast cancer or prostate cancer

_____ 2. Promotes secretory function in endometrium; influences contractile activity of the uterus; used with estrogens as oral contraceptives

_____ 3. Inhibits production of pituitary gonadotropins; used to treat endometriosis and fibrocystic breast disease

_____ 4. Initially increases and then decreases testosterone levels; used to treat endometriosis

_____ 5. Suppresses ovulation to prevent pregnancy

_____ 6. Prevents implantation of fertilized ovum; used as emergency postcoital contraceptive

_____ 7. Stimulates ovarian follicular growth; used to treat selected patients who have not responded to clomiphene citrate

A. Estrogen-progestin combinations

B. Danazol (Danocrine)

C. Urofollitropin (Metrodin)

D. Conjugated estrogens (Premarin)

E. Leuprolide acetate (Lupron)

F. Progesterone

G. Estrogen only (diethylstilbestrol)

XX. List 2 functions of the vagina that are made possible by the rugated walls of the vagina, which allow the vaginal walls to expand.

1.

2.

XXI. List 2 functions of the ovaries.

1.

2.

XXII. List the 3 parts of the pelvic exam.

1.

2.

3.

XXIII. List 3 purposes for endometrial biopsies.

1.

2.

3.

XXIV. List 4 functions of culdoscopy.

1.

2.

3.

4.

XXV. List 2 reasons why douching is a potentially dangerous procedure.

1.

2.

XXVI. List 4 teaching points to include when teaching the patient about appropriate vaginal hygiene.

1. Extrenal genitalia:

2. Genital area:

3. Underwear:

4. Douching:

XXVII. List 3 reasons why heat applications may be utilized as a therapeutic treatment for many reproductive system conditions.

1.

2.

3.

XXVIII. List 4 benefits of sitz baths, which provide heat to the perineal area.

1.

2.

3.

4.

XXIX. Explain what properties of the mucous membrane lead the nurse to use caution in the following areas when administering vaginal creams and suppositories.

1. Avoid injury:

2. Observe for systemic effects:

XXX. List 4 causes of vulvitis.

1.

2.

3.

4.

XXXI. List 2 reasons why estrogen deficiency frequently results in nonpathogenic vulvitis and vaginitis.

1.

2.

XXXII. List 2 reasons why moist heat is used in the treatment of bartholinitis.

1.

2.

XXXIII. List 3 characteristics of breast tissue in patients with symptomatic mastitis.

1.

2.

3.

XXXIV. List 2 complications of symptomatic mastitis.

1.

2.

XXXV. List 2 groups of women who are especially prone to developing non STD-associated pelvic inflammatory disease.

1.

2.

XXXVI. List 7 signs and symptoms of pelvic inflammatory disease.

1.   5.

2.   6.

3.   7.

4.

XXXVII. List 5 common side effects of danazol, which may be given to patients with endometriosis.

1.

2.

3.

4.

5.

XXXVIII. Explain why oral contraceptives may be prescribed for patients with endometriosis.

XXXIX. List 3 noninvasive methods of preliminary diagnosis of breast cysts.

1.

2.

3.

XL. List 3 indications for surgical biopsy of breast cysts in order to make a definitive diagnosis and to rule out cancer.

1.

2.

3.

XLI. List 3 methods of contraception that are difficult for women with fibroid tumors to use, and explain the potential difficulty.

1.

2.

3.

XLII. List 4 typical problems reported by patients who have rectoceles and cystoceles.

1.

2.

3.

4.

XLIII. In addition to stress incontinence and incomplete bladder emptying, list 3 symptoms that women with cystoceles are likely to experience.

1.

2.

3.

XLIV. List 5 factors that put a woman at risk to develop uterine displacement.

1.

2.

3.

4.

5.

XLV. Indicate how the following categories influence a person's chance for getting breast cancer.

1. Gender:

2. Family history:

3. Race:

4. Age:

5. Duration of menstruating life stage:

6. Radiation exposure:

XLVI. List 6 ways the nurse can intervene to prevent or minimize lymphedema in the mastectomy patient.

1.

2.

3.

4.

5.

6.

XLVII. List 2 ways that affected cervical tissue in patients with advanced cervical cancer may appear upon inspection.

1.

2.

XLVIII. List 3 ways ovarian cancer metastasizes.

1.

2.

3.

IL.   Internal radiation as a treatment for patients with ovarian cancer poses a nursing challenge; list 3 conditions related to internal radiation that make nursing interventions a challenge.

   1.

   2.

   3.

L.   List 3 types of medications that may be prescribed for cancer patients receiving internal radiation to moderate radiation side effects and facilitate patient comfort.

   1.

   2.

   3.

LI.   List 5 criteria by which achievement of the following nursing goals can be determined in patients with cancers of the female reproductive tract.

   1. Reduced anxiety and fear:

   2. Improved body image:

   3. Satisfactory sexual patterns

   4. Appropriate family-patient interactions:

   5. Absence of injury from radiotherapy:

LII.   Conception depends on the interaction of a number of factors: list the anatomic and physiologic conditions that must be present in the male and female reproductive tracts for conception to occur.

Female:

   1.

   2.

Male:

   1.

   2.

   3.

LIII.   List 4 reasons why the medical diagnosis for infertility starts with the male as the initial focus of diagnostic procedures.

   1.

   2.

   3.

   4.

LIV.   List 3 diagnostic tests that are part of infertility work-ups for females that provide data related to ovulation, cervical patency, and adequacy of the endometrium for ovum implantation.

   1.

   2.

   3.

LV. List 7 common symptoms of menopause that may occur in addition to hot flashes.

1.   5.

2.   6.

3.   7.

4.

LVI. Indicate how the following structures change after menopause without estrogen.

1. Uterus:

2. Vagina:

3. Vaginal tissues:

4. Breast tissue:

5. Pubic and axillary hair:

6. Bone mass:

LVII. List 3 contraindications of estrogen replacement therapy.

1.

2.

3.

LVIII. List 3 signs of circulatory disorders that patients receiving estrogen replacement therapy should report immediately to the physician.

1.

2.

3.

LIX. Choose the most appropriate answer.

1. The glands that secrete lubrication fluid in females are called:
   A. bulbourethral glands
   B. Bartholin's glands
   C. inguinal glands
   D. vulvar glands

2. The two main hormones produced by the ovaries are:
   A. estrogen and progesterone
   B. testosterone and prolactin
   C. thyroxine and oxytocin
   D. follicle-stimulating hormone and luteinizing hormone

3. When a patient comes to a clinic with a female reproductive problem, an opening question the nurse asks is:
   A. "What is wrong with you today?"
   B. "What is your problem that made you come in?"
   C. "Why did you come to the clinic today?"
   D. "What is the reason for your visit?"

4. The physical examination of women with reproductive system problems includes the assessment for the presence of Homans's sign in order to detect possible:
   A. vaginal infection
   B. thrombophlebitis
   C. abdominal distention
   D. breast lumps

5. In which position is the patient placed for a pelvic exam?
   A. lithotomy
   B. right side-lying
   C. knee-chest
   D. supine

6. The patient is advised by the nurse that air entering the pelvic cavity during the culdoscopy procedure may cause pain in the:
   A. abdomen
   B. heart
   C. thigh
   D. shoulder

7. A method of deliberate tissue destruction through use of heat, electricity, or chemicals is called:
   A. culdoscopy
   B. culposcopy
   C. cauterization
   D. dilation and curettage

8. Which of the following is a form of dry heat that may be applied to breasts or the abdomen to relieve pain?
   A. aquathermia (K-) pad
   B. hot compresses
   C. sitz baths
   D. whirlpools

9. A particularly helpful type of heat application for small areas such as the vulva or perineum is:
   A. sitz baths
   B. electric heating pad
   C. aquathermia (K-) pad
   D. hot compresses

10. Three signs for which the nurse must observe in patients taking sitz baths are severe pain, shock or:
    A. dyspnea
    B. faintness
    C. dermatitis
    D. headache

11. Dilation of large pelvic vessels during sitz baths may cause:
    A. hypertension
    B. hypotension
    C. pneumonia
    D. seizures

12. Following the administration of vaginal suppositories, the patient is asked to remain in which position for at least 15 minutes, to allow the medication to be absorbed?
    A. prone
    B. right side-lying
    C. sitting
    D. supine

13. Deviations from normal menstrual cycles are viewed as:
    A. uterine bleeding disorders
    B. vaginal hemorrhage problems
    C. endometrial cancers
    D. pelvic inflammatory disease

14. What laboratory test may be ordered for patients with uterine bleeding, if anemia is suspected?
    A. white blood cell count
    B. prothrombin
    C. hemoglobin
    D. electrolytes

15. The most common characteristics of vulvitis are inflammation and:
    A. bleeding
    B. pruritus
    C. cheesy discharge
    D. pain

16. A significant discharge may be seen in:
    A. vulvitis
    B. cystitis
    C. vaginitis
    D. pyelonephritis

17. Signs and symptoms of vaginitis include local swelling, itching and:
    A. redness
    B. pus
    C. hemorrhage
    D. ulcers

18. A potential complication of vulvitis and vaginitis is:
    A. hypotension
    B. ascending infection
    C. seizures
    D. thrombophlebitis

19. Bartholin's glands are vulnerable to a wide variety of infectious microorganisms due to their:
    A. size
    B. location
    C. structure
    D. secretions

20. When Bartholin's glands are infected, the resultant edema and pus formation occlude the duct and form:
    A. tumor
    B. cysts
    C. warts
    D. abscesses

21. The most noticeable symptoms to patients with bartholinitis, which causes them to seek medical attention, is:
    A. edema
    B. pain
    C. discharge
    D. itching

Introductory Nursing Care of Adults

22. The most serious complication of Bartholin's gland abscess is:
A. hypertension
B. dyspnea
C. systemic infection
D. kidney failure

23. Conservative treatment of bartholinitis is sitz baths and oral:
A. diuretics
B. anticholinergics
C. antispasmodics
D. analgesics

24. Cervicitis related to menopause is treated by:
A. estrogens
B. antiemetics
C. diuretics
D. analgesics

25. The portal of entry for organisms that cause mastitis is the:
A. areola
B. mammary gland
C. nipple
D. lactating duct

26. The main medical treatment for mastitis is:
A. antihistamines
B. antispasmodics
C. diuretics
D. antibiotics

27. Intrauterine devices used for contraception, multiple sexual partners, and vaginal douching are considered to be possible risk factors for:
A. menorrhagia
B. ovarian cysts
C. pelvic inflammatory disease
D. malignant neoplasms

28. The most serious complication of pelvic inflammatory disease is:
A. peritonitis
B. pneumonia
C. hemorrhage
D. hypertension

29. Treatment for pelvic inflammatory disease includes rest, application of heat, and administration of:
A. antiemetics
B. antibiotics
C. diuretics
D. antispasmodics

30. The major symptom of endometriosis is:
A. hemorrhage
B. pain
C. fever
D. tachycardia

31. Because the uterine endometrial tissue is bleeding simultaneously in endometriosis, pain appears as dysmenorrhea and may extend to a feeling of:
A. stabbing pain
B. sudden weakness
C. difficulty breathing
D. pelvic heaviness

32. A medical emergency in patients with endometriosis created by constriction of pelvic structures by adhesions is:
A. complete obstruction
B. anaphylactic shock
C. vaginal hemorrhage
D. difficulty breathing

33. The primary diagnostic procedure for endometriosis is the excision of endometrial implants via:
A. ultrasonography
B. culposcopy
C. dilation and curettage
D. laparoscopy

34. A preliminary diagnostic tool to determine the presence of pelvic masses, which may be found in endometriosis, is:
A. laparoscopy
B. ultrasonsography
C. culposcopy
D. dilation and curettage

35. The most common drug used to treat endometriosis is:
A. phenobarbital
B. danazol
C. amoxicillin
D. estrogen

36. Women who are given androgenic steroids for treatment of endometriosis often experience the common side effect of:
A. masculinizing characteristics
B. palpitations
C. insomnia
D. diuresis

37. Surgical management is commonly employed for patients with endometriosis and includes:
A. culposcopy
B. culdoscopy
C. laparoscopy
D. dilation and curettage

38. Three surgical means of removing endometrial implants include resection, electrocauterization, and:
A. laser excision
B. dilation and curettage
C. culposcopy
D. culdoscopy

39. The follicular ovarian cyst forms when the dominant follicle fails to rupture and release its ovum and:
    A. atrophies
    B. becomes malignant
    C. continues to grow
    D. causes gradually increasing pain

40. Severe and sudden abdominal pain may occur as a complication of follicular ovarian cysts due to:
    A. infection
    B. rupture
    C. muscle spasms
    D. vaginitis

41. Cysts that are usually resorbed spontaneously without treatment are:
    A. follicular cysts
    B. neoplasms
    C. breast cysts
    D. dermoid cysts

42. Which of the following cysts are usually removed surgically because of the potential for the development of malignancy?
    A. follicular
    B. corpus luteum
    C. fibroid
    D. dermoid

43. The only procedure for making a definitive diagnosis of cancer with breast cysts is:
    A. surgical biopsy
    B. mammography
    C. palpation
    D. ultrasound

44. A serious complication of a very large fibroid tumor is that it may compress the urethra, obstructing urine flow and causing secondary:
    A. vaginitis
    B. pelvic inflammatory disease
    C. hydronephrosis
    D. diuresis

45. For women with fibroid tumors who desire to become pregnant, a procedure that can be done by laser surgery to remove the tumor alone is:
    A. hysterectomy
    B. myomectomy
    C. dilation and curettage
    D. culdoscopy

46. Women at risk of developing rectoceles and cystoceles are those who have experienced a weakened pubococcygeal muscle due to:
    A. extended antibiotic treatment
    B. repeated pregnancies
    C. effects of herpes infection
    D. poor nutrition

47. Treatment of small cystoceles aimed at improving the tone of the pubococcygeal muscle is:
    A. pelvic floor (Kegel) exercises
    B. surgical intervention (A and P repair)
    C. vaginal hysterectomy
    D. increased fluid intake

48. Uterine prolapse is most apt to occur in postmenopausal women who have had:
    A. recurrent pelvic infections
    B. previous vaginal yeast infections
    C. hypertension
    D. multiple pregnancies

49. The most common surgical treatment for uterine prolapse is:
    A. vaginal hysterectomy
    B. lithotripsy
    C. culdoscopy
    D. dilation and curettage

50. The single best step toward detection of breast cancer in its early stage is:
    A. ultrasonography
    B. biopsy
    C. regular monthly BSE
    D. lumpectomy

51. Nearly one half of all malignant breast tumors are located in the:
    A. nipple-areolar complex
    B. lower outer quadrant
    C. upper outer quadrant
    D. lower inner quadrant

52. About what percentage of women diagnosed with breast cancer have no known risk factors?
    A. 10%
    B. 25%
    C. 50%
    D. 70%

53. The initial sign of breast cancer that can be palpated during SBE or visualized by mammogram is:
    A. nipple discharge
    B. painless breast lump
    C. ulceration
    D. dilated blood vessels

54. It is recommended that yearly mammograms be done every year beginning at age:
    A. 35
    B. 40
    C. 50
    D. 65

55. A synthetic nonsteroidal antiestrogen that acts as an estrogen antagonist and blocks circulating estrogen from reaching the cancer receptor cells is:
A. progesterone
B. tamoxifen
C. prednisone
D. adriamycin

56. A common nursing diagnosis for mastectomy patients is:
A. sleep pattern disturbance
B. decreased cardiac output
C. functional incontinence
D. body image disturbance

57. A radical mastectomy includes the removal of axillary:
A. blood vessels
B. nerves
C. lymph nodes
D. ganglia

58. An important aspect of postoperative care after mastectomy is directed toward the prevention and minimizing of:
A. lymphedema
B. hemorrhage
C. hypertension
D. nausea

59. Cervical cancer is usually diagnosed and treated in its early stage because it can be detected by:
A. Laparoscopy
B. Pap smears
C. culdoscopy
D. pelvic examination

60. Most types of cervical cancer are associated with microbes such as human papillomavirus and herpes simplex virus; therefore, it is thought that cervical cancer is related to:
A. high-fat diet
B. diabetes mellitus
C. sexually transmitted diseases
D. multiple pregnancies

61. Early cervical cancer is asymptomatic; symptoms of advanced cervical cancer may include:
A. recurrent urinary tract infections
B. bleeding after intercourse
C. hypotension when standing
D. dyspnea on exertion

62. Which type of cancer has the highest mortality rate of all female reproductive system cancers?
A. cervical
B. vulvar
C. breast
D. ovarian

63. Women who are at very high risk of developing ovarian cancer may have prophylactic surgery performed called:
A. total hysterectomy
B. radical mastectomy
C. bilateral oophorectomy
D. pelvic exenteration

64. A problem with making the diagnosis of ovarian cancer is that, in the early stages, ovarian cancer is:
A. hemorrhagic
B. asymptomatic
C. infectious
D. present with ascites

65. A particularly significant finding that could indicate a diagnosis of malignant ovarian cancer is:
A. CA-125 serum marker of 15 units per ml
B. history that includes late menarche
C. palpable bilateral masses
D. palpable unilateral mass

66. A blood test that is used to assess the progress or regression of ovarian tumor growth is:
A. hematocrit
B. CA-125
C. white blood cell count
D. hemoglobin

67. The most rare but the most visible type of cancer of the female reproductive system is cancer of the:
A. cervix
B. ovary
C. breast
D. vulva

68. In situ vaginal cancer is usually treated with:
A. laser surgery or cryosurgery
B. internal or external radiotherapy
C. partial or total vaginectomy
D. pelvic exenteration

69. In patients receiving internal radiation, effects on local tissue by the radioactive material produce a:
A. profuse, malodorous discharge
B. clear, watery discharge
C. frothy, gray discharge
D. white, cheesy discharge

70. The normal cessation of menstruation that marks the end of a woman's reproductive capacity is:
A. pregnancy
B. menstruation
C. dysmenorrhea
D. menopause

71. Diminished ovarian function associated with aging causes ovulation to cease as well as decreased production of:
    A. thyroxine
    B. estrogen
    C. epinephrine
    D. prolactin

72. With natural menopause, the woman's first sign may be:
    A. increased temperature
    B. loss of memory
    C. menstrual irregularity
    D. bone pain

73. A women is said to be postmenopausal when she has not had a menstrual period for:
    A. 3 months
    B. 1 year
    C. 2 years
    D. 5 years

74. Some women experience a surgical menopause brought on by the surgical removal of the:
    A. ovaries
    B. uterus
    C. vagina
    D. cervix

75. The type of drug therapy prescribed promptly for surgical menopause to decrease menopausal symptoms is:
    A. diuretics
    B. steroids
    C. estrogen
    D. analgesics

76. The symptom of hot flashes that may accompany menopause is due to:
    A. increased menstrual bleeding
    B. vasodilation
    C. abdominal cramps
    D. increased body temperature

77. Menopausal symptoms can usually be treated with:
    A. hormone replacement
    B. diuretics
    C. analgesics
    D. anticoagulants

78. Progesterone is added to estrogen replacement therapy in postmenopausal patients to decrease the risk of:
    A. breast cancer
    B. hot flashes
    C. endometrial cancer
    D. insomnia

79. The postmenopausal risk of osteoporosis may be reduced by taking supplements of:
    A. vitamin D
    B. thyroid hormone
    C. beta carotene
    D. calcium

LX. In the figure below, label the external female genitalia (A–K) from the terms provided (1–11) on the right. (Figure modified from Ignatavicius, D. D., & Bayne, M. V. [1991]. *Medical-surgical nursing: A nursing process approach* [p. 1628]. Philadelphia: W. B. Saunders.)

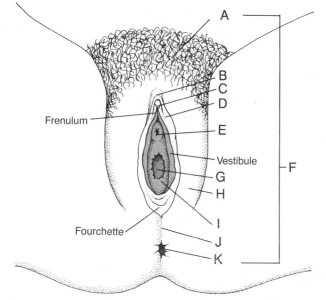

_____ 1. Labia minora

_____ 2. Hymen

_____ 3. Labia majora

_____ 4. Clitoris

_____ 5. Anus

_____ 6. Mons pubis

_____ 7. Introitus

_____ 8. Urethral meatus

_____ 9. Perineum

_____ 10. Prepuce

_____ 11. Vulva

Introductory Nursing Care of Adults

LXI. In the figure below, label the sites of endometriosis (A–K) from the terms provided (1–11).
(Figure from Ignatavicius, D. D., & Bayne, M. V. [1991]. *Medical-surgical nursing: A nursing process approach* [p. 1695]. Philadelphia: W. B. Saunders.)

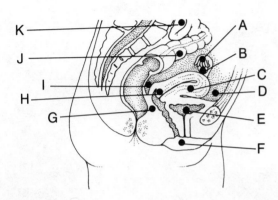

___ 1. Urinary bladder

___ 2. Small intestine

___ 3. Ovary

___ 4. Cervix

___ 5. Pelvic peritoneum

___ 6. Vulva

___ 7. Fallopian tube

___ 8. Cul-de-sac

___ 9. Large intestine

___ 10. Uterus

___ 11. Rectovaginal septum

CHAPTER

44

Male Reproductive Disorders

OBJECTIVES

1. Describe major structures and functions of the normal male reproductive system.
2. Identify data to be collected when assessing a patient with a disorder of the male reproductive system.
3. Discuss commonly used diagnostic tests and procedures and nursing implications of each.
4. Identify common therapeutic measures and nursing implications of each when patients are treated for disorders of the male reproductive system.
5. For selected disorders of the male reproductive system, explain the pathophysiology, signs and symptoms, complications, medical diagnosis, and medical treatment.
6. Apply the nursing process to design a care plan for a patient with a disorder of the male reproductive system.

LEARNING ACTIVITIES

I. Match the definition on the left with the most appropriate term on the right.

____ 1. Accumulation of blood in the tunica vaginalis, which is the membrane that lines the front and sides of the testis and the epididymis

____ 2. Prostatic and pelvic pain in the absence of infection or inflammation

____ 3. Inflammation of the epididymis

____ 4. Accumulation of clear fluid in the scrotum along the spermatic cord

____ 5. Sebaceous secretion found beneath the foreskin

____ 6. Inability to achieve and maintain an erection for sexual intercourse

____ 7. Inflammation of the prostate gland

____ 8. Involuntary discharge of semen

____ 9. Removal of all or part of the prostate gland

A. Ejaculation
B. Emission
C. Epididymitis
D. Erection
E. Hematocele
F. Hydrocele
G. Impotence
H. Infertility
I. Prostatectomy
J. Prostatitis
K. Prostatodynia
L. Smegma
M. Spermatocele
N. Sterile

I. *Continues*

I. *Continued*

____ 10. Swelling and rigidity of the penis

____ 11. A cystic mass on the epididymis that contains fluid and spermatozoa

____ 12. Reflexive expulsion of semen from the male urethra

____ 13. Free of microorganisms; infertile

____ 14. Inability to conceive and produce viable offspring

A. Ejaculation

B. Emission

C. Epididymitis

D. Erection

E. Hematocele

F. Hydrocele

G. Impotence

H. Infertility

I. Prostatectomy

J. Prostatitis

K. Prostatodynia

L. Smegma

M. Spermatocele

N. Sterile

II. Complete the statements on the left with the most appropriate term on the right.

____ 1. The _____ extends from the bladder to the urinary meatus at the end of the penis.

____ 2. The production of sperm is called _____.

____ 3. _____ is the hardening of an artery due to injury to the endothelial lining of the vessel and eventual scarring.

____ 4. The hardening of stiffening of an arterial wall due to systemic rather than localized insults is _____.

____ 5. _____ is a hormone necessary for the development of male reproductive organs, descent of the testicles, and production of sperm.

____ 6. The _____ provides outflow for semen during ejaculation.

____ 7. When the testes are located outside a dependent scrotal position, the condition is called _____.

____ 8. _____ is the surgical removal of a portion of the vas deferens.

A. Testosterone

B. Cryptorchidism

C. Urethra

D. Arteriosclerosis

E. Vasectomy

F. Spermatogenesis

G. Atherosclerosis

III. Complete the statements on the left with the most appropriate term on the right. Some terms may be used more than once, and some terms may not be used.

____ 1. Testosterone production begins at _____.

____ 2. Testosterone causes the testes to descend into the scrotum at _____.

____ 3. Spermatogenesis begins as a result of increased testosterone production at about _____, and continues throughout life.

____ 4. Sperm are produced in the testes in the _____.

____ 5. Sperm mature in about _____.

____ 6. The testes must descend into the _____ in order for optimal spermatogenesis.

____ 7. Spermatogenesis requires a body temperature which is _____.

A. Seminiferous tubules

B. Scrotum

C. 75 days

D. 7 weeks' gestation

E. 10 to 13 weeks' gestation

F. 7 to 9 months' gestation

G. 7 to 9 years of age

H. 10 to 13 years of age

I. Lower

J. Vas deferens

K. Higher

IV. Complete the statements on the left with the most appropriate term on the right. Some terms may be used more than once, and some terms may not be used.

____ 1. Sperm move into the _____, where maturation occurs.

____ 2. Sperm travel out of the scrotum through the abdominal wall to the pelvic cavity via the _____.

____ 3. Fluids and nutrients are added to seminal fluid along its anatomic pathway by the _____.

____ 4. The vas deferens serves as a major storage site for sperm and aids in propelling sperm during ejaculation through the _____.

____ 5. The normal flaccid penis is _____.

____ 6. To observe the glans in the uncircumcised male, one must retract the _____.

____ 7. The opening at the tip of the penis is the _____.

____ 8. Increased firmness and enlargement of the prostrate gland may indicate _____.

____ 9. A tender, boggy feeling on examination of the prostate may indicate _____.

____ 10. A hard prostate may indicate _____.

A. Benign prostatic hypertrophy

B. Urethral meatus

C. Epididymis

D. Foreskin

E. Cancer

F. Semisoft

G. Vas deferens

H. Prostate gland

I. Chronic prostatitis

J. Impotence

K. Ejaculation duct

V. Complete the statements on the left with the most appropriate term on the right. Some terms may be used more than once, and some may not be used.

____ 1. Below normal levels of testosterone result in abnormally high levels of _____.

____ 2. Above normal levels of serum prolactin may be caused by _____.

____ 3. Above normal levels of serum prolactin may cause _____.

____ 4. A hormone which is secreted by the anterior pituitary gland and causes stimulation of Sertoli's cells in the seminiferous tubules of the testes is _____ .

____ 5. Low thyroid hormone levels may result in _____.

____ 6. High levels of thyroid hormone may cause _____.

____ 7. Below normal levels of sperm result in increased secretion of the hormone called _____ .

____ 8. The most common inflammatory conditions of the male reproductive system are prostatitis and _____.

____ 9. Prostatitis may be caused by _____.

A. Decreased libido

B. Gynecomastia

C. Impotence

D. Orchitis

E. Bacteria

F. Serum luteinizing hormone

G. Follicle-stimulating hormone

H. Epididymitis

I. Testicular torsion

J. Benign pituitary tumor

VI. Complete the statements on the left with the most appropriate term on the right. Some terms may be used more than once, and some may not be used.

____ 1. In impotence, arteriosclerosis c compromises ability to fill because _____.

____ 2. Two conditions caused or enhanced by diabetes mellitus that may contribute to impotence are autonomic neuropathy and _____.

____ 3. The type of impotence likely to be caused by high blood pressure and its treatment is_____.

____ 4. Three treatments that may be recommended for treating impotence in the diabetic patient are behavioral therapy, papaverine self-injection, and _____.

____ 5. Spinal cord injuries that are more complete and more likely to cause impotence are those injuries which are _____.

____ 6. The most likely drugs to cause impotence are _____.

A. Failure to store

B. Lower

C. Antihypertensives

D. Failure to initiate

E. Atherosclerosis

F. Penile implant

G. Vascular surgery

H. High

I. Failure to fill

J. Antibiotics

K. Reduced blood supply

L. Neurologic disorders

VII. Complete the statements on the left with the most appropriate term on the right. Some terms may be used more than once, and some may not be used.

____ 1. _____ may be caused by infections, trauma, or the reflux of urine from the urethra through the vas deferens.

____ 2. _____ may be caused by injury to the penis, sickle cell crisis, medications, or papaverine injections.

____ 3. Inflammation of one of both testes is called _____.

____ 4. Enlargement of the prostate is called _____.

____ 5. _____ is the development of a hard, nonelastic fibrous tissue just under the skin of the penis.

____ 6. _____ is inflammation of the prostate gland.

____ 7. _____ is treated with bedrest, ice packs, sitz baths, analgesics, antibiotics, anti-inflammatory drugs, and scrotal support.

____ 8. Signs and symptoms of _____ include fever, tenderness, and scrotal redness.

____ 9. A prolonged penile erection not related to sexual desire is called _____.

____ 10. Signs and symptoms of _____ may include dysuria, frequency, hematuria, and foul-smelling urine.

____ 11. Acute _____ is treated with antimicrobials, analgesics, and sitz baths.

____ 12. Treatment of _____ may include topical or oral medications with vitamin E, oral aminobenzoic acid, radiation, surgical removal, and penile implants.

____ 13. Signs and symptoms of _____ include painful scrotal edema, nausea, vomiting, chills, and fever.

____ 14. Signs and symptoms of _____ include decreasing size and force of the urinary stream, inability to empty the bladder, frequency, and urinary retention.

A. Orchitis

B. Prostatitis

C. Phimosis

D. Epididymitis

E. Benign prostatic hypertrophy

F. Priapism

G. Prostate cancer

H. Peyronie's disease

VIII. Match the purpose/procedure on the left with the most appropriate diagnostic test/study on the right.

___ 1. An antigen is injected intradermally, marked with a waterproof pen, and examined after 48 hours to detect immune response

___ 2. Can determine susceptibility to various antimicrobials

___ 3. Assess the level of hormones that play a role in sexual development and/or function

___ 4. Detects sexually transmitted diseases

___ 5. Detects increases that may be associated with prostatic cancer and other conditions.

___ 6. Used to study the prostate for enlargement or lesions

___ 7. Used to assess testicular and prostatic tumors, may include intravenous injection of contrast dye

___ 8. Uses radioactive substances injected intravenously or given orally followed by imaging to assess testicular abnormalities

___ 9. Lighted instrument inserted through urethra to visualize urethra, bladder, and prostatic urethra; may detect prostatic hypertrophy

___ 10. Assesses male fertility or documents sterilization after vasectomy

___ 11. Detects elevations associated with metastatic prostate cancer; used to assess effects of treatment for prostate cancer

A. Cultures

B. Semen analysis

C. Mumps test

D. Tumor markers: serum prostatic-specific antigen

E. Ultrasonography

F. Computed tomography

G. Radionucleotide imaging procedures

H. Smears and stains

I. Cystoscopy

J. Serum acid phosphatase

K. Endocrinologic studies

IX. Match the "related to" statement on the left with the nursing diagnosis for the patient with testicular cancer on the right.

___ 1. Diminished or absent peristalsis caused by bowel manipulation during surgery

___ 2. Effects of anesthesia and abdominal surgery

___ 3. Diagnosis of cancer or anticipation of side effects of treatments

___ 4. Potential loss of reproductive capacity

___ 5. Surgical incision

___ 6. Surgery

A. Anxiety

B. Pain

C. Altered urinary elimination

D. High risk for injury (shock, infection, fluid and electrolyte imbalances)

E. Constipation

F. Situational low self-esteem

X. List 4 characteristics of the scrotum that enable it to keep a temperature lower than body temperature so that spermatogenesis can occur.

1.

2.

3.

4.

XI. List 2 main functions of the testes.

1.

2.

XII. On palpation, the epididymis should feel soft and tender. List 2 characteristics that should not normally be present.

1.

2.

XIII. List 6 systems other than the reproductive system that should be included in the review of systems for male patients with reproductive disorders.

1.

2.

3.

4.

5.

6.

XIV. List 5 important disease processes that should be included in assessment of the family history of male patients with reproductive disorders.

1.

2.

3.

4.

5.

XV. List 4 characteristics of semen that may be evaluated on gross analysis.

1.

2.

3.

4.

XVI. List 4 characteristics of semen that may be evaluated on microscopic analysis.

1.

2.

3.

4.

XVII. List directions to include in patient instructions for collecting a semen specimen at home in the following 5 areas.

1. Abstinence:

2. Container:

3. Condom:

4. Temperature:

5. Time frame for bringing specimen to lab:

XVIII. Explain why rubber condoms should not be used for collecting semen specimens.

XIX. List 3 hormones secreted by the anterior pituitary gland that stimulate the male reproductive system.

1.

2.

3.

XX. Clean catch urine samples may be used for urinalysis if they can be obtained without contamination. List 3 reasons why a patient might have trouble obtaining a clean catch.

1.

2.

3.

XXI. List 4 laboratory tests specific to diagnosing prostate cancer.

1.

2.

3.

4.

XXII. List 2 routes by which radioactive substances are given.

1.

2.

XXIII.   Before giving radioactive substances or dyes, what should the nurse do?

XXIV.   List 3 methods of treatment for benign prostatic hypertrophy.

1.

2.

3.

XXV.   List 4 indications for surgical intervention for benign prostatic hypertrophy.

1.

2.

3.

4.

XXVI.   List the nursing interventions for each of the following nursing diagnoses in the care plan of the patient with a prostatectomy:

1. High risk for fluid volume deficit related to hemorrhage:

2. Pain related to tissue trauma and bladder spasms:

3. High risk for infection related to invasive procedures of the urinary tract or catheterization:

4. High risk for injury related to obstructed urine flow, excessive absorption of irrigating fluids, or trauma to urinary sphincter:

XXVII.   Describe the causes and symptoms of the three types of impotence listed below:

1. Failure to initiate

   A. Causes:

   B. Symptoms:

2. Failure to fill

   A. Causes:

   B. Symptoms:

3. Failure to store

   A. Causes:

   B. Symptoms:

XXVIII. Treatment of impotence related to spinal cord injuries may include what 3 measures?

1.

2.

3.

XXIX. List 7 characteristics of testicular tumors.

1.

2.

3.

4.

5.

6.

7.

XXX. List 5 causes of male infertility.

1.

2.

3.

4.

5.

XXXI. List 3 parts of the male reproductive system that may be affected by cancer.

1.

2.

3.

XXXII. Choose the most appropriate answer.

1. Three normal changes that may occur in the male reproductive system due to aging are decreased testosterone, longer refractory period between erections, and:
   A. penile discharge
   B. pain with urination
   C. slower arousal
   D. descent of testicles

2. Impotence related to diabetes mellitus may be caused by:
   A. spinal cord injury
   B. atherosclerosis
   C. low hormone levels
   D. multiple sclerosis

3. Autonomic neuropathy inhibits muscle relaxation of lacunar spaces of the erectile chambers, which may make:
   A. the patient anxious about performance
   B. adequate filling of the penis with blood for an erection impossible
   C. testosterone levels abnormally low
   D. the patient sterile

4. The prostate is a walnut-sized secretory gland that:
   A. surrounds the urethra at the base of the bladder
   B. serves no function after puberty
   C. stores sperm, allowing them to mature
   D. secretes fluid that becomes part of the urine

5. Assessment of the male reproductive system may be difficult for some patients because of health beliefs, need for privacy, or:
   A. chronic disease
   B. advanced age
   C. defensiveness about behavior
   D. lack of sexual experience

6. The nurse should begin the patient's assessment by:
   A. exploring the family history
   B. inquiring about sexual function
   C. reviewing all systems
   D. obtaining a detailed description of the current problem

7. Past medical history helps link the current problem with previous problems and should include information about injuries, diseases, surgeries, allergies, treatments, and:
   A. marital status
   B. medications
   C. age and health of siblings
   D. age and health of parents

8. The health history should include information about medications the patient is taking because:
   A. they may impair his cognitive abilities
   B. they may make him too tired to participate in the assessment
   C. they may impair sexual function
   D. they may impair gastrointestinal function

9. Physical examination of the male reproductive system may be accomplished by:
   A. inspection and palpation
   B. auscultation and percussion
   C. percussion and palpation
   D. inspection and auscultation

10. Enlargement of male breasts is called:
    A. Peyronie's disease
    B. phimosis
    C. testicular torsion
    D. gynecomastia

11. Transurethral prostatectomy is the most common surgical procedure for benign prostatic hypertrophy. In this procedure:
    A. the prostate is approached through the bladder by way of a low abdominal incision
    B. portions of the prostate are cut away through a resectoscope inserted into the urethra
    C. access to the prostate is gained through an incision between the scrotum and the anus
    D. the surgeon reaches the prostate through a low abdominal incision and opens the front of the prostate

12. Nursing diagnoses for the patient with benign prostatic hypertrophy may include:
    A. high risk for infection
    B. sexual dysfunction
    C. pain
    D. altered urinary elimination

13. Nursing diagnoses for the patient immediately following a prostatectomy may include:
    A. anxiety
    B. fear
    C. high risk for fluid volume deficit
    D. altered urinary elimination

14. In impotence, failure to fill and failure to store often occur together because:
    A. of the psychological connection between the two functions
    B. they are both the result of atherosclerosis or aging
    C. failure to fill causes failure to store in many patients
    D. they are both the result of failure to initiate

XXXIII. In the figure below, label the parts of the male reproductive system (A–U) by using the terms below (1–21). (Figure from Ignatavicius, D. D., & Bayne, M. V. [1991]. *Medical-surgical nursing: A nursing process approach* [p. 1637]. Philadelphia: W. B. Saunders.)

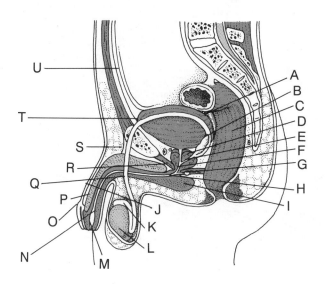

___	1.	Suspensory ligament	
___	2.	Corpus cavernosum	
___	3.	Root of penis	
___	4.	Seminal vesicle	
___	5.	Prostatic urethra	
___	6.	Corpus (body) of penis	
___	7.	Bladder	
___	8.	Vas deferens	
___	9.	Rectovesical pouch	
___	10.	Membranous urethra	
___	11.	Urogenital diaphragm	

___ 12. Peritoneum

___ 13. Corona

___ 14. Rectum

___ 15. Corpus spongiosum

___ 16. Testis

___ 17. Prostate gland

___ 18. Penile urethra

___ 19. Epididymis

___ 20. Bulbourethral (Cowper's glands)

___ 21. Ejaculatory ducts

Sexually Transmitted Diseases

OBJECTIVES

1. List infectious diseases classified as sexually transmitted diseases.
2. Explain why the nurse's approach is important when dealing with patients who have sexually transmitted diseases.
3. Identify therapeutic communication strategies.
4. Describe tests used to diagnose sexually transmitted diseases and the nursing considerations associated with each.
5. Explain why sexually transmitted diseases must be reported to the health department.
6. For selected sexually transmitted diseases, describe the pathophysiology, signs and symptoms, complications, and medical treatment.
7. List information to be included when teaching patients how to prevent sexually transmitted diseases.
8. List nursing considerations when a patient is on drug therapy for a sexually transmitted disease.
9. Identify data to be collected when assessing a patient with a sexually transmitted disease.
10. Develop a nursing care plan for a patient with a sexually transmitted disease.

LEARNING ACTIVITIES

I. Match the definition on the left with the most appropriate term on the right.

___ 1. A papule that breaks down into a painless ulcer at the site of entry of the organism that causes syphilis

___ 2. A condition in which the blood has antibodies for the human immunodeficiency virus (HIV), meaning the individual has been infected with this virus

___ 3. Inflammation of the vagina; can be caused by chemical irritants, dryness, estrogen deficiency, or infectious agents

___ 4. An infection of the ovaries, fallopian tubes, and pelvic area

___ 5. Dormant; during the latency period of a disease, there are no signs or symptoms of the disease

___ 6. Inflammation of the cervix (narrow, lower end of the uterus)

___ 7. A disease that can be transmitted by intimate genital, oral, or rectal contact

___ 8. An infection caused by an organism that usually does not cause a disease but becomes pathogenic when body defenses are impaired

A. Vaginitis

B. Cervicitis

C. Opportunistic infection

D. HIV positive

E. Sexually transmitted disease

F. Pelvic inflammatory disease

G. Chancre

H. Latent

II. Complete the statements on the left with the most appropriate term on the right. Some terms may be used more than once, and some terms may not be used.

____ 1. Erythromycin ophthalmic ointment may be ordered for the newborn to prevent eye infection caused by exposure during delivery to _____ .

____ 2. A papule that becomes a painless, red ulcer within a week is a sign of _____.

____ 3. Treatment with ceftriaxone sodium (Rocephin) and doxycycline calcium (Vibramycin) or tetracycline cures most cases of _____.

____ 4. _____ is caused by the spirochete *Treponema pallidum.*

____ 5. If gonorrhea is untreated, the bacteria remain in the body and the person remains _____.

____ 6. When the chancre disappears, patients may erroneously assume they are cured; in fact, the infecting organism has moved into the _____.

____ 7. Infections that may lead to heart tissue and joint damage are complications of _____.

____ 8. Pustules, fever, sore throat, and generalized aching are symptoms that occur in the secondary stage of _____.

____ 9. A typical lesion, called a chancre, is the first sign of _____.

____ 10. If untreated, gonorrhea can cause _____.

A. Gonorrhea

B. Sterility

C. Infectious

D. Digestive system

E. Syphilis

F. *Chlamydia trachomatis*

G. Blood

H. Gonococci

I. Liver failure

J. *Treponema pallidum*

III. Complete the statements on the left with the most appropriate term on the right. Some terms may be used more than once, and some terms may not be used.

____ 1. An eye ointment that is recommended because it is effective against chlamydia as well as gonorrhea is _____.

____ 2. An antibody test called the Herp-Check can detect active _____.

____ 3. In females with venereal warts, the warts generally appear around the urethra, vagina, cervix, perineum, anal canal, and the _____.

____ 4. A penile discharge that is initially thin and then creamy, accompanied by painful urination, is a symptom of _____.

____ 5. A sexually transmitted disease caused by a protozoan parasite is _____.

A. Chlamydia

B. Condylomata acuminata (venereal warts)

C. Erythromycin

D. Metronidazole (Flagyl)

E. Heart damage

F. Vulva

G. Acyclovir (Zovirax)

H. Trichomoniasis

I. Tetracycline

J. Herpes

K. Sterility

___ 6. The drug of choice for the treatment of trichomoniasis is _____.

___ 7. If left untreated, chlamydia can result in _____.

___ 8. A condition caused by the human papilloma virus is _____.

___ 9. There is an increased risk of cervical cancer in women who have _____.

___ 10. The drug of choice for treatment of bacterial vaginosis is _____.

___ 11. Premature births and miscarriages are high among women with _____.

A. Chlamydia
B. Condylomata acuminata (venereal warts)
C. Erythromycin
D. Metronidazole (Flagyl)
E. Heart damage
F. Vulva
G. Acyclovir (Zovirax)
H. Trichomoniasis
I. Tetracycline
J. Herpes
K. Sterility

IV. Complete the statements on the left with the most appropriate term on the right. Some terms may be used more than once, and some terms may not be used.

___ 1. Complaints of flu-like symptoms and a burning sensation during urination are symptoms of _____.

___ 2. Condyloma warts are generally pink and soft, with a _____.

___ 3. A frothy, yellowish vaginal discharge with a foul odor is a sign of _____.

___ 4. Males with venereal warts generally present with warts on the glans, foreskin, urethral opening, penile shaft, or _____.

___ 5. _____ is transmitted by contact with the mucous membranes in the mouth, eyes, urethra, vagina, or rectum.

___ 6. Painful, itching sores on or around the genitals that appear about 2 to 20 days after infection are symptoms of _____.

___ 7. Genital irritation, a thin gray discharge and a fishy odor are symptoms of _____.

___ 8. Newborns with eye damage or infant pneumonia may have been exposed to _____.

___ 9. A drug that is helpful in minimizing symptoms of HSV is the antiviral drug called _____.

___ 10. Cryosurgery may be used in the treatment of _____.

A. Acyclovir (Zovirax)
B. Trichomoniasis
C. Chlamydia
D. Strawberry-like
E. Metronidazole (Flagyl)
F. Herpes
G. Bacterial vaginosis
H. Cauliflower-like
I. Anus
J. Condyloma acuminata (venereal warts)
K. Scrotum

V. Match the symptoms on the left with the most appropriate stage of syphilis on the right. Some stages may be used more than once, and some may not be used.

___ 1. The disease is not spread by sexual contact during this stage, but may be transmitted by blood exposure

___ 2. Occurs 1 to 6 months after contact

___ 3. Arthritis, numbness of the extremities, ulcers, and pain

___ 4. No symptoms in this stage, which follows the secondary stage

___ 5. A reddish papule appears where the organism entered the body, usually the genitals, anus, or mouth

___ 6. Pustules, fever, sore throat, and generalized aching

___ 7. This stage occurs 3 years after contact and may not appear for decades

___ 8. The papule becomes a painless, red ulcer

___ 9. Rash on extremities, chest or back, hands or feet

___ 10. A chancre appears

A. Primary

B. Secondary

C. Middle

D. Latent

E. Late

VI. Match the purpose of the HIV test on the left with the most appropriate test on the right. Some tests may be used more than once, and some tests may not be used.

___ 1. Detects the presence or absence of an immune response to HIV infection

___ 2. Test done if the second ELISA is positive

___ 3. Usual examination of choice because it is less expensive

___ 4. Most accurate screening test for HIV

___ 5. HIV screening test that can be done at home and analyzed in 5 minutes

A. Rapid plasma reagin test

B. Latex agglutination test

C. Western blot test

D. ELISA

VII. Match the sexual practices on the left with their relative safety (in transmission of disease) on the right.

_____ 1. Oral sex with properly used condom

_____ 2. Contact with blood

_____ 3. Oral sex without condom

_____ 4. Opened-mouth kissing

_____ 5. Vaginal or anal intercourse without condom

_____ 6. Body massage

_____ 7. Oral/anal contact

_____ 8. Ingestion of urine or semen

_____ 9. Mutual masturbation

_____ 10. Vaginal or anal intercourse with properly used condom

_____ 11. Closed-mouth kissing

A.   Safe

B.   Possibly safe

C.   Unsafe

VIII. List 2 reasons why there is such a high incidence of sexually transmitted diseases (STDs).

1.

2.

IX. List 4 modes of transmission of HIV.

1.

2.

3.

4.

X. List the 3 primary risk factors for the transmission of HIV to women.

1.

2.

3.

XI. List the infection control guidelines related to the areas below that were issued by the Centers for Disease Control and Prevention. The guidelines were initially intended to be used when working with persons infected with HIV but are now required for all patients.

1. Handling body fluid:

2. Possibility of blood splattering exists:

3. Handling of needles:

4. Disposal of needles:

5. Accidental spill of body fluids:

XII. When a patient has an HIV infection, patient teaching is critical. The teaching responsibilities may be shared by the physician and the nurse. Explain what should be taught for each of the topics listed below, which are part of the teaching plan.

1. Explain how the infection is transmitted and how to reduce the risk of transmission. List 6 areas to be covered.

   A. Sexual partners:

   B. Needles:

   C. Blood, plasma, or body tissue:

   D. Sex:

   E. Sexual or needle-sharing partners:

   F. Females and pregnancy:

2. The patient should report for periodic blood tests to monitor:

3. Explain the prognosis with an HIV infection:

XIII. List one example for each of the following factors that could place a person at risk for STDs.

1. Age:

2. Sexual preference:

3. Habits:

4. Occupation:

XIV. List the factors to be observed in each of the following categories when a nurse is doing a physical examination of a person with STD.

1. Skin:

2. Head and neck:

3. Neck:

4. Abdomen:

XV. List 3 relevant aspects of the functional assessment in the areas below for which the nurse needs to obtain information regarding the care of patients with STDs.

1. Sexual behaviors:

2. Drug use:

3. Past infections:

XVI. List 10 nursing diagnoses that may apply to the patient with a sexually transmitted disease.

1.

2.

3.

4.

5.

6.

7.

8.

9.

10.

XVII. Patients with STDs may experience sexual dysfunction; list 3 factors that may be related to altered sexuality patterns.

1.

2.

3.

XVIII. List 4 behaviors associated with ineffective coping of individuals with STD.

1.

2.

3.

4.

XIX. List the key points to teach the patient with STD regarding the following topics.

1. Antibiotic therapy:

2. Transmission of STDs:

3. Sexual activity:

4. Condoms;

5. Patients with HSV infections:

XX. Choose the most appropriate answer.

1. A total of 85% of all cases of sexually transmitted diseases involve people between the ages of:
   A. 12 and 20
   B. 15 and 30
   C. 20 and 40
   D. 30 and 50

2. Serologic tests for STDs are designed to detect infectious diseases by measuring:
   A. white blood cells
   B. red blood cells
   C. clotting factors
   D. antigens or antibodies

3. Patients with gonococcal, chlamydial, herpes simplex, trichomoniasis, or yeast infections often have:
   A. vaginal or penis discharge
   B. increased temperature or tachycardia
   C. generalized infection and rash
   D. mouth sores and pharyngitis

4. When collecting a sample of vaginal discharge for culture and sensitivity tests, the person collecting the sample always wears:
   A. goggles
   B. masks
   C. gloves
   D. gowns

5. If males have a whitish- or greenish-colored discharge from the penis and complain of a burning sensation during urination, this is suggestive of:
   A. herpes simplex
   B. chlamydia
   C. gonorrhea
   D. syphilis

6. Female patients with gonorrhea are apt to have vaginal discharge, a burning sensation during urination, abnormal menstruation, and:
   A. dyspnea
   B. abdominal pain
   C. hypotension
   D. edema

7. Severe neurologic problems, blindness, and even death may occur as complications of:
   A. herpes simplex
   B. cervicitis
   C. syphilis
   D. gonorrhea

8. Two screening tests for syphilis include the rapid plasma reagin (RPR) and the:
   A. VDRL
   B. RBC
   C. WBC
   D. BUN

9. The treatment of choice for syphilis is:
   A. Vibramycin
   B. erythromycin
   C. tetracycline
   D. penicillin

10. After completing treatment for primary or secondary syphilis, the patient is advised not to engage in sexual activity for:
    A. 5 days
    B. 2 weeks
    C. 1 month
    D. 6 months

11. Chlamydial infection is sometimes labeled:
    A. nongonoccal urethritis
    B. herpes simplex
    C. trichomoniasis
    D. condylomata acuminata

12. Human immunodeficiency virus gradually destroys cells that are essential for resisting pathogens called:
    A. neutrophils
    B. T4 cells
    C. B cells
    D. eosinophils

13. HIV is passed from person to person primarily through:
    A. air droplet contact
    B. hand to mouth contact
    C. sexual contact
    D. mouth to mouth contact

14. Early symptoms of HIV include fever, night sweats, anorexia, and:
    A. edema
    B. hypertension
    C. confusion
    D. weight loss

15. The most common infection seen in persons with AIDS is
    A. herpes zoster
    B. dermatitis
    C. *Pneumocystis carinii* pneumonia
    D. Kaposi's sarcoma

16. For many women, one of the first symptoms of HIV is:
    A. vaginal candidiasis
    B. burning on urination
    C. menstrual irregularities
    D. hemorrhoids

17. A type of skin cancer that has dramatically increased as a result of AIDS is:
    A. *Pneumocystis carinii* pneumonia
    B. melanoma
    C. Kaposi's sarcoma
    D. venereal warts

18. A positive test for HIV means a person:
    A. has AIDS now
    B. has been exposed to AIDS
    C. will develop AIDS in the future
    D. was exposed to AIDS within the last 4 weeks

19. The medical treatment for HIV infection includes the use of zidovudine (AZT, Retrovir), which is given to:
    A. cure AIDS
    B. prevent transmission to sexual partners
    C. treat the secondary infections of AIDS
    D. slow the progress of AIDS

20. Drugs such as Pentam and Septra are used to:
    A. prevent or treat the opportunistic infections
    B. slow the progress of AIDS
    C. decreased the dermatitis associated with AIDS
    D. increase T4 lymphocytes

21. The best way to prevent transmission of HIV is to:
    A. use condoms during all sexual contact
    B. wash hands thoroughly following contact with HIV-positive persons
    C. abstain from sexual contact
    D. get plenty of rest and eat a nutritious diet

22. The risk of transmission of HIV during sexual contact is reduced by the use of:
    A. antibiotics
    B. condoms
    C. antiviral agents
    D. birth control pills

23. It is recommended that gloves be worn when handling body fluids of:
    A. HIV-positive patients
    B. infectious patients
    C. patients with opportunistic infections
    D. all patients

24. Results of HIV testing are:
    A. reported to the hospital administrator
    B. reported to the family
    C. kept strictly confidential
    D. given to the legal guardian

25. A discussion of sexual behavior can be awkward for the nurse and the patient; before nurses can deal with patients' sexuality, they must:
    A. present the patient with written information
    B. be aware of their own values
    C. ask the patient to demonstrate understanding of the material presented by stating information in their own words
    D. check the patient's chart to see if the patient has sexually transmitted diseases

26. With a sexually transmitted disease, common reasons that patients give for seeking medical care include pain, fever, lesions, or genital:
    A. itching
    B. edema
    C. bleeding
    D. discharge

27. Specimens collected during a pelvic exam are handled as:
    A. infective material
    B. clean specimens
    C. sterile specimens
    D. chemically unstable material

28. A nursing diagnosis related to lesions or inflammation for patients with STD is:
    A. anxiety
    B. pain
    C. self-esteem disturbance
    D. noncompliance

29. A nursing diagnosis related to possible effects of STD or reaction of partner is:
    A. pain
    B. high risk for injury
    C. anxiety
    D. impaired tissue integrity

30. A nursing diagnosis related to stigma associated with STD, shame, or anger is:
    A. high risk for injury
    B. pain
    C. ineffective individual coping
    D. knowledge deficit

31. Some sexually transmitted diseases are painless, but patients may have pain associated with oral lesions, rectal lesions, or:
    A. vaginal bleeding
    B. genital edema
    C. nerve irritation
    D. pelvic infection

32. Untreated STDs can lead to serious complications such as PID and:
    A. edema
    B. sterility
    C. shock
    D. kidney failure

33. The patient with AIDS is at high risk for secondary infections because of impaired:
    A. skin integrity
    B. immune function
    C. physical mobility
    D. airway clearance

34. Patients with AIDS pose a threat to their:
    A. children
    B. parents
    C. sexual partners
    D. siblings

35. Emergency drugs for possible hypersensitivity reactions that need to be kept on hand when administering drug therapy to patients with STD include epinephrine, corticosteroids, and:
    A. acyclovir (Zovirax)
    B. diphenhydramine hydrochloride (Benadryl)
    C. didanosine (Videx)
    D. pentamidine isethionate (Pentam)

36. Chronic infections, such as HSV and HIV, require permanent alterations in:
    A. sexual activity
    B. menstrual periods
    C. skin integrity
    D. nutritional habits

37. Related to altered sexuality patterns in patients with STD, the nurse explains that sexual dysfunction may be overcome by dealing with:
    A. adverse drug effects of prescribed medications
    B. need for more exercise
    C. emotional reactions to the disease
    D. conflict resolution

38. The nurse can show support for the patients with HIV infection by being sensitive, courteous, and:
    A. reassuring
    B. positive
    C. nonjudgmental
    D. authoritarian

39. Females with HSV infections are advised to have annual Papanicolaou smears because they are at increased risk of:
    A. pyelonephritis
    B. cervical cancer
    C. kidney failure
    D. AIDS

40. Herpes simplex virus can be transmitted by sexual contact, but unlike most other STDs, it can also be transmitted by:
    A. air droplets
    B. mouth to nose contact
    C. fecal contamination
    D. hand contact

41. Most STDs respond to antimicrobial agents; an exception is HSV, which is minimized but not cured by:
    A. penicillin G
    B. tetracycline hydrochloride (Achromycin)
    C. acyclovir sodium (Zovirax)
    D. metronidazole (Flagyl)

42. Although most STDs respond to antimicrobial agents, one STD that may be slowed by the use of zidovudine (AZT) is:
    A. HSV
    B. HIV
    C. syphilis
    D. chlamydia

43. In order to identify and treat infected individuals so that transmission of the sexually transmitted disease can be slowed, partners may be notified and confirmed cases of certain STDs must be reported to the:
    A. United States Department of Health
    B. hospital administrator
    C. Department of Public Safety
    D. local public health department

44. In children between the ages of 10 and 14, more than 10,000 cases of which STD are reported annually?
    A. herpes simplex
    B. chlamydia
    C. gonorrhea
    D. trichomoniasis

45. Gonorrhea can be found in the penis, cervix, throat, and:
    A. kidney
    B. anus
    C. heart
    D. lungs

46. Gonorrhea is transmitted through:
    A. toilet seats
    B. doorknobs
    C. sexual contact
    D. towels and linens

CHAPTER

46

Skin Disorders

OBJECTIVES

1. Describe the structure and functions of the skin.
2. List the components of the nursing assessment of the skin.
3. Define terms used to describe the skin and skin lesions.
4. Explain the tests and procedures used to diagnose skin disorders.
5. Explain the nurse's responsibilities regarding the tests and procedures for diagnosing skin disorders.
6. Explain the therapeutic benefits and nursing considerations for patients who receive dressings, soaks, and wet wraps, phototherapy, and drug therapy for skin problems.
7. For selected skin disorders, describe the pathophysiology, signs and symptoms, diagnostic tests, and medical treatment.
8. Apply the nursing process to plan care for the patient with a skin disorder.

LEARNING ACTIVITIES

I.   Match the definition on the left with the most appropriate term on the right.

____ 1. Chronic autoimmune condition characterized by blisters on the face, back, chest, groin, and umbilicus

____ 2. Capable of dissolving keratin, the outer surface of the epidermis

____ 3. Small, soft, raised lesion (skin tag)

____ 4. Itching

____ 5. To remove debris, including necrotic tissue

____ 6. Inflammatory skin disorder characterized by comedones, pustules, and cysts

____ 7. Skin condition characterized by scaly lesions and caused by rapid proliferation of epidermal cells

____ 8. Skin inflammation where two skin surfaces touch

____ 9. Mole

____ 10. Inflammation of the skin

____ 11. Benign tumor composed of blood vessels

____ 12. Pigmented spot on sun-exposed skin

A.   Débride

B.   Psoriasis

C.   Acrochordon

D.   Lentigo

E.   Acne

F.   Pemphigus

G.   Nevus

H.   Pruritus

I.   Dermatitis

J.   Keratolytic

K.   Angioma

L.   Intertrigo

II. Complete the statements on the left with the most appropriate term on the right. Some terms may be used more than once, and some terms may not be used.

____ 1. The secretion that coats the skin and creates an oily barrier that holds in water is _____.

____ 2. A result of the thinning of the skin layers and degeneration of elastin fibers is _____.

____ 3. The dissipation of heat from the skin occurs through _____.

____ 4. Sweating helps cool the body through _____.

____ 5. Ultraviolet rays in sunlight activate a substance in the skin that is eventually converted into _____.

____ 6. The secretion that plays a minor role in excretion of wastes is _____.

____ 7. Heat is retained through _____.

____ 8. Two skin secretions are sweat and _____.

____ 9. The skin is endowed with sensory receptors for touch, pain, temperature, and _____.

____ 10. The secretion that promotes the loss of body heat through evaporation is _____.

A. Evaporation
B. Vasoconstriction
C. Sebum
D. Melanin
E. Vasodilation
F. Sweat
G. Lymph
H. Wrinkling
I. Pressure
J. Lactic acid
K. Vitamin D

III. Complete the statements on the left with the most appropriate term on the right. Some terms may be used more than once, and some terms may not be used.

____ 1. A test used to diagnose viral skin infections is _____.

____ 2. When a skin lesion is thought to be caused by scabies, the top of the lesion is excised with a _____.

____ 3. An examination in which in the patient's skin is inspected under black light in a darkened room is called _____.

____ 4. A test used to identify allergens in which common irritants are applied to the skin is called _____.

____ 5. The removal of skin for microscopic examination is called _____.

____ 6. The type of biopsy in which the skin is cleansed and the specimen obtained with a scalpel is _____.

____ 7. The type of biopsy in which a circular tool cuts around the lesions, which is then lifted up and severed, is _____.

____ 8. The type of biopsy indicated for deep specimens in which sutures are required to close the site is _____.

A. Biopsy
B. Aspiration biopsy
C. Scalpel
D. Punch biopsy
E. Gram's stain
F. Wood's light
G. Shave biopsy
H. Surgical excision
I. Tzanck's smear
J. Patch testing

IV. Complete the statements on the left with the most appropriate term on the right. Some terms may be used more than once, and some terms may not be used.

____ 1. _____ are used to soothe, soften, and remove crusts, debris, and necrotic tissue.

____ 2. Following photochemotherapy (PUVA), which is used to treat psoriasis and cutaneous T-cell lymphoma, patients are instructed to wear sunscreen and dark glasses to decrease exposure to other sources of _____.

____ 3. After phototherapy, the patient may have dry skin and _____.

____ 4. A type of phototherapy used for atopic dermatitis in which the patient bathes first in a tar emulsion bath is _____.

____ 5. For topical application to skin disorders, drugs are combined with various substances in forms called _____.

____ 6. The use of ultraviolet light in combination with photosensitive drugs to promote shedding of the epidermis is called _____.

____ 7. A type of dressing that is usually covered by a dry dressing and left in place for 15 to 20 minutes is _____.

____ 8. Signs and symptoms of phototoxicity include vesicles, pain, and _____.

____ 9. Phototherapy may be employed in the treatment of _____.

____ 10. Phototherapy is contraindicated in patients with a history of _____.

A. Vehicles

B. Psoriasis

C. Phototherapy

D. Ultraviolet light

E. Occlusive dressings

F. Redness

G. Pallor

H. Wet wrap

I. Pruritus

J. Herpes simplex infection

K. Soaks and wet wraps

L. Goeckerman regimen

V. Complete the statements on the left with the most appropriate term on the right. Some terms may be used more than once, and some terms may not be used.

____ 1. Abnormally dry, itchy skin that becomes inflamed and is prone to infections is _____.

____ 2. Medications that are often ordered for pruritus include local anesthetics, corticosteroids, and _____.

____ 3. Applications that may be helpful if the patient has dry skin are lubricants or _____.

____ 4. Pruritus may be present with a number of systemic conditions such as _____.

____ 5. A chronic inflammatory disease of the skin caused by excess production of sebum is _____.

____ 6. _____ may become chronic and lead to thickening and discoloration of the affected skin.

____ 7. A prominent symptom with psoriasis, dermatitis, eczema, and insect bites is _____.

____ 8. Seborrheic dermatitis of the scalp is called _____.

____ 9. Topical medications used to treat atopic dermatitis include moisturizers, corticosteroids, and _____.

____ 10. Areas with fine powdery scales, thick crusts, or oily patches are symptomatic of _____.

____ 11. An inflammatory condition caused by contact with a substance that triggers an allergic response is _____.

____ 12. The presence of white, yellowish, or reddish scales is a symptom of _____.

A. Emollients

B. Lupus erythematosus

C. Pruritus

D. Anticholinergics

E. Seborrheic dermatitis

F. Tar preparations

G. Cardiovascular disease

H. Atopic dermatitis

I. Dandruff

J. Liver disease

K. Contact dermatitis

L. Antihistamines

VI. Complete the statements on the left with the most appropriate term on the right. Some terms may be used more than once, and some terms may not be used.

____ 1. Patients with mild psoriasis are usually treated with topical medications including keratolytics, tar derivatives, and _____.

____ 2. Cornstarch is contraindicated as a powder for patients with intertrigo, because it supports the growth of _____ .

____ 3. Bright-red lesions that may be covered with silvery scales are characteristic of _____.

____ 4. Topical medications that are commonly used for intertrigo are corticosteroids and _____.

____ 5. A chronic condition caused by rapid proliferation of epidermal cells is _____.

____ 6. Patient complaints of pain, irritation, or redness in body folds are common in _____.

____ 7. A drug that was used in the past to remove heavy scales in patients with psoriasis and that stains skin, hair, and furniture is _____.

____ 8. Inflammation of the skin where two skin surfaces touch is called _____.

____ 9. Joint pain or stiffness is documented in patients with psoriasis because psoriasis can cause _____.

A.   Anthralin (Anthra-Derm)

B.   Antihistamines

C.   Psoriasis

D.   Methotrexate

E.   Intertrigo

F.   Arthritis

G.   Corticosteroids

H.   Antifungals

I.   *Candida albicans*

VII. Complete the statements on the left with the most appropriate term on the right. Some terms may be used more than once, and some terms may not be used.

____ 1. Candidiasis infections, which are manifested as red lesions with white plaques, are found on the _____.

____ 2. Lesions with scaly patches and raised borders, along with pruritus, are associated with _____ infections.

____ 3. Three common sites for candidiasis include the mouth, skin, and the _____.

____ 4. Moist red lesions associated with *C. albicans* are seen on the _____.

____ 5. A yeast infection, caused by *C. albicans*, is known as _____.

____ 6. Oral candidiasis is treated with _____.

____ 7. In addition to the mouth and vagina, an area which is susceptible to candidiasis, owing to the constant moisture found there, is _____.

____ 8. Creamy white lesions are commonly found in the mouths of patients with _____.

A.   Nystatin

B.   Vagina

C.   Candidiasis

D.   Toes

E.   Mucous membranes

F.   Skin

G.   Ostomy site

H.   Tinea

I.   Scalp

VIII. Complete the statements on the left with the most appropriate term on the right. Some terms may be used more than once, and some terms may not be used.

____ 1. Mild cases of acne respond well to antibiotics and _____.

____ 2. A skin condition that affects the hair follicles and sebaceous glands is _____.

____ 3. The problem with taking Accutane for acne is that it may cause _____.

____ 4. A drug that may be prescribed to counteract the effects of androgenic hormones in acne patients is _____.

____ 5. Comedones (whiteheads and blackheads), pustules, and cysts are characteristics of _____.

____ 6. Two oral antibiotics that are frequently given for acne are tetracycline and _____.

____ 7. If acne is severe and unresponsive to antibiotics, _____ may be prescribed.

____ 8. A condition in which androgenic hormones cause increased sebum production and bacteria proliferate, causing hair follicles to block and become inflamed, is _____.

A. Herpes simplex

B. Acne

C. Tretinoin (Retin-A)

D. Acyclovir (Zovirax)

E. Estrogen

F. Erythromycin

G. Fetal deformities

H. Isotretinoin (Accutone)

IX. Complete the statements on the left with the most appropriate term on the right. S

____ 1. The elderly are especially susceptible to complications from herpes zoster, which include _____ involvement.

____ 2. The first symptoms of herpes zoster are heightened sensitivity along a nerve pathway, pain, and _____.

____ 3. Cold sores or fever blisters are oral lesions caused by _____.

____ 4. Sites most often infected by the herpes simplex virus (HSV) are the nose, lips, cheeks, ears, and _____.

____ 5. Wet dressings soaked in _____ may be used to treat lesions associated with herpes zoster.

____ 6. Diagnostic tests used to identify herpes infections include _____.

____ 7. When the mucous membranes are affected with herpes zoster, _____ develop.

A. Genitalia

B. Crusts

C. Ophthalmic

D. Acyclovir (Zovirax)

E. Itching

F. Burow's solution

G. Ulcers

H. Immunosuppressed

I. HSV

J. Shingles

K. Tzanck's smear

___ 8. Herpes simplex infections are treated with _____.

___ 9. Herpes zoster infection is commonly called _____.

___ 10. When the skin is infected with herpes zoster, _____ form.

___ 11. _____ patients are especially susceptible to herpes infections and must be protected from infected people.

A. Genitalia
B. Crusts
C. Ophthalmic
D. Acyclovir (Zovirax)
E. Itching
F. Burow's solution
G. Ulcers
H. Immunosuppressed
I. HSV
J. Shingles
K. Tzanck's smear

X. Complete the statements on the left with the most appropriate term on the right.

___ 1. Squamous cell carcinomas, unlike basal cell carcinomas, grow rapidly and _____.

___ 2. A chronic autoimmune condition in which bullae (blisters) develop on the face, back, chest, groin, and umbilicus is _____.

___ 3. The use of liquid nitrogen to freeze and destroy lesions found in actinic keratosis is called _____.

___ 4. A condition with painless, nodular lesions that have a pearly appearance is _____.

___ 5. The drug of choice for actinic keratosis is _____.

___ 6. The use of electrical current to destroy the le-sions found in actinic keratosis is called _____.

___ 7. Scaly ulcers or raised lesions are characteristics of _____.

___ 8. Although basal cell carcinomas grow slowly and rarely metastasize, they should be removed because they can cause local _____.

___ 9. A malignancy of the blood vessels is _____.

___ 10. A precancerous lesion most often found on areas exposed to sunlight, such as the face, neck, forearms, and backs of the hands is _____.

___ 11. A condition in which malignant T cells migrate to the skin is _____.

___ 12. Skin cancers are most common among light-skinned people who have had repeated _____ exposure.

___ 13. Squamous cell carcinomas are usually caused by overuse of alcohol and _____.

A. Electrodesiccation
B. Sun
C. Kaposi's sarcoma
D. Metastasize
E. Squamous cell carcinoma
F. Cryotherapy
G. Actinic keratosis
H. 5FU
I. Pemphigus
J. Tobacco
K. Tissue destruction
L. Basal cell carcinoma
M. Cutaneous T-cell lymphoma

XI. Complete the statements on the left with the most appropriate term on the right.

___ 1. A burn that affects the epidermis and the dermis is _____.

___ 2. First-degree burns that are pink to red, like a sunburn, are called _____.

___ 3. An accurate estimate of burn size based on differences in body proportions is the _____.

___ 4. Burns are classified by the size and depth of the tissue injury; extent is often defined as the percentage of _____ affected.

___ 5. Third-degree burns involving the epidermis, dermis, and underlying tissues, including fat, muscle, and bone, are called _____.

___ 6. Tissue injuries caused by heat are referred to as _____.

___ 7. Full-thickness burns that extend into deep tissue layers are classified as _____.

___ 8. The _____ does not take age into account in estimating burn size.

___ 9. Second-degree burns that are painful and sensitive to cold are called _____.

___ 10. A superficial burn affecting only the epidermis is classified as _____.

A. First degree
B. Second degree
C. Third degree
D. Burns
E. Superficial burns
F. Superficial partial-thickness burns
G. Deep partial-thickness burns
H. Full-thickness burns
I. Body surface area
J. Rule of nines
K. Lund and Browder method

XII. Match the definition or description on the left with the most appropriate term on the right. Some terms may be used more than once, and some may not be used.

___ 1. Pigmented spots on sun-exposed areas; commonly called "liver spots," although they have nothing to do with the liver

___ 2. Large purplish bruises that resolve very slowly; can result from minor trauma

___ 3. Bright-red papules

___ 4. Waxy, raised lesions; flesh-colored to dark brown or black and variously sized from small and nearly flat to large and prominent

___ 5. Small, soft, raised lesions; flesh-colored or pigmented

A. Senile angiomas
B. Acrochordons
C. Nevi
D. Senile purpura
E. Lentigines
F. Seborrheic keratoses

XIII. Match the color change on the left with the most appropriate cause on the right.

_____ 1. Cyanosis

_____ 2. Jaundice

_____ 3. Pallor

_____ 4. Erythema

A. Vasoconstriction due to acute anxiety or fear, cold, some drugs, cigarette smoking, edema

B. Increased local blood flow due to inflammation, fever, or emotions such as embarrassment or anger

C. Inadequate oxygenated blood in the tissue due to anemia, respiratory disorders, or cardiovascular disorders

D. Reflects increased bilirubin in the blood due to liver disease or destruction of red blood cells

XIV. Match the example or description on the left with the most appropriate type of lesion on the right.

_____ 1. Freckle, petechia, hypopigmentation

_____ 2. Mole, wart

_____ 3. Herpes simplex, herpes zoster

_____ 4. Acne, impetigo

_____ 5. Vitiligo

_____ 6. Psoriasis

_____ 7. Fibroma, xanthone

_____ 8. Allergic response, insect bite

A. Plaque
B. Wheal
C. Papule
D. Patch
E. Pustule
F. Vesicle
G. Nodule
H. Macule

XV. Match the example or description on the left with the most appropriate type of lesion on the right.

_____ 1. Lipoma, hemangioma

_____ 2. Blister

_____ 3. Impetigo, weeping ezcematous dermatitis

_____ 4. Psoriasis, seborrheic dermatitis, eczema

_____ 5. Cheilosis, tinea pedis

_____ 6. Pressure sore, chancre

_____ 7. Scratching with insect bites, scabies, dermatitis

_____ 8. Sebaceous cyst

_____ 9. Flat or raised, color darker than surrounding skin

_____ 10. Shallow, superficial depression

A. Fissure
B. Nevus
C. Erosion
D. Tumor
E. Excoriation
F. Scale
G. Crust
H. Bulla
I. Cyst
J. Ulcer

XVI. Match the use/action on the left with the most appropriate drug group on the right.

___ 1. Interfere with viral replication

___ 2. Decreases proliferation of epidermal cells in psoriasis

___ 3. Reduce inflammation in various skin disorders

___ 4. Kill parasites and their eggs; used to treat pediculosis (lice) and scabies (mite) infestations

___ 5. Dissolve keratin and slow bacterial growth; used to treat acne and psoriasis

___ 6. Effective against fungi; used to treat fungal infections

___ 7. Used to treat psoriasis

___ 8. Destroy microorganisms; used to treat skin infections

___ 9. Reduces formation of comedones; increases mitosis of epithelial cells; used to treat acne

A. Keratolytics (for example, coal tar)

B. Topical anti-infectives (for example, bacitracin)

C. Antiviral agents (for example, acyclovir)

D. Photosensitivity drugss (for example, methoxsalen)

E. Topical antifungal agents (for example, nystatin)

F. Topical anti-inflammatories (for example, hydrocortisone)

G. Vitamin A derivatives (for example, Retin-A)

H. Pediculicides and scabicides (for example, Kwell)

I. Antipsoriatics (for example, anthralin)

XVII. Match the description or anatomic location on the left with the most appropriate fungal infection on the right.

___ 1. Beard

___ 2. Scalp

___ 3. Skin, mouth, vagina, gastrointestinal tract, lungs

___ 4. Groin

___ 5. Athlete's foot

___ 6. Hand

A. Tinea pedis

B. Tinea manus

C. Tinea cruris

D. Tinea corporis

E. Tinea barbae

F. Candidiasis

XVIII. Match the signs or symptoms on the left with the most appropriate skin infection on the right.

___ 1. Vesicle or pustule that ruptures, leaving a thick crust

___ 2. Inflamed hair follicles with white pustules

___ 3. Inflamed skin and subcutaneous tissue with deep, inflamed nodules

___ 4. Clustered, interconnected furuncles

___ 5. Local tenderness and redness at first, then malaise, chills, and fever. Site becomes more erythematous. Nodules and vesicles may form. Vesicles may rupture, releasing purulent material.

___ 6. At first, small shiny lesions. They enlarge and become rough.

A. Furuncle (boil)

B. Verruca (wart)

C. Folliculitis

D. Cellulitis

E. Impetigo

F. Carbuncle

Introductory Nursing Care of Adults

XIX. Match the definition or description on the left with the most appropriate stage of burn injury on the right. Some terms may be used more than once, and some may not be used.

___ 1. Lasts as long as efforts continue to promote improvement or adjustment; follows acute stage

___ 2. Begins with the injury and ends when fluid shifts have stabilized

___ 3. Begins with fluid stabilization

A. Chronic

B. Emergent

C. Rehabilitation

D. Acute

XX. Match the appearance characteristics on the left with the sensations experienced in the same depth of burn on the right.

___ 1. Large thick-walled blisters covering extensive area (vesiculation); edema; mottled red base; broken epidermis; wet, shiny, weeping surface

___ 2. Variable e.g., deep red, black, white, brown; dry surface; edema; fat exposed; tissue disrupted

___ 3. Mild to severe erythema; skin blanches with pressure

A. Little pain; insensate

B. Painful; sensitive to cold air

C. Painful; hyperesthetic; tingling; pain eased by cooling

XXI. Match the characteristics on the left with the (A) open care or (B) closed care on the right.

___ 1. Uses topical medications covered by dressings

___ 2. Less restrictive and simpler

___ 3. Uses topical antimicrobials but not dressings

___ 4. Provides greater opportunity for loss of fluid and heat through the wound surface

A. Open care

B. Closed care

XXII. Match the definition or description on the left with the most appropriate term on the right. Some terms may be used more than once, and some may not be used.

___ 1. Removal of necrotic tissue from a wound

___ 2. Covering a wound with skin

___ 3. Can be reduced by use of pressure dressings in early stages of care

___ 4. May be accomplished by mechanical means, surgical excision, or enzymes

___ 5. Can be reduced by use of custom-fitted garments that apply continuous pressure 23 hours a day

A. Skin grafting

B. Scarring

C. Débridement

XXIII. Match the conditions treated with plastic surgery on the left with the type of surgery used on the right.

___ 1. Birthmarks

___ 2. Excess tissue around the eyes

___ 3. Developmental defects

___ 4. Disfiguring scars

___ 5. Receding chin

___ 6. Facial wrinkles

A. Aesthetic surgery

B. Reconstructive surgery

XXIV. Match the signs and symptoms of skin infestations on the left with infestation on the right.

___ 1. Thin, red lines on skin, itching

___ 2. Itching of hairy areas of body (head, pubis); nits (eggs) seen as tiny white particles attached to hair shafts

A. Lice

B. Scabies

XXV. List 5 functions of the skin.

1.

2.

3.

4.

5.

XXVI. List 3 protective functions of the skin.

1.

2.

3.

XXVII. List 2 ways the skin regulates temperature.

1.

2.

XXVIII. List 5 age-related changes in the skin.

1.

2.

3.

4.

5.

XXIX. List 11 sources of data that should be included in assessment data as part of a review of the skin system.

1.

2.

3.

4.

5.

6.

7.

8.

9.

10.

11.

XXX. List 7 characteristics of the skin that can be evaluated by palpation.

1.

2.

3.

4.

5.

6.

7.

XXXI. List 12 classifications of drugs that may be used as topical agents to treat skin disorders and skin manifestations of other conditions.

1.	7.
2.	8.
3.	9.
4.	10.
5.	11.
6.	12.

XXXII. List 6 forms of topical medication vehicles used to treat skin disorders.

1.

2.

3.

4.

5.

6.

XXXIII. List 6 groups of patients who are at risk of developing candidiasis.

1.   4.

2.   5.

3.   6.

XXXIV. List the 5 criteria for a major burn in an adult.

1.

2.

3.

4.

5.

XXXV. Indicate the complications that may occur following burns in the following 3 areas.

1. Gastrointestinal function:

2. Immune system:

3. Respiratory system:

XXXVI. List 5 functions of wound care after a burn injury.

1.

2.

3.

4.

5.

XXXVII. List 10 nursing diagnoses for patients with burns.

1.

2.

3.

4.

5.

6.

7.

8.

9.

10.

XXXVIII. List 6 common nursing diagnoses for patients after plastic surgery.

1.

2.

3.

4.

5.

6.

XXXIX. List 5 skin changes associated with malnutrition.

1.

2.

3.

4.

5.

XL. Choose the most appropriate answer.

1. The outermost layer of the skin is the:
   A. dermis
   B. subcutaneous
   C. corium
   D. epidermis

2. The layer of the skin that contains nerve endings, sweat glands, and hair roots is the:
   A. epidermis
   B. stratum germinativum
   C. dermis
   D. stratum corneum

3. Epidermal cells produce a dark pigment that helps determine the color of the skin called:
   A. sebum
   B. cerumen
   C. keratin
   D. melanin

4. The dermis is well supplied with blood vessels, causing the skin to redden when surface vessels:
   A. dilate
   B. constrict
   C. multiply
   D. stimulate

5. The layer beneath the dermis is the:
   A. stratum corneum
   B. stratum germinativum
   C. subcutaneous tissue
   D. epidermis

6. The two types of glands found in the skin are sweat glands and:
   A. ceruminous glands
   B. sebaceous glands
   C. endocrine glands
   D. thymus glands

7. Scalp hair thins in older men and women, but there may be an increase in:
   A. elastic tissue
   B. facial hair
   C. subcutaneous tissue
   D. capillaries

8. Nevi (moles) are carefully inspected for pigmentation, ulcerations, or changes in surrounding skin, and:
   A. vascular irregularities
   B. amount of edema
   C. amount of pus
   D. irregularities in shape

9. When assessing capillary refill, after applying pressure to cause blanching and then releasing the pressure, the nurse should observe that the color returns to normal within:
   A. 1 to 2 minutes
   B. 3 to 5 seconds
   C. 30 to 40 seconds
   D. 50 to 60 seconds

10. The potassium hydroxide (KOH) examination is used in combination with a culture to diagnose infections of the skin, hair, or nails that are:
    A. viral
    B. bacterial
    C. caused by parasites
    D. fungal

11. When a skin biopsy is scheduled, the physician may advise the patient to avoid which drug before the procedure to reduce bleeding?
    A. diphenhydramine
    B. tetracycline
    C. aminophylline
    D. aspirin

12. Two assessments of the fingernails and toenails include noting the color of the nail bed and assessing:
    A. capillary refill
    B. edema
    C. hemorrhage
    D. mobility

13. Two functions of dressings for skin disorders are to protect healing wounds and to retain surface moisture to:
    A. increase vasoconstriction
    B. improve clotting
    C. promote healing
    D. decrease edema

14. The most common nursing diagnosis for patients with pruritus is high risk for:
    A. altered tissue perfusion
    B. impaired skin integrity
    C. injury
    D. infection

15. Nursing diagnoses for the patient with atopic dermatitis may include impaired skin integrity related to:
    A. decreased resistance to infection
    B. self-care practices
    C. hypertension
    D. excessive dryness

16. Measures that decrease itching and moisturize the skin help to maintain:
    A. tissue perfusion
    B. hyperthermia
    C. airway clearance
    D. skin integrity

17. Patients with any break in the skin are at high risk for infection, because the break in the skin presents a portal for:
    A. pathogens
    B. blood
    C. pus
    D. sweat

18. The assessment of patients with seborrheic dermatitis includes inspecting affected areas for:
    A. bleeding and exudate
    B. edema and redness
    C. scales and crusts
    D. yellow skin and ascites

19. Patients with psoriasis are told to report signs of secondary infection to the physician; these signs include increased redness, purulent discharge, and:
    A. fever
    B. numbness
    C. pain in calf
    D. shortness of breath

20. The organisms that cause tinea infections take advantage of trauma in:
    A. tough, connective tissue
    B. dry, scaly tissue
    C. toenails and fingernails
    D. warm, moist tissue

21. An important risk factor for developing candidiasis is:
    A. hypertension
    B. antibiotic therapy
    C. emotional stress
    D. tachycardia

22. A primary nursing diagnosis for patients with candidiasis is:
    A. activity intolerance
    B. altered oral mucous membrane
    C. decreased cardiac output
    D. self-care deficit

23. Acne is caused by:
    A. eating too much chocolate
    B. fatty foods
    C. poor hygiene
    D. blocked hair follicles

24. The nurse advises the patient with shingles that the condition is communicable to people who have never been exposed to:
    A. measles
    B. pertussis
    C. chickenpox
    D. polio

25. The most serious form of skin cancer is:
    A. basal cell carcinoma
    B. melanoma
    C. squamous cell carcinoma
    D. cutaneous T-cell lymphoma

26. The health history of patients with a nail disorder needs to include the diagnoses of peripheral vascular disease or:
    A. diabetes mellitus
    B. hypertension
    C. kidney disease
    D. pneumonia

27. Burn-injured tissue releases chemicals that cause increased:
    A. heart rate
    B. capillary permeability
    C. hypertension
    D. hemoglobin

28. Following a burn, plasma leaks into the tissue due to increased capillary:
    A. constriction
    B. dilation
    C. production
    D. permeability

29. Burn injury to cell membranes permits excess sodium to enter the cell and allows potassium to escape into the extracellular compartment; these shifts in fluids and electrolytes cause local edema and a decrease in:
    A. respiratory rate
    B. CNS stimulation
    C. cardiac output
    D. red blood cell production

30. The shift of plasma proteins from the capillaries may result in:
    A. hypoproteinemia
    B. increased blood volume
    C. dehydration
    D. increased urine output

31. A complication of untreated fluid shifts in burn patients is:
    A. hypovolemic shock
    B. kidney failure
    C. pneumonia
    D. convulsions

32. Common complications of plastic surgery procedures are:
    A. fluid volume excess and edema
    B. hematoma and hemorrhage
    C. numbness and shortness of breath
    D. fever and purulent discharge

33. Vitamin A is essential for:
    A. blood clotting
    B. bone formation
    C. wound healing
    D. healthy skin

34. Food allergies can cause:
    A. scabies
    B. basal cell carcinoma
    C. psoriasis
    D. atopic dermatitis

XLI. In the figure below, label the parts of the skin (A–P) from the terms provided (1-16).

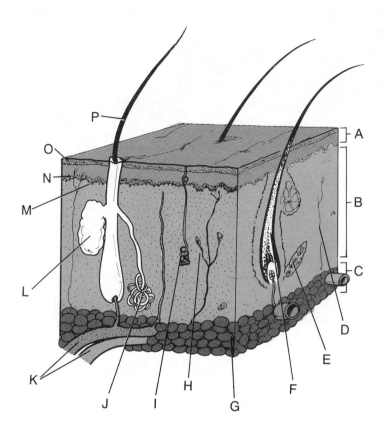

____ 1. sebaceous gland

____ 2. nerves

____ 3. hair follicle

____ 4. dermis

____ 5. hair shaft

____ 6. stratum corneum

____ 7. blood vessels

____ 8. epidermis

____ 9. arrector pili muscle

____ 10. melanocyte

____ 11. stratum germinativum

____ 12. apocrine sweat gland

____ 13. adipose tissue

____ 14. connective tissue

____ 15. eccrine sweat gland

____ 16. subcutaneous tissue

Eye and Vision Disorders

OBJECTIVES

1. Identify the data to be collected in the nursing assessment of the eye and vision.
2. Identify the nursing responsibilities for patients having diagnostic tests or procedures to diagnose eye disorders.
3. Describe the nursing care of patients who require common therapeutic measures for eye disorders: irrigation, application of ophthalmic drugs, and surgery.
4. Describe the pathophysiology, signs and symptoms, diagnosis, and treatment of selected eye conditions.
5. Apply the nursing process to plan care for the patient with an eye disorder.

LEARNING ACTIVITIES

I.   Match the definition on the left with the most appropriate term on the right.

____ 1. Farsightedness; ability to see distant objects better than near objects

____ 2. Measurement of pressure such as intraocular pressure

____ 3. Agent that causes the pupil to constrict

____ 4. Error of refraction caused by uneven curvature of the cornea or lens; causes visual distortion

____ 5. Inflammation of the cornea

____ 6. Inflammation of the membrane lining the eyelids and the eyeball

____ 7. A visual impairment associated with older age in which the lens becomes more rigid and less able to change shape, resulting in a decreased ability to focus on near objects

____ 8. Clouding or opacity of the normally transparent lens within the eye; causes blurred vision and objects to take on a yellowish hue

____ 9. Removal of an intact organ, such as the eyeball

____ 10. Agent that paralyzes the ciliary muscle so that the eye does not accommodate

____ 11. Nearsightedness; ability to see near objects better than distant objects

____ 12. Bending of light rays

____ 13. In relation to the eyelid, outward turning of the lid

____ 14. Agent that causes the pupil to dilate

____ 15. In relation to the eyelid, inward turning of the lid

A.   Keratitis

B.   Presbyopia

C.   Ectropion

D.   Tonometry

E.   Cycloplegic

F.   Hyperopia

G.   Enucleation

H.   Conjunctivitis

I.   Refraction

J.   Entropion

K.   Miotic

L.   Mydriatic

M.   Cataract

N.   Astigmatism

O.   Myopia

II.   Match the definition on the left with the most appropriate term on the right.

____ 1. Inflamed, enlarged meibomian gland

____ 2. Yellow color of the sclera caused by excess bilirubin in the blood; jaundice

____ 3. Excessive sensitivity to light

____ 4. Inflammation of the hair follicles and glands on the margins of the eyelids

____ 5. Inflammation of a sebaceous gland of the eyelid; commonly called a stye

A.   Photophobia

B.   Hordeolum

C.   Icterus

D.   Chalazion

E.   Blepharitis

III.   Complete the statements on the left with the most appropriate term on the right. Some terms may be used more than once, and some terms may not be used.

____ 1. The eyelids and eyelashes protect the eye by shielding it from foreign substances and by keeping the eye _____.

____ 2. The eyelids are lined with a mucous membrane called the palpebral _____.

____ 3. The portion of the mucous membrane that covers the anterior sclera is called _____.

____ 4. The glands located above the eyes that secrete tears into the eyes are called _____.

____ 5. The structures in the upper eyelids through which tears are secreted into the eyes are called _____.

____ 6. A process that occurs about 15 times a minute and that bathes the eyeballs in fluid is called spontaneous _____.

____ 7. Tear fluid provides oxygen and some nutrients to the _____.

____ 8. Normally, tear fluid drains from the eye through the lacrimal sac into the _____.

____ 9. Decreased tear production occurs to some extent with _____.

____ 10. Severe deficiencies in tear fluid cause "dry eyes"; the part of the eye that is then made susceptible to injury by dry eyes is the _____.

____ 11. The simultaneous movement of both eyes in the same direction is called _____.

A.   Cornea

B.   Lacrimal glands

C.   Eversion

D.   Conjugate movement

E.   Lacrimal ducts

F.   Nose

G.   Conjunctiva

H.   Dry

I.   Blinking

J.   Pharynx

K.   Moist

L.   Aging

M.   Bulbar conjunctiva

IV. Complete the statements on the left with the most appropriate term on the right. Some terms may be used more than once, and some terms may not be used.

___ 1. The eyeball consists of three layers of tissue: the sclera, the choroid and the _____.

___ 2. The tough outer layer of the eyeball is the _____.

___ 3. The sclera is mostly white except for the clear part of the eye in front; called the _____.

___ 4. The cornea is covered by a protective membrane called the _____.

___ 5. The middle layer of the eyeball is the _____.

___ 6. The colored part of the eye is the _____.

___ 7. The hole in the center of the iris is the _____.

___ 8. The muscular part of the eye that contracts and relaxes to control the amount of light entering the eye is the _____.

___ 9. Dim light causes the iris to _____.

___ 10. Dim light causes the pupil to _____.

___ 11. Bright light causes the iris to _____.

___ 12. The part of the eyeball that is rich in blood vessels is the _____.

___ 13. The back of the eye, which receives nourishment from the blood supply in the middle layer, is the _____.

___ 14. The inner lining of the eyeball is the _____.

A. Pupil
B. Cornea
C. Vitreous humor
D. Relax
E. Conjunctiva
F. Iris
G. Sclera
H. Aqueous humor
I. Contract
J. Choroid
K. Macula
L. Dilate
M. Retina

V. Complete the statements on the left with the most appropriate term on the right. Some terms may be used more than once, and some terms may not be used.

___ 1. A clear, gelatinous material that helps hold the retina in place is the _____.

___ 2. A transparent structure behind the iris is the _____.

___ 3. The process that permits the eye to focus on objects at different distances is called _____.

___ 4. The anterior chamber is filled with a clear, watery fluid called the _____.

___ 5. Aqueous humor is produced in the _____.

___ 6. The function of aqueous humor is to moisturize and nourish the lens and the _____.

___ 7. The larger posterior chamber behind the lens is filled with _____.

___ 8. The retina contains light-sensitive receptors called rods and _____.

___ 9. The receptors most important for vision in dim light are the _____.

___ 10. An area of the eye that has no blood vessels and that is dependent on the choroid for nourishment is the _____.

___ 11. The cranial nerve that sends visual messages to the brain for interpretation is the _____.

___ 12. When the eye is examined with an ophthalmoscope, the part of the optic nerve that can be seen is referred to as the _____.

___ 13. The anterior chamber is located between the iris and _____.

___ 14. The receptors used for daylight vision and color perception are the _____.

___ 15. The area of sharpest vision on the retina is the _____.

A. Retina

B. Accommodation

C. Cones

D. Sclera

E. Ciliary body

F. Optic nerve

G. Vitreous humor

H. Rods

I. Iris

J. Lens

K. Optic disk

L. Cornea

M. Macula

N. Aqueous humor

VI. Complete the statements on the left with the most appropriate term on the right. Some terms may be used more than once, and some terms may not be used.

____ 1. If untreated, glaucoma may result in _____.

____ 2. A procedure that measures the approximate pressure in the blood vessels of the eye is _____.

____ 3. Having the patient read a chart through a series of lenses is a measure of _____.

____ 4. Having the patient read a Snellen chart with rows of progressively smaller letters is a measure of _____.

____ 5. The area a person can see while looking straight ahead without moving the head is called _____.

____ 6. The measurement of pressure in the anterior chamber of the eye is _____.

____ 7. A condition in which the pressure in the eye is increased is called _____.

____ 8. Differences in pressure from one eye to the next reflect insufficiency of the _____.

____ 9. Since the retina is composed of nerve tissue, a characteristic that can be measured is _____.

____ 10. Many patients report a feeling of warmth, nausea, or vertigo following _____.

____ 11. A procedure that is done to detect abrasions of the cornea is the application of _____.

____ 12. To obtain images of the eye for diagnostic purposes, the physician may order computed tomography scanning, ultrasonography, or _____.

____ 13. As light enters the eye, the light rays bend so that they focus on the retina; this bending is called _____.

____ 14. Two procedures used to measure electrical potential in the retina are electroretinography and _____.

____ 15. A test used to detect abnormal blood vessels or blood flow by injecting a dye and photographing the retina is _____.

A. Fluorescein angiography

B. Carotid artery

C. Visual acuity

D. Blindness

E. Pain

F. Glaucoma

G. Topical dyes

H. Visual field

I. Visual evoked response

J. Ophthalmodynamometry

K. Magnetic resonance imaging

L. Electrical potential

M. Refraction

N. Eye irrigation

O. Tonometry

VII. Complete the statements on the left with the most appropriate term on the right. Some terms may be used more than once, and some terms may not be used.

_____ 1. When irrigating a patient's eye, the nurse should position the patient with affected eye down so that contaminated fluid does not run into the _____.

_____ 2. The irrigating fluid should be directed to the lower _____.

_____ 3. When administering eye drops, the medication should be at _____.

_____ 4. When administering topical eye drops, the lower eyelid is gently pulled down to expose the _____.

_____ 5. Following administration of topical eye drops, the nurse or the patient should apply gentle pressure to the _____.

_____ 6. A procedure that is done to remove irritating chemicals from the eye is _____.

A. Room temperature

B. Irrigation

C. Lacrimal sac

D. Eye drop administration

E. Unaffected eye

F. Upper eyelid

G. Conjunctival sac

VIII. Complete the statements on the left with the most appropriate term on the right. Some terms may be used more than once.

_____ 1. The transparent portion of the eye that has no blood vessels, making it vulnerable to infections, is called the _____.

_____ 2. Itching, burning, and photophobia are symptoms of _____.

_____ 3. The application of warm, moist compresses several times a day is a treatment for _____.

_____ 4. _____ causes considerable pain but produces no noticeable drainage.

_____ 5. An inflammation of the glands in the eyelids is called _____.

_____ 6. The medical treatment of keratitis includes topical antibiotics and _____.

_____ 7. Untreated blepharitis could lead to inflammation of the cornea or _____.

_____ 8. The cleansing of the eyelids with baby shampoo is a treatment for _____.

_____ 9. Redness, mild irritation, and mucopurulent drainage are symptoms of _____.

_____ 10. _____ is commonly called a stye.

_____ 11. _____ is commonly called pinkeye.

A. Hordeolum

B. Corticosteroids

C. Chalazion

D. Blepharitis

E. Bacterial conjunctivitis

F. Cornea

G. Keratitis

IX. Complete the statements on the left with the most appropriate term on the right.

____ 1. Because eye pads provide a dark, damp environment for microorganisms to grow, they are not used for _____.

____ 2. The type of conjunctivitis that may persist a long time and is likely to produce severe eye damage is _____.

____ 3. A red, swollen, tender area in the affected part of the eye is a sign of _____.

____ 4. Organisms other than bacteria and viruses that can cause conjunctivitis include chlamydia and _____.

A.   Keratitis

B.   Viral conjunctivitis

C.   Parasites

D.   Hordoleum

X. Complete the statements on the left with the most appropriate term on the right.

____ 1. The recommended treatment for entropion and ectropion is _____.

____ 2. Foreign bodies that are embedded in the eye should be removed only by a _____.

____ 3. A tissue that forms when the cornea is injured by infection or trauma is _____.

____ 4. The only treatment for corneal opacity is a surgical treatment called _____.

____ 5. A condition in which the lower eyelid droops and turns out is called _____.

____ 6. _____ tissue is easier to preserve than other body tissues.

____ 7. A keratoplasty can be done under _____.

____ 8. A condition in which eyelashes rub against the eye, causing pain and possibly scratching the cornea is _____.

____ 9. If lens extraction is necessary for cloudy lenses due to injury or age-related changes, the preoperative eye drops that are ordered to dilate the pupils and allow access to the lens are _____.

____ 10. During a keratoplasty, the surgeon first removes the patient's damaged cornea and replaces it with a _____.

____ 11. Eye drops that are used to constrict the pupil before a keratoplasty are _____.

A.   Local anesthesia

B.   Scar

C.   Graft

D.   Ectropion

E.   Mydriatics

F.   Surgery

G.   Antibiotics

H.   Entropion

I.   Physician

J.   Miotics

K.   Eye

L.   Keratoplasty

XI. Complete the statements on the left with the most appropriate term on the right.

___ 1. An important disadvantage of contact lens is the risk of _____.

___ 2. The condition in which the lens is situated too far from the retina is _____.

___ 3. The adjustment of the lens for near and distant vision is _____.

___ 4. The primary treatment of errors of refraction is _____.

___ 5. The result of irregularities in the cornea or lens is _____.

___ 6. When the lens is too close to the retina, light rays come together behind the retina; this condition creates _____.

___ 7. Tiny plastic disks made to fit over the patient's cornea are _____.

___ 8. A normal age-related change that often develops after age 40 is _____.

A. Corrective lenses
B. Hyperopia
C. Astigmatism
D. Contact lenses
E. Corneal injury
F. Accommodation
G. Presbyopia
H. Myopia

XII. Complete the statements on the left with the most appropriate term on the right. Some terms may be used more than once.

___ 1. Timolol maleate (Timoptic) is a _____ used in glaucoma to lower intraocular pressure.

___ 2. A condition in which intraocular pressure is increased above normal is _____.

___ 3. Excess pressure impairs blood flow to the optic nerve, resulting in _____.

___ 4. _____ vision is lost first in glaucoma.

___ 5. Patients with glaucoma have fields of vision that gradually narrow until the patient has _____.

___ 6. A type of acute glaucoma that is considered a medical emergency is _____.

___ 7. Acetazolamide (Diamox) is a _____ used to reduce intraocular pressure by decreasing the production of aqueous humor.

___ 8. _____ is a surgical procedure for glaucoma.

___ 9. Chronic glaucoma is also called _____.

___ 10. A person who can only see a small circle, as if looking through a tube, has _____.

___ 11. A surgical procedure in which a window is cut to permit aqueous humor to flow through the pupil normally in angle-closure glaucoma is _____.

___ 12. Open-angle glaucoma is usually treated first with drug therapy, which includes _____.

___ 13. Adrenergics decrease _____ by decreasing the formation of aqueous humor and increasing its outflow.

A. Open-angle glaucoma
B. Iridotomy
C. Intraocular pressure
D. Miotic(s)
E. Carbonic anhydrase inhibitor
F. Peripheral
G. Phacoemulsification
H. Glaucoma
I. Angle-closure glaucoma
J. Tunnel vision
K. Trabeculoplasty
L. Vision impairment
M. Beta blocker(s)

XIII. Complete the statements on the left with the most appropriate term on the right. Some terms may be used more than once, and some terms may not be used.

___ 1. Cataracts may be congenital, degenerative, or _____.

___ 2. The _____ is located behind the iris and changes shape to focus on images of various sizes.

___ 3. When the lens becomes opaque so that it is no longer transparent, it is called a _____.

___ 4. Once the lens is removed, the eye is said to be _____.

___ 5. _____ cataracts are more common with aging, but may occur earlier with diabetes or Down's syndrome.

___ 6. The _____ is a clear flexible structure encased in an elastic capsule.

___ 7. Signs and symptoms of cataracts include cloudy vision, seeing spots, and _____.

___ 8. The only treatment for cataracts is removal of the _____.

___ 9. The surgical treatment for cataracts that involves the use of sound waves to break up the lens is _____.

A. Floaters

B. Cataract

C. Degenerative

D. Phacoemulsification

E. Traumatic

F. Lithotripsy

G. Aphakic

H. Lens

I. Cornea

XIV. Complete the statements on the left with the most appropriate term on the right.

___ 1. _____ is a separation of the sensory layer of the eyeball from the pigmented layer.

___ 2. A part of the retina that is responsible for central vision is the _____.

___ 3. Regular eyeglasses do not improve vision with _____.

___ 4. The term used for removal of the eye is _____.

___ 5. The _____ is sutured over the muscle during enucleation.

___ 6. _____ uses a cold probe applied to the eyeball beneath the tear in retinal detachment.

___ 7. Signs and symptoms of retinal detachment may include seeing flashes of light or _____.

___ 8. _____ is often used as an additional treatment for retinal detachment along with laser treatment or cryotherapy.

___ 9. In _____, intense light burns the detached portion of the retina.

___ 10. In retinal detachment, vision may be _____.

A. Cryotherapy

B. Enucleation

C. Macula

D. Conjunctiva

E. Floaters

F. Laser surgery

G. Retinal detachment

H. Scleral buckling

I. Cloudy

J. Macular degeneration

XV.   Match the definition or description on the left with the most appropriate term on the right. Some terms may be used more than once.

____   1.   Physician with specialized training in diagnosing and treating eye conditions

____   2.   Individual who prescribes corrective lenses for refractive errors as well as treats other eye conditions with medications and surgery

____   3.   Individual trained to diagnose errors of refraction and to prescribe corrective lenses

____   4.   Individual who fills prescriptions written by an ophthalmologist or optometrist and fits the prescribed lenses

A.   Optometrist

B.   Ophthalmologist

C.   Optician

XVI. Match the use/action on the left with the most appropriate drug classification on the right.

____   1.   Treatment or prevention of eye infections

____   2.   Treatment of herpes simplex keratitis

____   3.   Dilate pupil; used in open-angle glaucoma; decreases corneal congestion; controls hemorrhage

____   4.   Prevent redness and swelling caused by inflammation due to causes other than bacterial infection

____   5.   Primarily used to treat glaucoma

____   6.   Block sensation in external eye for tonometry, removal of sutures or foreign bodies, some surgical procedures

____   7.   Effective against some fungal infections of eye

____   8.   Dilate pupil; used before eye exams and for uveitis; decrease lacrimal gland secretion

A.   Antibiotics

B.   Anti-inflammatory agents

C.   Miotics

D.   Antifungals

E.   Topical anesthetics

F.   Antimuscarinics

G.   Antivirals

H.   Sympathomimetics

XVII. Match the "related to" statements on the right with the most appropriate nursing diagnoses for patients following eye surgery on the left.

____   1.   Pain

____   2.   Anxiety

____   3.   High risk for injury

____   4.   Sensory perceptual alteration (vision)

A.   Tissue trauma

B.   Temporary vision impairment

C.   Disease process, trauma to the eye, patching

D.   Pressure or trauma

XVIII. List interventions in the following areas that relate to lighting for patients who are partially sighted.

1. Glare:

2. Windows:

3. Floors:

4. Furniture color:

5. Light switches, handrails, and steps:

6. Dishes and cups:

XIX. Match the purpose/procedure on the left with the appropriate diagnostic test for eye disorders on the right.

____ 1. Allows diagnosis of abnormalities of retina, optic disk, and blood vessels

____ 2. Series of pictures of blood vessels in eye taken after injection of dye into vein in hand or arm

____ 3. Identifies area person can see while looking straight ahead

____ 4. Measures intraocular pressure

____ 5. Identifies refractive errors and corrective lens needed

A. Fluorescein anigiography

B. Tonometry

C. Ophthalmoscopy

D. Refraction

E. Visual fields

XX. Match the use/action on the left with the classification of drugs used to treat glaucoma on the right. Some classifications may be used more than once.

____ 1. Treatment of acute glaucoma

____ 2. Initial treatment of acute and chronic glaucoma

____ 3. Preoperative preparation for glaucoma surgery

____ 4. Treatment of chronic glaucoma

A. Direct acting miotics

B. Osmotic diuretics

C. Beta-adrenergic blocking agents

XXI. List 3 causes of increased tear production.

1.

2.

3.

XXII.   Indicate the age-related changes that occur in the eye related to the following areas.

1. Skin around the eye:

2. Eyelids:

3. Amount of fat around the eye:

4. Tear secretion:

5. Size of pupil:

6. Pupillary response to light:

XXIII.   Indicate the age-related changes that occur with respect to vision in the following areas.

1. Lens (list 3 changes):

    A.

    B.

    C.

2. Ability to focus:

3. Sensitivity to glare:

XXIV.   List 10 changes in vision that the nurse should record when assessing patients with eye disorders.

1.   6.

2.   7.

3.   8.

4.   9.

5.   10.

XXV.   If the patient reports eye pain, the nurse inquires about its location and nature; list 3 words frequently used to describe eye pain.

1.

2.

3.

XXVI.   List 3 words to describe drainage from the eye.

1.

2.

3.

XXVII.   List 4 non–eye-related medical conditions that often have accompanying eye problems.

1.

2.

3.

4.

XXVIII.   List 4 drugs that are especially likely to be related to vision disturbances.

1.

2.

3.

4.

XXIX.   List 3 medical conditions which may cause loss of parts of the visual field.

1.

2.

3.

XXX.   List 6 types of drugs commonly used as topical medications for eye disorders.

1.   4.

2.   5.

3.   6.

XXXI.   List 5 common goals of nursing care after eye surgery.

1.

2.

3.

4.

5.

XXXII.   List the 2 main nursing diagnoses following cataract surgery.

1.

2.

XXXIII.   List 5 factors to teach the patient following cataract surgery.

1.

2.

3.

4.

5.

XXXIV.   List 4 common nursing diagnoses for patients with glaucoma.

1.

2.

3.

4.

XXXV. List 5 infectious and inflammatory conditions of the eye.

1.

2.

3.

4.

5.

XXXVI. List 3 errors of refraction.

1.

2.

3.

XXXVII. List 12 signs of possible eye problems.

1.   7.

2.   8.

3.   9.

4.   10.

5.   11.

6.   12.

XXXVIII. List the associated eye disorders that may be present with the following diseases.

1. Diabetes:

   A. Elevated blood glucose:

   B. Changes in retina due to diabetes:

2. Neurologic disorders (brain tumors, head injuries, and strokes)

   A. Vision:

   B. Movement of eyes:

3. Thyroid disease

   A. Hyperthyroidism:

4. Hypertension

   A. Changes in blood vessels of the eye:

XXXIX. Choose the most appropriate answer.

1. As light enters the eye, it passes through the transparent cornea, aqueous humor, lens, and the:
   A. conjunctiva
   B. sclera
   C. vitreous humor
   D. lacrimal glands

2. The refractive media (cornea, aqueous humor, lens, and vitreous humor) bend horizontal and vertical light rays so that they focus on the:
   A. iris
   B. optic nerve
   C. choroid
   D. retina

3. The age-related change of impaired ability to focus in the elderly is called:
   A. presbyopia
   B. myopia
   C. mydriasis
   D. photophobia

4. Dark spots that are actually bits of debris in the vitreous are called:
   A. flashes
   B. floaters
   C. blind spots
   D. cataracts

5. Sensitivity to light is called:
   A. photophobia
   B. presbyopia
   C. myopia
   D. hyperopia

6. When the nurse is doing a physical assessment of the eyes, the lids should cover the eyeball completely when closed; when the eyes are open, the lower lid should be at the level of the:
   A. conjunctiva
   B. retina
   C. iris
   D. lacrimal gland

7. The eyeball is inspected for color and moisture; the sclera should be clear:
   A. yellow
   B. white
   C. gray
   D. black

8. Excessive redness of the sclera may be an indication of:
   A. hypertension
   B. exophthalmos
   C. liver dysfunction
   D. irritation

9. The pupils are assessed for size, equality, and reaction to light; pupils that are unequal, dilated, or do not respond to light suggest:
   A. diabetes
   B. liver dysfunction
   C. inflammation
   D. neurologic problems

10. When the patient is asked to focus on the nurse's finger as it is moved slowly toward the patient's nose, the nurse is assessing:
    A. presbyopia
    B. astigmatism
    C. accommodation
    D. refraction

11. Visual acuity is commonly tested using the:
    A. Snellen chart
    B. accommodation test
    C. tonometry
    D. fluorescein angiography

12. If more than one eye medication is being given, the nurse must wait how long between each medication?
    A. 60 seconds
    B. 5 minutes
    C. 30 minutes
    D. 60 minutes

13. Eye surgery may involve surgical incisions, the application of cold probes (cryotherapy), or the use of:
    A. tonometry
    B. lasers
    C. fluorescein angiography
    D. topical dyes

14. Following eye surgery, the patient is usually positioned:
    A. flat in bed
    B. prone position
    C. side-lying position, on affected side
    D. head of bed elevated

15. An important aspect of the care of postoperative eye patients is to prevent increased:
    A. blood pressure
    B. cardiac output
    C. intraocular pressure
    D. ocular movement

16. Nurses can teach people how to care for their eyes in order to protect their vision; it is important to tell people that:
    A. burning sensations in the eyes should be reported to the physician
    B. watching too much television or sitting too close to the television injures the eyes
    C. eating foods with high vitamin A content will improve vision
    D. eyes need to be rinsed regularly to protect vision

17. The most frequently performed eye operation in the United States is:
    A. enucleation
    B. cryotherapy
    C. cataract extraction
    D. vitrectomy

18. Symptoms of cataracts include:
    A. inflammation
    B. cloudy vision
    C. redness
    D. swelling

19. Following cataract surgery, the most important thing is to prevent:
    A. conjunctivitis
    B. hypertension
    C. pain
    D. strain on the operative eye

20. Medications prescribed after cataract surgery usually include antibiotics and:
    A. miotics
    B. antihistamines
    C. anticholinergics
    D. corticosteroids

21. One of the leading causes of blindness in the United States is:
    A. conjunctivitis
    B. retinal detachment
    C. glaucoma
    D. cataracts

22. After an enucleation, a prosthesis can be fitted by an optician after:
    A. 24 hours
    B. 5 days
    C. 1 month
    D. 6 months

XL. In the figure below, match the internal structures of the eye (A–Q) with the labels provided (1–17).

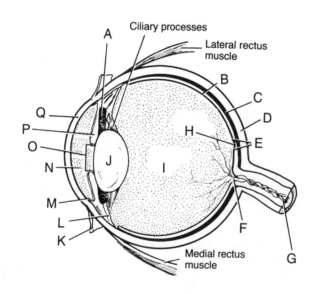

_____ 1. Anterior chamber

_____ 2. Canal of Schlemm

_____ 3. Choroid

_____ 4. Ciliary body

_____ 5. Conjunctiva

_____ 6. Cornea

_____ 7. Fovea centralis

_____ 8. Iris

_____ 9. Lens

_____ 10. Macula lutea

_____ 11. Optic disk

_____ 12. Optic nerve

_____ 13. Posterior chamber

_____ 14. Pupil

_____ 15. Retina

_____ 16. Sclera

_____ 17. Vitreous body

Ear and Hearing Disorders

OBJECTIVES

1. Identify the data to be collected when assessing a patient with a disorder affecting the ear, hearing, or balance.
2. Describe the tests and procedures used to diagnose disorders of the ear, hearing, or balance.
3. Explain the nursing considerations for each of the tests and procedures.
4. Explain the nursing involvement for patients receiving common therapeutic measures for disorders of the ear, hearing, or balance.
5. For selected disorders, describe the pathophysiology, signs and symptoms, complications, and medical or surgical treatment.
6. Write a nursing care plan for a patient with a disorder of the ear, hearing, or balance.
7. Identify measures the nurse can take to reduce the risk of hearing impairment and to detect problems early.

LEARNING ACTIVITIES

I. Match the definition on the left with the most appropriate term on the right.

____ 1. Capable of injuring the eighth cranial (acoustic) nerve or other structures involved in hearing and balance

____ 2. Eardrum; the membrane that separates the external and middle portions of the ear

____ 3. Waxy secretion in the external auditory canal; earwax

____ 4. Ringing, buzzing, or roaring noise in the ears

____ 5. State of balance needed for walking, standing, and sitting

____ 6. Feeling of unsteadiness

____ 7. Hearing loss associated with aging

____ 8. Sensation that one's body or one's surrounding are rotating

____ 9. Pertaining to the ear

____ 10. Pain in the ear

A. Tinnitus

B. Otalgia

C. Cerumen

D. Presbycusis

E. Typanic membrane

F. Otic

G. Equilibrium

H. Vertigo

I. Ototoxic

J. Dizziness

II. Complete the statements on the left with the most appropriate term on the right. Some terms may be used more than once, and some terms may not be used.

____ 1. The reason that pain in the ear can sometimes be traced to disorders of the nose, mouth, or neck is that the auricle is innervated by many _____.

____ 2. A structure at the end of the auditory canal that is shiny and pearl gray in color is the _____.

____ 3. Sound waves entering the external auditory canal cause the tympanic membrane to _____.

____ 4. The external auditory canal is lined with cells that secrete _____.

____ 5. The visible part of the ear is the _____.

____ 6. The external auditory canal extends from the external opening of the ear to the _____.

____ 7. The external ear contains the auricle and the _____.

A. Auricle (pinna)

B. External auditory canal

C. Blood vessels

D. Cerumen (earwax)

E. Nerves

F. Soften

G. Typanic membrane

H. Vibrate

III. Complete the statements on the left with the most appropriate term on the right. Some terms may be used more than once.

____ 1. The bony structure behind the auricle is called the _____.

____ 2. The membranous labyrinth and the bony labyrinth make up the _____.

____ 3. The middle ear is an air-filled space in the _____.

____ 4. The eustachian tube is an important structure in the _____.

____ 5. A structure that extends from the middle ear to the nasopharynx is the _____.

____ 6. The function of the three small bones in the middle ear (ossicles) is to forward the sound waves transmitted by the tympanic membrane to the _____.

____ 7. The structure that separates the middle ear from the inner ear is the _____.

____ 8. The portion of the ear that contains three small bones called ossicles is the _____.

____ 9. A structure that equalizes air pressure on both sides of the tympanic membrane is the _____.

A. Eustachian tube

B. Oval window

C. Mastoid process

D. Middle ear

E. Temporal bone

F. Inner ear

IV. Complete the statements on the left with the most appropriate term on the right. Some terms may be used more than once, and some terms may not be used.

___ 1. The receptor end organ of hearing is the _____.

___ 2. The parts of the bony labyrinth are the vestibule, semicircular canals, and the _____.

___ 3. Receptors in the vestibule monitor the position of the head to maintain posture and _____.

___ 4. The organ of Corti transmits stimuli from the oval window to the _____.

___ 5. Receptors in the semicircular canals monitor changes in rate of direction of movement to maintain _____.

___ 6. The membranous labyrinth contains fluid called _____.

___ 7. A coiled tube, found in the inner ear, that looks like a snail, is called the _____.

___ 8. The oval window opens into the _____.

A. Balance

B. Oval window

C. Endolymph

D. Cochlea

E. Temporal bone

F. Organ of Corti

G. Vestibule

H. Acoustic (auditory) nerve

V. Complete the statements on the left with the most appropriate term on the right. Some terms may be used more than once, and some terms may not be used.

___ 1. A procedure in which a receiver is surgically placed behind the ear is _____.

___ 2. The _____ determines which type of hearing aid is needed.

___ 3. Electrodes attached to the receiver in a cochlear implant stimulate nerve fibers in the cochlea to produce _____.

___ 4. Most hearing aids use transistors, which allow the device to be very small; in order to work, transistors require _____.

___ 5. A procedure that allows the profoundly deaf to recognize some environmental sounds, such as sirens, doorbells, and telephones, is the _____.

___ 6. Hearing aids that are worn in the external ear canal are called _____.

___ 7. A microphone, a processor, a transmitter, and a receiver make up the _____.

___ 8. A hearing-impaired person who cannot benefit from regular hearing aids may benefit from a(n) _____.

___ 9. Hearing aids that are worn behind the ear against the skull are called _____.

A. Batteries

B. Bone conduction receivers

C. Audiologist

D. Computer chips

E. Air conduction receivers

F. Cochlear implant

G. Otologist

H. Sound

I. Electronystagmography

Introductory Nursing Care of Adults

VI.   Complete the statements on the left with the most appropriate term on the right. Some terms may be used more than once, and some terms may not be used.

____ 1.   Patients who hear better in noisy settings than in quiet settings have _____.

____ 2.   Congenital problems, noise trauma, aging, Meniere's syndrome, ototoxicity, diabetes, and syphilis may all be causes of _____.

____ 3.   A condition in which the stapes in the middle ear does not vibrate is _____.

____ 4.   A hearing loss that results from interference with the transmission of sound waves from the external or middle ear to the inner ear is _____.

____ 5.   A disturbance of the neural structures in the inner ear or the nerve pathways to the brain results in _____.

____ 6.   Patients who either cannot perceive or cannot interpret sounds that are heard may have _____.

____ 7.   Otosclerosis can be treated surgically with a procedure called _____.

____ 8.   A combination of conductive and sensorineural losses results in _____.

____ 9.   Persons with conductive hearing losses are usually helped to hear by _____.

____ 10. Obstruction of the external canal or eustachian tube or otosclerosis may cause _____.

____ 11. Sensorineural hearing loss is sometimes called _____.

____ 12. Problems in the central nervous system may result in _____.

____ 13. Patients who can hear sounds but have difficulty understanding speech have _____.

____ 14. Patients with conductive hearing loss do not speak loudly because _____ allows them to hear their own voices.

A.   Mixed hearing loss

B.   Otosclerosis

C.   Cochlear implants

D.   Nerve deafness

E.   Central hearing loss

F.   Otitis media

G.   Cholesteatoma

H.   Sensorineural loss

I.   Hearing aids

J.   Labyrinthitis

K.   Conductive hearing loss

L.   Bone conduction

M.   Stapedectomy

VII. Complete the statements on the left with the most appropriate term on the right. Some terms may be use more than once, and some terms may not be used.

___ 1. A type of ear infection which usually develops with colds is _____.

___ 2. The treatment for cholesteatoma is _____.

___ 3. Soreness, headache, malaise and an elevated white blood cell count are symptoms of _____.

___ 4. If fluid remains in the middle ear following serous otitis media _____ may develop.

___ 5. A very serious infection that can lead to a brain abscess, meningitis, or paralysis of the facial muscles is _____.

___ 6. The usual treatment for acute otitis media is _____.

___ 7. An infection of the middle ear is called _____.

___ 8. A condition that produces disturbances in both hearing and balance is _____.

___ 9. An ear infection characterized by hearing loss and continuous or intermittent drainage is _____.

___ 10. Sterile fluid accumulates behind the tympanic membrane in _____.

___ 11. _____ is the creation of a small opening in the tympanic membrane to reduce pressure and allow fluid to drain.

___ 12. _____ is characterized by thickening and scarring in the middle ear structures.

___ 13. An ear infection that is usually not painful but in which the eardrum is usually perforated is _____.

___ 14. Edema in acute otitis media leads to blockage of the _____.

___ 15. Inflammation of the labyrinth is _____.

___ 16. A growth in the middle ear is called a _____.

A. Meningitis
B. Mastoiditis
C. Serous otitis media
D. Labyrinthitis
E. Anti-inflammatories
F. Chronic otitis media
G. Eustachian tube
H. Acute otitis media
I. Electronystagmography
J. Antibiotics
K. Adhesive otitis media
L. Cholesteatoma
M. Chemotherapy
N. Surgical removal
O. Myringotomy
P. Otitis media

VIII. Complete the statements on the left with the most appropriate term on the right. Some terms may be used more than once, and some terms may not be used.

____ 1. "Swimmer's ear" is also called _____.

____ 2. An inflamed area in the external auditory canal caused by infection of a hair follicle is a _____.

____ 3. Treatment for external otitis includes topical corticosteroids and _____.

____ 4. Infection or inflammation of the lining of the external ear canal is called _____.

____ 5. Swimming can lead to otitis by washing out protective _____.

____ 6. Drainage in external otitis may be blood tinged or _____.

____ 7. _____ may be caused by scratching or cleaning the ear with sharp objects.

____ 8. When infection is present in external otitis, it is frequently caused by streptococcus or _____.

____ 9. The most characteristic symptom of external otitis is _____.

A. Cerumen

B. Pain

C. Furuncle

D. Otitis media

E. Purulent

F. Antibiotics

G. Redness

H. Staphylococcus

I. External otitis

IX. Match the description on the left with the most appropriate hearing specialist on the right.

____ 1. A person trained to diagnose types of hearing loss

____ 2. A person who carries out tests to determine whether a hearing aid will help a particular patient

____ 3. A physician who specializes in diseases of the ears and throat

A. Audiologist

B. Otologist

C. Otolaryngologist

X.   Match the definition or description on the left with the most appropriate term on the right. Some terms may be used more than once, and some may not be used.

____ 1.   A test used to detect lesions in the vestibule by placing electrodes around the eyes, and measuring eye movements as ears are irrigated

____ 2.   An instrument used to examine the external auditory canal

____ 3.   The use of a tuning fork placed on the patient's mastoid bone to assess the patient's ability to hear sound waves conducted through the air

____ 4.   Test in which the ear is irrigated with warm or cold water followed by observation of the patient for reactions that suggest vestibular problems

____ 5.   The assessment of the ability to hear simple sound waves

____ 6.   A gross assessment of hearing

____ 7.   The use of a tuning fork placed on the midline of the skull in which the patient is asked to identify the side in which the sound is loudest

____ 8.   A precise measure of hearing acuity

____ 9.   An examination that permits diagnosis of inflammatory and infectious processes as well as obstructions of the external canal

____ 10. Test used to diagnose disorders in the vestibular system or its CNS connections

____ 11. Purpose of test is to examine the external auditory canal and tympanic membrane

____ 12. A test whose results are altered by CNS depressants, barbiturates and alcohol

A.   Caloric test

B.   Weber's test

C.   Vestibulography

D.   Rinne's test

E.   Otoscopic examination

F.   Whisper test

G.   Electroencephalography

H.   Electronystagmography

I.   Challenge test

J.   Audiometry

K.   Shout test

L.   Otoscope

XI.   In these nursing diagnoses of patients having ear surgery, match the "related to" statements on the right with the nursing diagnoses on the left.

Causes

____ 1.   High risk for infection

____ 2.   High risk for impaired skin integrity

____ 3.   Sensory perceptual alteration (auditory)

____ 4.   Pain

____ 5.   High risk for injury

Nursing Diagnoses

A.   Tissue trauma or edema

B.   Dizziness or vertigo

C.   Pressure in the ear or delayed wound healing

D.   Surgical incision

E.   Packing and edema in affected ear

XII. Match the nursing interventions on the left with the nursing diagnoses on the right for patients who have had ear surgery. Some nursing diagnoses may be used more than once, and some may not be used.

____ 1. Encourage patient to avoid crowds and people with colds

____ 2. Administer analgesics as ordered

____ 3. Do not shampoo for 2 weeks

____ 4. Avoid straining; give stool softeners as ordered

____ 5. Keep ear canal dry for 2 to 4 weeks

____ 6. Avoid nose blowing, coughing, sneezing

____ 7. Raise side rails and leave bed in low position

____ 8. Encourage balanced diet with adequate protein and vitamin C

A. High risk for impaired skin integrity

B. High risk for infection

C. Sensory perceptual alterations

D. Pain

E. Anxiety

F. High risk for injury

G. Self-care deficit

XIII. Match the "related to" statements on the left with the most appropriate nursing diagnosis for the hearing-impaired patient on the right. Some nursing diagnoses may be used more than once, and some may not be used.

____ 1. Altered social interaction, threat to body image, or denial

____ 2. Inability to hear

____ 3. Inability to communicate verbally

A. Social isolation

B. Knowledge deficit

C. Ineffective individual coping

D. Impaired verbal communication

XIV. Match the "related to" statements on the left with the most appropriate nursing diagnoses for the patient with labyrinthitis on the right.

____ 1. Anorexia and nausea

____ 2. Acute illness

____ 3. Vomiting

____ 4. Vertigo

A. High risk for fluid volume deficit

B. Anxiety

C. Altered nutrition: less than body requirements

D. High risk for injury

XV.   Match the use/action on the left with the most appropriate drug classification on the right.

_____ 1.   Dry external canal after swimming or bathing. Decrease risk of infection.

_____ 2.   Prevent or treat nausea, vomiting, motion sickness.

_____ 3.   Broad-spectrum drugs used to treat infections of lining of external auditory canal.

_____ 4.   Soften earwax. Treat aphthous ulcers.

_____ 5.   Treat inflammation, pruritus, and allergic response. Usually combined with antibacterial or antifungal drug.

A.   Topical corticosteroids

B.   Drying agents

C.   Antibacterial and softening agents

D.   Antibiotics

E.   Antiemetics

XVI.   Match the ototoxic drugs on the left with their most appropriate classification on the right. Some classifications may be used more than once, and some may not be used.

_____ 1.   Aspirin

_____ 2.   Erythromycin estolate (Ilosone)

_____ 3.   Furosemide (Lasix)

_____ 4.   Cisplatin (Platinol)

_____ 5.   Indomethacin (Indocin)

_____ 6.   Streptomycin sulfate

_____ 7.   Ethacrynic acid (Edecrin)

_____ 8.   Quinidine

_____ 9.   Tetracycline

_____ 10.   Bleomycin (Blenoxane)

A.   Antiarrhythmics

B.   Antibiotics

C.   Antineoplastics

D.   Antihistamines

E.   Anti-inflammatories/Analgesics

F.   Diuretics

XVII.   List 5 structures in the middle ear through which sound waves travel, beginning with the tympanic membrane and ending with the oval window.

1.

2.

3.

4.

5.

XVIII. List age-related changes in the ear in the 6 areas below.

1. Skin or auricle:

2. External canal:

3. Cerumen:

4. Hairs in the canal:

5. Eardrum:

6. Bony joints in the middle ear:

XIX. List 8 symptoms that may reflect problems with the ear.

1.

2.

3.

4.

5.

6.

7.

8.

XX. List three uses of otic drops.

1.

2.

3.

XXI. List 4 areas to assess in patients following ear surgery.

1.

2.

3.

4.

XXII. List 5 complications of chronic otitis media.

1.

2.

3.

4.

5.

XXIII. List 6 signs and symptoms of labyrinthitis.

1.

2.

3.

4.

5.

6.

XXIV. List 4 potential complications of surgery for Meniere's disease.

1.

2.

3.

4.

XXV. List 4 signs and symptoms of ototoxicity.

1.

2.

3.

4.

XXVI. Choose the most appropriate answer.

1. Age-related changes in the inner ear affect sensitivity to sound, understanding of speech, and:
   A. balance
   B. infection
   C. cerumen production
   D. blood pressure

2. The type of hearing loss usually associated with aging is:
   A. otitis media
   B. cholesteatoma
   C. otosclerosis
   D. presbycusis

3. Pain in the ear is called:
   A. otosclerosis
   B. otitis
   C. ototoxicity
   D. otalgia

4. Continuous or intermittent ringing in the ears is called:
   A. presbycusis
   B. tinnitus
   C. otalgia
   D. vertigo

5. One cause of congenital hearing loss in an infant occurs when, during the mother's pregnancy, she contracted:
   A. pneumonia
   B. gonorrhea
   C. rubella
   D. herpes

6. When taking a history from patients with hearing disorders, one should identify any drugs taken that might be:
   A. otosclerotic
   B. otic
   C. ototoxic
   D. hypertensive

7. Ototoxicity means a drug can damage the eighth cranial nerve or the organs of:
   A. hearing and balance
   B. vision and sight
   C. smell and taste
   D. movement and coordination

8. Examples of drugs that can have ototoxic effects are:
   A. aspirin and antibiotics
   B. anticoagulants and corticosteroids
   C. central nervous system stimulants and adrenergics
   D. diuretics and antihypertensives

9. When assessing the position of the auricles, the nurse should observe that the top of the auricle normally will be at about the level of the:
   A. nostrils
   B. forehead
   C. eye
   D. mouth

10. The external auditory canal is inspected for obvious obstructions or:
    A. edema
    B. cyanosis
    C. drainage
    D. jaundice

11. The only normal secretion in the external auditory canal is:
    A. sebum
    B. purulent drainage
    C. cerumen
    D. mucus

12. Otic drops, or ear drops, are intended to be placed directly into the:
    A. middle ear canal
    B. inner ear canal
    C. tympanic membrane
    D. external ear canal

13. The use of a solution to cleanse the external ear canal or to remove something from the canal is called:
    A. audiometry
    B. irrigation
    C. débridement
    D. electronystagmography

14. A common indication for irrigation is:
    A. clot formation
    B. impacted cerumen
    C. purulent drainage
    D. bleeding

15. A device that amplifies sound is:
    A. audiometer
    B. tuning fork
    C. hearing aid
    D. otoscope

16. Persons who benefit the most from hearing aids are those with:
    A. sensorineural loss
    B. mixed hearing loss
    C. conductive hearing loss
    D. Meniere's disease hearing loss

17. Postoperative dizziness or vertigo following ear surgery may put the patient at risk for:
    A. injury
    B. impaired skin integrity
    C. infection
    D. pain

18. Patients who have had ear surgery may have altered auditory sensory perception due to:
    A. dizziness or vertigo
    B. knowledge deficit
    C. self-care deficit
    D. packing and edema in affected ear

19. Postoperative patients following ear surgery often complain of the sensation that the room is spinning or that their bodies are spinning; this is charted as:
    A. dizziness
    B. otalgia
    C. edema
    D. vertigo

20. After ear surgery, patients are advised to move slowly and carefully to avoid sudden movement, which may cause:
    A. hemorrhage
    B. vertigo
    C. infection
    D. edema

21. Of all the sensory disorders, people who probably suffer the most severe social isolation are those with:
    A. hearing impairment
    B. sight impairment
    C. smell impairment
    D. taste impairment

22. To prevent one form of congenital hearing impairment, all women of childbearing age should be immunized for:
    A. pertussis
    B. influenza
    C. rubella
    D. hepatitis B

23. One of the most common causes of obstruction of the external ear canal is:
    A. hemorrhage
    B. infection
    C. impacted cerumen
    D. blood clots

24. Patients with impacted cerumen may complain of hearing loss or:
    A. sharp pain
    B. tinnitus
    C. bloody discharge
    D. headache

25. When a large amount of hardened cerumen is present in the ear canal, the physician may order ear drops before irrigation to:
    A. decrease inflammation
    B. anesthetize the area
    C. soften the cerumen
    D. stop internal bleeding

26. The primary diagnosis for patients with impacted cerumen is:
    A. high risk for infection
    B. self-esteem alteration
    C. sensory perceptual alteration
    D. high risk for injury

27. A very common problem after mastoidectomy or middle ear surgery is:
    A. nausea
    B. constipation
    C. oliguria
    D. seizures

28. Because the fixed stapes cannot vibrate in otosclerosis, sound waves cannot be transmitted to the:
    A. middle ear
    B. tympanic membrane
    C. inner ear
    D. external auditory canal

29. Slow progressive hearing loss in the absence of infection is the primary symptom of:
    A. acute otitis media
    B. labyrinthitis
    C. perforated eardrum
    D. otosclerosis

30. The most common treatment for otosclerosis is a surgical procedure called:
    A. myringotomy
    B. stapedectomy
    C. mastoidectomy
    D. incision and drainage

31. A hereditary condition in which an abnormal growth causes the footplate of the stapes to become fixed is:
    A. cholesteatoma
    B. otosclerosis
    C. labyrinthitis
    D. conductive hearing loss

32. An inner ear infection that usually follows an upper respiratory infection, and that may lead to Meniere's disease, is:
    A. otitis media
    B. otosclerosis
    C. mastoiditis
    D. labyrinthitis

33. The treatment for labyrinthitis is:
    A. antiemetics
    B. analgesics
    C. corticosteroids
    D. beta blockers

34. Patients with labyrinthitis often have vomiting, which puts them at high risk for:
    A. infection
    B. anxiety
    C. fluid volume deficit
    D. injury

35. A major concern for a patient with vertigo is:
    A. infection
    B. safety
    C. nutrition
    D. edema

36. The primary symptom of ototoxicity with salicylates is:
    A. vertigo
    B. tinnitus
    C. dizziness
    D. anorexia

37. The classic symptoms of Meniere's disease include hearing loss and:
    A. edema
    B. hemorrhage
    C. confusion
    D. vertigo

38. A low buzzing sound that sometimes becomes a roar and that is a symptom of Meniere's disease is documented as:
    A. vertigo
    B. tinnitus
    C. dizziness
    D. otitis

39. When the caloric test or electronystagmography is done on patients with Meniere's disease, they will experience severe:
    A. vertigo
    B. seizures
    C. headache
    D. flushing

40. Following surgery for Meniere's disease, the nurse needs to assess the patient for:
    A. facial nerve damage
    B. fluid volume excess
    C. decreased cardiac output
    D. urinary retention

41. Presbycusis is the result of changes in one or more parts of the:
    A. middle ear
    B. external auditory canal
    C. eustachian tube
    D. cochlea

42. Damage to the ear or eighth cranial nerve caused by specific chemicals, including some drugs, is called:
    A. otosclerosis
    B. Meniere's disease
    C. ototoxicity
    D. cholesteatoma

43. A labyrinth disorder in which there is an accumulation of fluid in the inner ear is:
    A. otosclerosis
    B. otitis media
    C. Meniere's disease
    D. presbycusis

44. Drugs that can cause permanent hearing loss are:
    A. antihypertensives
    B. aminoglycosides (antibiotics)
    C. anticholinergics
    D. diuretics

45. Patients who are at special risk of developing ototoxicity because their bodies excrete drugs more slowly are those with:
    A. renal failure
    B. pneumonia
    C. myocardial infarction
    D. liver disease

XXVII. In the figure below, label all parts of the ear (A–K), using the labels provided (1-11).

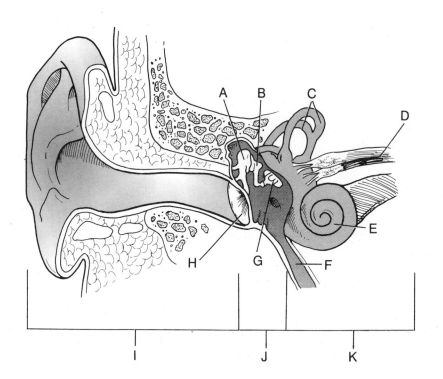

____ 1. Eighth cranial (vestibulocochlear) nerve

____ 2. External ear

____ 3. Stapes

____ 4. Malleus

____ 5. Inner ear

____ 6. Semicircular canals

____ 7. Eustachian tube

____ 8. Incus

____ 9. Middle ear

____ 10. Tympanic membrane

____ 11. Cochlea

XXVIII. Trace the sound waves from the external ear to the brain in the figure below. Label each step (A–F), using the labels below (1-6)

Sound
waves   Brain

→ A → B → C → D → E → F →

_____ 1. Oval window

_____ 2. Sensory receptors in inner ear

_____ 3. External canal

_____ 4. Tympanic membrane

_____ 5. Acoustic nerve

_____ 6. Malleus, incus, and stapes

Nose, Sinus, and Throat Disorders

OBJECTIVES

1. Describe the nursing assessment of the nose, sinuses, and throat.
2. Identify nursing responsibilities for patients undergoing tests or procedures to diagnose disorders of the nose, sinuses, or throat.
3. Describe the nurse's role when the following common therapeutic measures are instituted for disorders of the nose, sinuses, or throat: administration of topical medications, irrigations, humidification, suctioning, tracheostomy care, and surgery.
4. Explain the pathophysiology, signs and symptoms, complications, and medical or surgical treatment of selected disorders of the nose, sinuses, and throat.
5. Apply the nursing process to plan care for patients with disorders of the nose, sinuses, or throat.

LEARNING ACTIVITIES

I. Match the definition on the left with the most appropriate term on the right.

____ 1.	Agent that reduces swelling, especially of the nasal mucous membranes	A. Epistaxis
____ 2.	Inflammation of the tonsils	B. Antihistamine
____ 3.	Growth that protrudes from a mucous membrane	C. Coryza
____ 4.	Solid or liquid particles suspended in a gas	D. Polyp
____ 5.	Inflammation of the paranasal sinuses	E. Allergen
____ 6.	Nosebleed	F. Decongestant
____ 7.	Surgical removal of the larynx	G. Laryngectomy
____ 8.	Drug that blocks the effects of histamine, a body chemical that causes allergic symptoms	H. Laryngitis
____ 9.	Inflammation of the nasal mucous membrane	I. Tonsillitis
____ 10.	Substance capable of initiating an allergic or hyper-sensitivity response	J. Aerosol
____ 11.	Inflammation of the larynx	K. Rhinitis
____ 12.	Discharge from the nasal mucous membranes	L. Sinusitis

II. Complete the statements on the left with the most appropriate term on the right. Some terms may be used more than once, and some terms may not be used.

____ 1. The terms maxillary, frontal, ethmoid, and sphenoid refer to _____.

____ 2. _____ are projections that increase the surface area that inspired air crosses.

____ 3. In _____, the nurse shines a special light into the patient's mouth to see if the sinus cavities are filled with air.

____ 4. Mucus protects the nasal airway because it is _____.

____ 5. Spaces in the bones of the skull are called _____.

____ 6. The sinuses are lined with _____.

____ 7. Particles that are trapped in the mucus are swept toward the throat by _____.

____ 8. The _____ cells line the roof of the nasal cavity.

____ 9. Specialized sensory cells detect odors and relay information about odors to the brain by way of the _____.

____ 10. The side walls of the internal nose have folds of tissue called _____.

____ 11. A layer of mucus covers the membrane inside the nose; the mucus traps particles and _____ dry air.

____ 12. The sinuses produce mucus that drains into the _____.

____ 13. The _____ are air spaces that act as sound chambers for the voice and reduce the weight of the skull.

A. Acidic

B. Optic nerve

C. Cilia

D. Nasal cavity

E. Olfactory nerve

F. Turbinates

G. Nares

H. Mucous membrane

I. Moisturizes

J. Sinuses

K. Alkaline

L. Tonsils

M. Transillumination

N. Olfactory

III. Complete the statements on the left with the most appropriate term on the right. Some terms may be used more than once, and some terms may not be used.

____ 1. The epiglottis is located on top of the _____.

____ 2. A flap that operates like a trapdoor, closing during swallowing to prevent food from entering the respiratory tract, is the _____.

____ 3. Loss of voice is referred to as _____.

____ 4. The pharynx is also called the _____.

____ 5. The pharynx extends from the back of the nasal cavities to the _____.

____ 6. The larynx is commonly referred to as the _____.

____ 7. The masses of lymphatic tissue that guard against bacterial invasion of the respiratory and digestive tracts are adenoids and _____.

____ 8. The passageway between the throat and the trachea is the _____.

____ 9. The pharynx provides passageways from the nose and mouth to the digestive and _____ tracts.

____ 10. The eustachian tubes originate in the middle ear and open into the _____.

____ 11. Two bands of tissue that stretch across the interior of the larynx are the _____.

____ 12. The tube that prevents excessive pressure from building up in the middle ear is the _____.

____ 13. Masses of lymphatic tissue that are found in the throat are tonsils and _____.

A. Throat

B. Respiratory

C. Tonsils

D. Vocal cords

E. Esophageal sphincter

F. Aphonia

G. Eustachian tube

H. Larynx

I. Adenoids

J. Esophagus

K. Nares

L. Epiglottis

M. Nasopharynx

N. Voice box

O. Digestive tube

IV.   Complete the statements on the left with the most appropriate term on the right. some terms may be used more than once, and some terms may not be used.

___ 1. Until the patient with a tracheostomy adjusts to the inspiration of air directly into the trachea, _____ is necessary to prevent excessive drying of the mucosa.

___ 2. Nasal surgery may be indicated for various obstructions, injuries, and _____.

___ 3. The washing of secretions from the nasal cavity is called _____.

___ 4. Following nasal or sinus surgery, a bedside room humidifier may be ordered; a more effective option is a face tent or _____.

___ 5. _____ water should be used in aerosol humidifiers.

___ 6. A washing out procedure that is done to treat congestion or pain in the throat is called _____.

___ 7. If a tracheostomy tube is in place, _____ nebulizers, are used.

___ 8. _____ is done to remove secretions from the upper airway.

___ 9. _____ water should be used in steam humidifiers.

___ 10. An _____ dispenses tiny droplets of water into the room.

___ 11. _____ create an aerosol or steam.

A.   Nasal irrigation

B.   Humidifiers

C.   Sterile distilled water

D.   Tapwater

E.   Aerosol

F.   Throat irrigation

G.   Chronic infections

H.   Oxygen mask

I.   Plain distilled water

J.   Humidification

K.   Suctioning

L.   Aerosol mask

V.   Complete the statements on the left with the most appropriate term on the right.

___ 1. Pain or a feeling of heaviness over the frontal or maxillary area is a common symptom of _____.

___ 2. Sinus infection usually spreads into the sinuses from the _____.

___ 3. _____ sinusitis follows obstruction of the flow of secretions from the sinus.

___ 4. Two findings related to assessment of the sinuses, that may be observed when palpating the frontal and maxillary sinuses, include _____.

___ 5. Toothache-like pain is a common symptom of sinusitis that involves the _____.

___ 6. Potential complications of sinusitis include brain abscess, osteomyelitis, orbital cellulitis, and _____.

A.   Pain and tenderness

B.   Chronic

C.   Meningitis

D.   Maxillary sinuses

E.   Nasal passages

F.   Chronic sinusitis

G.   Redness and fever

H.   Acute

I.   Skull

J.   Acute sinusitis

K.   Sinusitis

L.   Streptococcus

Introductory Nursing Care of Adults

___ 7. Repeated infections often result in _____.

___ 8. Inflammation of the sinuses, usually the maxillary and frontal sinuses, is called _____.

___ 9. The most common causative organisms of sinusitis are staphylococcus and _____.

___ 10. _____ sinusitis is a permanent thickening of the mucous membranes in the sinuses.

___ 11. The possibility of brain infection exists in patients with sinusitis because the sinuses are located in the _____.

___ 12. Allergic rhinitis, deviated septum, nasal polyps, tumors, airborne pollution, and inhaled drugs such as cocaine are causes of _____.

A. Pain and tenderness
B. Chronic
C. Meningitis
D. Pharynx
E. Nasal passages
F. Chronic sinusitis
G. Redness and fever
H. Acute
I. Skull
J. Acute sinusitis
K. Sinusitis
L. Streptococcus
M. Maxillary sinuses

VI. Complete the statements on the left with the most appropriate term on the right.

___ 1. To decrease the patient's reaction to offending allergens, the allergist may recommend injections for _____.

___ 2. Nasal polyps tend to grow, and they eventually obstruct the _____.

___ 3. Medical treatment for epistaxis includes the use of silver nitrate or _____.

___ 4. The priority assessment when a patient has severe epistaxis is for evidence of excessive _____.

___ 5. A common respiratory condition, which is classified as acute (seasonal) or chronic (perennial), is _____.

___ 6. Swollen masses of sinus or nasal mucosa and connective tissue that extend into the nasal passages are called _____.

___ 7. The drugs used to treat allergic rhinitis are primarily decongestants and _____.

___ 8. Two methods used to apply pressure in patients with epistaxis include placement of a nasal balloon catheter and _____.

___ 9. Three symptoms that are normal following the Caldwell-Luc procedure are swelling, bruising, and _____.

___ 10. Following nasal polyp surgery, the patient is advised not to take _____.

___ 11. Complications related to posterior packing include infection, blockage of the eustachian tube, and _____.

___ 12. Chronic allergic rhinitis is often due to exposure to allergens in the environment such as _____.

___ 13. Nursing care of patients with epistaxis includes monitoring vital signs to detect signs of _____.

A. Numbness
B. Allergic rhinitis
C. Hypovolemia
D. Nasal airways
E. Antihistamines
F. Airway obstruction
G. Nasal packing
H. Electric cautery
I. Desensitization
J. Coryza
K. Nasal polyps
L. Aspirin
M. House dust
N. Blood loss

VII. Complete the statements on the left with the most appropriate term on the right. Some terms may be used more than once, and some terms may not be used.

___ 1. In an effort to limit new growth of polyps, sinus surgery is done; two surgical procedures include the Caldwell-Luc procedure or _____.

___ 2. The release of chemicals, including histamine, following exposure to an allergen, causes increased capillary permeability and _____.

___ 3. _____ resemble white grapes in size and shape.

___ 4. Acute allergic rhinitis is most often due to exposure to _____.

___ 5. Patients with triad disease have asthma, aspirin allergy, and _____.

___ 6. Removing allergens or treating the allergic responses may reduce the size of _____.

___ 7. The overuse of decongestant nose drops or sprays may result in _____.

___ 8. A condition that follows exposure to an allergen is _____.

___ 9. Swelling of the nasal mucosa occurs as a result of fluid leaks from the _____.

___ 10. The cause of nasal polyps is unknown, but patients often have a history of infections or _____.

A. Allergic rhinitis
B. Vasodilation
C. Vasoconstriction
D. Capillaries
E. Pollens
F. Rhinitis
G. Coryza
H. Nasal polyps
I. Ethmoidectomy

VIII. Complete the statements on the left with the most appropriate term on the right.

___ 1. Growths of tissue that may develop in the nasal passages and sinuses and that may be benign or malignant are called _____.

___ 2. The primary symptom of nasal tumors is _____.

___ 3. External nasal tumors are usually either basal cell or _____ carcinomas.

___ 4. The common cold is known as _____.

___ 5. Acute viral coryza is contagious and spread by _____.

___ 6. Signs and symptoms of the common cold include fever, fatigue, sore throat and _____.

___ 7. Complications of acute viral coryza include otitis media, sinusitis, bronchitis, and _____.

A. Nasal discharge
B. Resistance
C. Septoplasty
D. Biopsy
E. Squamous cell
F. Viruses
G. Droplet infection
H. Acute viral coryza
I. Septum
J. Nasal obstruction
K. Bacteria
L. Pneumonia
M. Decongestants
N. Tumors
O. Saddle deformity

____ 8. Septal deviations are corrected by a surgical procedure called a submucosal resection or nasal _____.

____ 9. The two major complications of submucosal resection are tears of the septum and _____.

____ 10. A diagnosis of cancer of the nose is made by taking a _____.

____ 11. The nose is divided into two passages by a cartilaginous wall called the _____.

____ 12. Complications of acute viral coryza are more common in people with lowered _____.

____ 13. Drug therapy for acute common coryza includes antipyretics, antihistamines, and _____.

____ 14. Antibiotics are not effective against infections caused by _____.

____ 15. Inappropriate use of antibiotics promotes the development of resistant strains of _____.

A. Nasal discharge
B. Resistance
C. Septoplasty
D. Biopsy
E. Squamous cell
F. Viruses
G. Droplet infection
H. Acute viral coryza
I. Septum
J. Nasal obstruction
K. Bacteria
L. Pneumonia
M. Decongestants
N. Tumors
O. Saddle deformity

IX. Complete the statements on the left with the most appropriate term on the right.

____ 1. Pharyngitis is treated with rest, fluids, analgesics, and _____.

____ 2. As long as the patient has fever, the level of activity that is often recommended is _____.

____ 3. A soft or liquid diet may be ordered because of _____.

____ 4. A treatment that may be ordered to increase moisture in the room air is _____.

____ 5. The recommended daily fluid intake for patients with pharyngitis is _____.

____ 6. Fluids must be increased slowly in the elderly because they do not adjust well to sudden changes in _____.

____ 7. Inflammation of the mucous membranes of the throat is called _____.

____ 8. _____ is a complication of bacterial pharyngitis that occurs 7 to 10 days after the throat infection.

____ 9. A usual course of antibiotic therapy is _____.

____ 10. If bacterial infection is confirmed, the antibiotic is usually continued for _____ after all signs and symptoms disappear.

____ 11. The physician often orders antibiotics for pharyngitis, usually erythromycin or _____.

____ 12. Before an antibiotic is ordered, a _____ should be taken.

____ 13. _____ is a complication of bacterial pharyngitis that occurs 3 to 5 weeks after the initial throat infection.

A. 48 hours
B. Humidification
C. Acute glomerulonephritis
D. Dysphagia
E. Blood volume
F. Culture specimen
G. Rheumatic fever
H. Bedrest
I. 10 days
J. Pharyngitis
K. Throat gargles (irrigations)
L. Penicillin
M. 2000–3000 ml
N. Temperature

X. Complete the statements on the left with the most appropriate term on the right.

____ 1. Common causative organisms of tonsillitis include streptococcus, staphylococcus, *Haemophilus influenza*, and _____.

____ 2. Tonsillitis is a contagious infection spread by food or _____.

____ 3. A patient with tonsillitis usually reports a sore throat, difficulty swallowing, fever, chills, muscle aches, and _____.

____ 4. If swollen tissue blocks the eustachian tubes in patients with tonsillitis, there may also be pain in the _____.

____ 5. An elevated white blood cell count in patients with tonsillitis suggests a _____.

____ 6. Inflammation of lymphatic tissue in the throat is called _____.

____ 7. The throat culture identifies the _____.

____ 8. The medical treatment of tonsillitis usually includes the use of _____.

____ 9. A serious complication of tonsillitis caused by streptococcus is _____.

A. Headache

B. Peritonsillar abscess

C. Tonsillitis

D. Airborne routes

E. Bacterial infection

F. Pathogenic organisms

G. Ears

H. Antibiotics

I. Pneumococcus

XI. Complete the statements on the left with the most appropriate term on the right.

____ 1. Following laryngectomy, many patients are able to learn to control and use air to produce sounds, which is called _____.

____ 2. Following larnyngectomy, some patients use an electronic device to produce sound, which is called _____.

____ 3. A procedure done during total laryngectomy to create a connection between the pharynx and trachea is called _____.

____ 4. A procedure in which the surgeon creates a fistula between the trachea and the esophagus is called _____.

A. Laryngoplasty

B. Artificial larynx

C. Esophageal speech

D. Tracheoesophageal prosthesis

II.   Match the definition or description on the left with the most appropriate term on the right.

____   1.   Tests done to isolate and identify infective mechanisms

____   2.   Inspection of the larynx to aid in diagnosis of abnormalities or to remove foreign bodies

____   3.   Instrument used in direct laryngoscopy

____   4.   Instrument used to visualize the larynx in indirect laryngoscopy

A.   Laryngoscopy

B.   Fiberoptic laryngoscope

C.   Mirrors

D.   Throat culture

XIII.   Match the actions and uses of the drugs on the left with the classification of drugs on the right.

____   1.   Anesthetic effect on skin and mucous membranes

____   2.   Reduce body temperature; treat fever

____   3.   Decongestion, vasoconstriction

____   4.   Treat allergic reactions, prevent motion sickness

____   5.   Reduce pain

____   6.   Kill or suppress growth of microorganisms

____   7.   Decrease salivary and respiratory secretions

A.   Sympathomimetics

B.   Anticholinergics

C.   Antihistamines

D.   Antipyretics

E.   Analgesics

F.   Anesthetics

G.   Anti-infectives

XIV.   Match the "related to" statements on the left with the nursing diagnoses for patients with epistaxis on the right. Some diagnoses may be used more than once, and some may not be used.

____   1.   Hypovolemia secondary to hemorrhage

____   2.   Threat of excessive bleeding or unpleasant procedures

____   3.   Pressure (of packing or nasal balloon) and possible airway obstruction

____   4.   Presence of nasal packing

A.   High risk for injury

B.   High risk for infection

C.   Anxiety

D.   Decreased cardiac output

XV. Indicate for each characteristic on the left whether it refers to (A) viral or (B) bacterial pharyngitis.

   ___   1.   Positive culture   A.   Viral

   ___   2.   Dysphagia   B.   Bacterial

   ___   3.   Normal CBC

   ___   4.   Rhinorrhea

   ___   5.   Abrupt onset of symptoms

   ___   6.   Malaise

   ___   7.   Mild elevation of temperature

   ___   8.   Gradual onset of symptoms

   ___   9.   Joint and muscle pain

   ___   10.   Rare complications

XVI. List 11 observations to be made when collecting data for an assessment of patients who seek medical attention for symptoms that affect the nose, sinuses, and throat.

1.

2.

3.

4.

5.

6.

7.

8.

9.

10.

11.

XVII. List 10 age-related changes of the nose, throat and sinuses in the following areas.

1. Size of nose:

2. Nasal obstruction:

3. Cartilage of the external nose:

4. Effect of nasal decongestants:

5. Mucous membrane:

6. Production of mucus:

7. Occurrence of epistaxis (nosebleed):

8. Sense of smell:

9. Tissues of the larynx:

10. Esophageal sphincter:

XVIII. List 6 adverse effects of drugs used to treat nasal congestion or nasal discharge in the elderly.

1.   4.

2.   5.

3.   6.

XIX. List interventions in preparing patients for laryngoscopy in the following 3 areas.

1. Oral intake:

2. Drugs:

3. Allergies:

XX. Suctioning should be done only when there is evidence that it is necessary; list 4 signs that indicate a need for suctioning.

1.

2.

3.

4.

XXI. List 5 complications of suctioning that may occur if it is done too often or if it is done incorrectly.

1.

2.

3.

4.

5.

XXII. List 4 common nursing diagnoses for the patient who has had nasal surgery.

1.

2.

3.

4.

XXIII. List 3 points to teach patients following nasal surgery to reduce the risk of bleeding.

1.

2.

3.

XXIV. List 4 ways to reduce the pain and promote drainage of patients with sinusitis.

1.

2.

3.

4.

XXV.   List 5 signs and symptoms of allergic rhinitis.

1.

2.

3.

4.

5.

XXVI.   List 5 problems that may lead to epistaxis.

1.

2.

3.

4.

5.

XXVII.   List 4 signs and symptoms of pharyngitis.

1.

2.

3.

4.

XXVIII.   List 6 indications for tonsillectomies.

1.

2.

3.

4.

5.

6.

XXIX.   Indicate how the tonsillectomy patient is positioned (1) after local anesthesia and (2) after general anesthesia.

1.

2.

XXX.   List 6 factors that may cause laryngitis.

1.

2.

3.

4.

5.

6.

XXXI. List 3 symptoms of laryngitis.

1.

2.

3.

XXXII. List 7 signs and symptoms of cancer of the larynx.

1.

2.

3.

4.

5.

6.

7.

XXXIII. List 10 nursing diagnoses for patients with total laryngectomy.

1.

2.

3.

4.

5.

6.

7.

8.

9.

10.

XXXIV. List 3 reasons why patients with laryngectomy may experience anxiety.

1.

2.

3.

XXXV. Nutrition is often a problem after laryngectomy; explain why the patient's sense of smell is impaired.

XXXVI. List 2 reasons why patients with total laryngectomies may experience ineffective individual coping and why they need to make considerable adjustments in their lives.

1.

2.

XXXVII. The tracheostomy permits unfiltered air to enter the respiratory tract in patients who have had total laryngectomies; list 3 effects on the patient of unfiltered air entering the respiratory tract.

1.

2.

3.

XXXVIII. Match the description on the left with the complications of total laryngectomy on the right.

_____ 1. An emergency that must be corrected surgically; patients at highest risk for this complication are those who had radiation prior to surgery

_____ 2. A drainage pathway that forms when saliva leaks through a defect in the suture line in the pharynx; complication which requires that the patient be fed through a nasogastric tube

_____ 3. Nnarrowing of the trachea that develops weeks or months after surgery

A. Salivary fistula

B. Carotid artery blowout

C. Tracheal stenosis

XXXIX. Choose the most appropriate answer.

1. The mucous membranes and tonsils of the throat are inspected for redness, drainage, swelling, or:
   A. cyanosis
   B. lesions
   C. pallor
   D. coolness

2. Inspection and palpation of the neck may reveal enlarged:
   A. lymph nodes
   B. tonsils
   C. adenoids
   D. vocal cords

3. Epistaxis (nosebleed) is more common in older people, especially in those taking:
   A. antibiotics
   B. analgesics
   C. anticoagulants
   D. diuretics

4. Elderly patients with a weakened esophageal sphincter, which may allow gastric contents to flow back into the throat when the patient lies down, may experience a burning sensation in the:
   A. larynx
   B. nares
   C. trachea
   D. stomach

5. Following laryngoscopy, the patient takes nothing by mouth until:
   A. respirations are normal
   B. vomiting has stopped
   C. the gag reflex returns
   D. a 24-hour period has gone by

6. Before suctioning a patient, it is important to:
   A. administer antiemetics as ordered
   B. ambulate the patient
   C. oxygenate the patient
   D. administer antibiotics as ordered

7. Key points to remember when suctioning a patient include:
   A. keep vent closed when inserting the catheter
   B. apply suction continuously as the catheter is withdrawn
   C. suction for no longer than 30 seconds
   D. use of sterile procedure

8. Key points to remember when doing tracheostomy care include:
   A. use of universal precautions
   B. suction the tracheostomy after removing the old dressings
   C. use a sterile solution of iodine to clean the inner cannula
   D. cut a new pad to fit around the tracheostomy site

9. After nasal surgery, the nurse assesses for pain, pressure, anxiety, and:
   A. tachycardia
   B. dyspnea
   C. hypotension
   D. pallor

10. After nasal surgery, the patient's vital signs are monitored to detect signs of:
    A. hypokalemia
    B. hypernatremia
    C. hypovolemia
    D. inadequate circulation

11. The patient who has had nasal surgery may be at high risk for fluid volume deficit due to:
    A. blood loss from nasal passageways
    B. nasal packing
    C. airway obstruction
    D. facial bruising

12. Because the nasal cavity has an extensive blood supply, following nasal surgery there is a risk of:
    A. hemorrhage
    B. infection
    C. hypertension
    D. confusion

13. Laxatives or stool softeners may be ordered for patients following nasal surgery in order to prevent:
    A. diarrhea
    B. vomiting
    C. hypertension
    D. straining

14. The best position for patients following nasal surgery to help control swelling is:
    A. flat bed
    B. elevated head of bed
    C. side-lying position
    D. supine position

15. When the nasal cavity is packed following surgery, the patient breathes through the mouth; a measure that helps decrease dryness of the mucous membranes is use of:
    A. frequent oral hygiene
    B. humidifiers
    C. oral fluids high in vitamin C
    D. ice packs

16. Patients may experience body image disturbance following nasal surgery due to:
    A. airway obstruction
    B. blood loss
    C. hypovolemia
    D. facial bruises

17. Serious neurologic complications should be suspected in patients with sinusitis if the patient develops:
    A. tachycardia and restlessness
    B. high fever and seizures
    C. confusion and cyanosis
    D. dyspnea and anxiety

18. The type of surgery performed for chronic maxillary sinusitis is:
    A. laryngoscopy
    B. tonsillectomy and adenoidectomy
    C. the Caldwell-Luc procedure
    D. nasal septoplasty

19. Desensitizing injections, or "allergy shots," are composed of dilute solutions of:
    A. allergens
    B. histamines
    C. antihistamines
    D. plasma

20. Deviated septum may obstruct the nasal passage and block:
    A. sinus drainage
    B. eustachian tube drainage
    C. pharyngeal drainage
    D. jugular vein drainage

21. Patients with deviated septum may complain of epistaxis, sinusitis, and:
    A. palpitations
    B. headaches
    C. insomnia
    D. sweating

22. The medical term for a nosebleed is:
    A. septoplasty
    B. coryza
    C. rhinitis
    D. epistaxis

Introductory Nursing Care of Adults

23. When epistaxis occurs, the patient should sit down and lean forward; direct pressure should be applied for:
    A. 1 to 2 minutes
    B. 3 to 5 minutes
    C. 7 to 10 minutes
    D. 15 to 20 minutes

24. With facial trauma or nasal fracture, the recommended treatment initially is application of:
    A. ice pack
    B. warm compress
    C. direct pressure
    D. heat

25. Patients with severe epistaxis may be at high risk for infection due to:
    A. possible airway obstruction
    B. nasal packing
    C. hypotension
    D. hypovolemia

26. The two major problems that may develop in the postoperative phase of tonsillectomy are respiratory distress and:
    A. infection
    B. hemorrhage
    C. hypersensitivity reaction
    D. cardiac dysrhythmia

27. Early signs of inadequate oxygenation in the postoperative tonsillectomy patient include restlessness, increased pulse rate, and:
    A. cyanosis
    B. pallor
    C. numbness
    D. confusion

28. Following a tonsillectomy, a treatment that may be applied to the neck to decrease swelling and pain is:
    A. heating pad
    B. TENS unit
    C. antibiotic ointment
    D. ice collar

29. Which foods should be avoided in patients following a tonsillectomy?
    A. frozen liquids
    B. ice cream
    C. applesauce
    D. citrus juices

30. Which of the following symptoms should be reported to the physician if the nurse observes them in the postoperative tonsillectomy patient who has been discharged?
    A. bleeding
    B. earache
    C. white patches in throat (surgical site)
    D. sore throat

31. In order to reduce irritation of the larynx in patients with laryngitis, a treatment usually prescribed is:
    A. surgery
    B. voice rest
    C. intravenous fluids
    D. application of heat

32. A primary nursing diagnosis for patients with laryngitis due to aphonia is:
    A. high risk for infection
    B. high risk for injury
    C. impaired verbal communication
    D. altered tissue perfusion

33. Benign masses of fibrous tissue that result primarily from overuse of the voice, but that can also follow infections, are called:
    A. nodules
    B. myomas
    C. fibromas
    D. tumors

34. The only symptom of laryngeal nodules is:
    A. pain
    B. fever
    C. dysphagia
    D. hoarseness

35. A swollen mass of mucous membrane attached to the vocal cord is called a:
    A. nodule
    B. tumor
    C. cancer
    D. polyp

36. Individuals who both smoke and use alcohol are at particularly high risk for:
    A. tonsillitis
    B. pneumonia
    C. cancer of the larynx
    D. nasal polyps

37. Malignancies in the larynx tend to spread fairly early; the most common site of metastasis is the:
    A. liver
    B. colon
    C. lung
    D. brain

38. Total laryngectomy causes permanent loss of:
    A. voice
    B. cough
    C. sternocleidomastoid muscle
    D. swallow reflex

39. A total laryngectomy involves removal of the entire larynx, vocal cords, and:
    A. pharynx
    B. epiglottis
    C. tonsils
    D. esophagus

40. Gently closing one naris at a time and instructing the patient to breathe through the other naris is a way to assess:
A. lung sounds
B. aphonia
C. sense of smell
D. patency of the nostrils

41. Normally, the frontal and maxillary sinuses are filled with:
A. fluid
B. air
C. polyps
D. cysts

42. In the immediate postoperative period with total laryngectomy, the nurse's assessment focuses on comfort, circulation, and:
A. fluid balance
B. oxygenation
C. infection
D. hypovolemia

43. In the laryngectomy patient, the nurse assesses the need for suctioning by observing audible or visible mucus, increased pulse, and:
A. pallor
B. swelling
C. pain
D. restlessness

44. Factors that affect the respiratory status of laryngectomy patients include positioning, fluids, and:
A. nutrition
B. verbal communication
C. humidification
D. personal hygiene

45. A position that promotes maximal lung expansion in the laryngectomy patient is:
A. semiprone
B. flat
C. semi-Fowler's
D. side-lying

46. To prevent pooling of secretions in the lungs of laryngectomy patients, the nurse should encourage:
A. coughing and deep breathing
B. increased fluid intake
C. early ambulation
D. avoidance of dusty places

XL. In the figure below, label the structures of the nose and throat (A–V) from the list of terms provided (1–22).

____ 1. Tongue
____ 2. Thyroid cartilage
____ 3. Oropharynx
____ 4. Middle turbinate
____ 5. Vocal cord
____ 6. Esophagus
____ 7. Adenoids (pharyngeal tonsils)
____ 8. Epiglottis
____ 9. Hard palate
____ 10. Superior turbinate
____ 11. Glottis
____ 12. Opening of eustachian tube
____ 13. Inferior turbinate
____ 14. Palatine tonsil
____ 15. Hyoid bone
____ 16. Uvula
____ 17. Laryngopharynx
____ 18. Nose
____ 19. Nasopharynx
____ 20. Lingual tonsils
____ 21. Soft palate
____ 22. Larynx

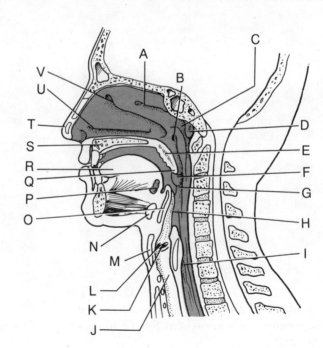

Psychological Responses to Illness

OBJECTIVES

1. Define mental illness.
2. Discuss a continuum for mental health and illness.
3. Discuss personality development from the psychoanalytic, social, behavioral, and cognitive perspectives.
4. Discuss the concepts of stress, anxiety, adaptation and homeostasis, and depression.
5. Identify some basic coping strategies (defense mechanisms).
6. Differentiate between conflict and motivation.
7. Discuss how age and cultural and spiritual beliefs affect an individual's ability to cope with illness.
8. Discuss the concepts of anxiety, fear, stress, loss, grief, hopelessness, and powerlessness in relation to illness.
9. Describe several factors that may precipitate adaptive or maladaptive coping behaviors in response to illness.
10. Discuss implementation of the nursing process to enhance a patient's mental health as the patient deals with the stresses of illness.

LEARNING ACTIVITIES

I. Match the definition on the left with the most appropriate term on the right.

_____ 1. A model used to demonstrate the range of mental health on a line between health at one end and illness at the opposite extreme

_____ 2. A condition of lack of hope, which may hinder action

_____ 3. Attempts to cope using strategies that ultimately do not return the individual to homeostasis

_____ 4. A vague sense of impending doom or apprehension that appears to have no clearly identifiable cause

_____ 5. The point on the health continuum at which the individual moves toward illness and disequilibrium occurs

A. Crisis
B. Maladaptive
C. Coping strategy
D. Depression
E. Stressor
F. Conflict
G. Stress
H. Mental health continuum
I. Feelings
J. Anxiety
K. Adaptation
L. Self-esteem
M. Hopelessness
N. Eustress
O. Defense mechanism

I. *Continues*

I. *Continued*

_____ 6. Psychological struggle that results when two incompatible possibilities occur at the same time

_____ 7. The organism's attempt to return to homeostasis

_____ 8. A conscious or unconscious mechanism used to relieve or diminish anxiety

_____ 9. Any physiologic or psychological tension that threatens a person's equilibrium

_____ 10. A mood of sadness; a withdrawal from usual commitments

_____ 11. Stress that is perceived as helpful (e.g., graduation, vacation)

_____ 12. An adaptive or maladaptive mental attitude, behavior, or both that is consciously or unconsciously perceived as helping to reduce stress, anxiety, or fear

_____ 13. The perception of self as having a sense of worth

_____ 14. All emotional and physical responses and sensations

_____ 15. A factor that causes stress

A. Crisis
B. Maladaptive
C. Coping strategy
D. Depression
E. Stressor
F. Conflict
G. Stress
H. Mental health continuum
I. Feelings
J. Anxiety
K. Adaptation
L. Self-esteem
M. Hopelessness
N. Eustress
O. Defense mechanism

II. Match the definition on the left with the most appropriate term on the right.

_____ 1. Physical, cognitive, and psychological development that is predictable and sequential

_____ 2. A tendency toward equilibrium or a steady state

_____ 3. A feeling that one's actions do not affect an outcome or that one lacks personal control over certain events or situations

_____ 4. Persons, items, or organizations that can be drawn on for a sense of support (e.g., family, money, skills, beliefs)

_____ 5. Analogous to anxiety; however, is related to dread of a specific or real occurrence

_____ 6. Actions that occur intentionally or spontaneously and are observable and measurable

_____ 7. The individual's physical and psychological experiences that influence how the body is perceived

_____ 8. The idea that an object or person will continue to exist when no longer in sight.

A. Fear
B. Compulsion
C. Instinct
D. Illusion
E. Homeostasis
F. Behavior
G. Cognition
H. Ego
I. Powerlessness
J. Body image
K. Object permanence
L. Resources
M. Loss
N. Growth and development
O. Libido

_____ 9. The inborn source of bodily need or impulse

_____ 10. Psychic energy used to operate the id, ego, and superego in psychoanalytic theory

_____ 11. The workings of the mind; language, memory, intellect, and reasoning

_____ 12. Act carried out, to some degree against a person's conscious will, to avoid anxiety

_____ 13. The removal of a highly valued person, object, or situation

_____ 14. False perception or belief

_____ 15. In psychoanalytic theory, the "rational self" or "reality" principle of personality; mediates between the id and the superego

A. Fear
B. Compulsion
C. Instinct
D. Illusion
E. Homeostasis
F. Behavior
G. Cognition
H. Ego
I. Powerlessness
J. Body image
K. Object permanence
L. Resources
M. Loss
N. Growth and development
O. Libido

III. Match the definition on the left with the most appropriate term on the right.

_____ 1. A sense of comfort and satisfaction derived from the fulfillment of one's needs

_____ 2. An emotional response to a perceived loss of someone or something of value

_____ 3. In psychoanalytic theory, occurs during the phallic stage when the child unconsciously desires the parent of the opposite sex; conflict is resolved when the child identifies with the parent of the same sex

_____ 4. A group of people with whom the individual identifies and derives a sense of belonging

_____ 5. The belief that one is at the center of the universe

_____ 6. Resources that are used to cope with stress

_____ 7. Personal standards for decision making

_____ 8. Inner drive that leads an individual to complete a task or meet a goal

_____ 9. Expected function or behaviors; one may have more than one (e.g., mother, daughter, teacher, wife)

_____ 10. One's mental image or picture of oneself

_____ 11. In psychoanalytic theory the "pleasure principle" of the personality

_____ 12. Stress that is perceived as harmful (e.g., death, loss of a job)

_____ 13. Deeply ingrained patterns of behavior that include the way one relates to, perceives, and thinks about the environment and self

_____ 14. Feeling that arises when there is interference with goal-directed activity

_____ 15. False belief that is held as true despite evidence to the contrary

A. Value system
B. Distress
C. Oedipus complex
D. Frustration
E. Delusion
F. Support system
G. Peer group
H. Self-concept
I. Gratification
J. Personality
K. Motivation
L. Egocentric
M. Id
N. Grief
O. Role

IV.   Complete the statements on the left with the most appropriate term on the right. Some terms may not be used.

____ 1.   The individual level of health is directly related to one's ability to adjust to a variety of internal and external _____.

____ 2.   The first priority of human needs according to Maslow is _____.

____ 3.   Mental health and illness is viewed as a _____.

____ 4.   The type of stress involved in graduating from an educational program is called _____.

____ 5.   The loss of a job is an example of the type of stress called _____.

____ 6.   Mental health can be facilitated by mild _____.

____ 7.   Stress, response, and adaptation can be thought of as an individual's attempt to maintain _____.

____ 8.   A condition that results in inner tension and anxiety that may affect an individual's ability to function is _____.

____ 9.   Deeply ingrained patterns of behavior which include the way people relate, perceive, and think about the environment and themselves are called _____.

A.   Distress

B.   Illness

C.   Life, safety, and security

D.   Crisis

E.   Stress

F.   Self-actualization

G.   Eustress

H.   Personality

I.   Stressors

J.   Homeostasis

K.   Continuum

V.   Complete the statements on the left with the most appropriate term on the right. Some terms may be used more than once.

____ 1.   When a person finds a suspicious lump in her breast and does not keep appointments for a breast biopsy, this action could be called _____.

____ 2.   When anxiety intensifies to an excessive level, perception of reality becomes solely focused on the _____.

____ 3.   When a student fails to complete an assignment correctly and complains about the objectives for the assignment, this action is _____.

____ 4.   Transferring feelings associated with one person or event to another that is considered less threatening is _____.

A.   Introjection

B.   Rationalization or intellectualization

C.   Anxiety

D.   Compensation

E.   Denial

F.   Identification

G.   Isolation

H.   Crisis

I.   Displacement

___ 5. An attempt to make up for real or imagined weakness is _____.

___ 6. The use of logic, reasoning, and analysis to avoid unacceptable feelings is _____.

___ 7. A painful emotion that results from one's perception of danger is _____.

___ 8. Internalizing or taking on the values and beliefs of another person is _____.

___ 9. A boy who is angry with a teacher and comes home and yells at his dog is an example of _____.

___ 10. When a man appears apathetic as he discusses a fire fight in which he participated in Vietnam, it is an example of _____.

___ 11. When a child dresses and uses mannerisms similar to those of a movie star, this action is called _____.

___ 12. Refusal to acknowledge a real situation is _____.

___ 13. When an adolescent perceived as unattractive becomes an outstanding athlete, this action could be called _____.

___ 14. When a child takes on the values and beliefs of a parent, it is called _____.

___ 15. Emulation of admirable qualities in another to enhance one's self esteem is _____.

___ 16. The separation of emotion from an associated thought or memory is _____.

A. Introjection

B. Rationalization or intellectualization

C. Anxiety

D. Compensation

E. Denial

F. Identification

G. Isolation

H. Crisis

I. Displacement

VI. Complete the statements on the left with the most appropriate term on the right. Some terms may be used more than once.

___ 1. The transformation of unacceptable impulses or drives into constructive or more acceptable behavior is _____.

___ 2. Actually or symbolically attempting to cancel out an action that was unacceptable is _____.

___ 3. When an individual who witnesses a murder and then experiences sudden blindness without an organic cause, it is called _____.

___ 4. When a patient who unconsciously hates his father continuously tells the nurses how great his father is, it is an example of _____.

___ 5. Unacceptable feelings or impulses are transferred to another in _____.

A. Substitution

B. Projection

C. Sublimation

D. Repression

E. Conversion

F. Regression

G. Reaction formation

H. Undoing

I. Suppression

VI.   *Continues*

Introductory Nursing Care of Adults

VI. *Continues*

___ 6. _____ is a conscious or voluntary inhibition of unacceptable ideas, impulses, and memories.

___ 7. Sprinkling salt over one's left shoulder to prevent bad luck after spilling salt on the table is an example of _____.

___ 8. When the person who has a strong unconscious sexual attraction to a parent marries someone who resembles that parent, it is called _____.

___ 9. When a child starts sucking her thumb when her new baby brother comes home from the hospital, it is an example of _____.

___ 10. When a child who fails an algebra class forgets to show his report card to his parents, this action is called _____.

___ 11. An emotional conflict is turned into a physical symptom, which provides the individual with some sort of benefit (secondary gain), in _____.

___ 12. Avoidance of unacceptable thoughts and behaviors by expressing opposing thoughts or behaviors is _____.

___ 13. When a wife who is jealous of her husband accuses him of jealousy, this is called _____.

___ 14. An unconscious defense mechanism in which unacceptable ideas, impulses, and memories are kept out of consciousness is _____.

___ 15. In _____, an individual replaces a highly valued, unattainable object with a less valued, attainable object.

___ 16. _____ is withdrawing to an earlier level of development to benefit from the associated comfort levels.

___ 17. When a woman cannot remember a sexual assault, it is an example of _____.

___ 18. When a person who has aggressive tendencies becomes a football star, it is an example of _____.

A. Substitution

B. Projection

C. Sublimation

D. Repression

E. Conversion

F. Regression

G. Reaction formation

H. Undoing

I. Suppression

VII. Match the description on the left with the most appropriate dimension of self on the right. Some terms may be used more than once.

_____ 1. Depressed individual is unable to develop a repertoire of successful coping behaviors

_____ 2. An individual is genetically predisposed to depression

_____ 3. An individual grows up in a family and within a culture in which exercise and diet are valued

_____ 4. Individual does not believe he has the ability to cope, and depression results

_____ 5. A person is predisposed to diabetes mellitus

_____ 6. Depressed individual grows up in a family in which maladaptive coping or poor problem-solving practices are practiced

_____ 7. Successful coping abilities have been acquired

_____ 8. An individual's perception of a stressful event related to religion

A. Community-society

B. Body-physiology

C. Soul-spirituality

D. Mind-emotion

VIII. Match the description on the left with the most appropriate component of personality in Freud's theory on the right. Some components may be used more than once, and some may not be used.

_____ 1. The component that functions to inhibit impulses of the id

_____ 2. The component that may be called the rational self or the reality principle

_____ 3. Develops as the baby experiences some degree of frustration and discomfort

_____ 4. The component that decides what instincts will be satisfied and how

_____ 5. The subjective reality of this component is the pursuit of pleasure and the relief or avoidance of pain

_____ 6. The moral or judicial branch of personality

A. Oral

B. Ego

C. Phallic

D. Superego

E. Anal

F. Id

G. Genital

IX. Match the description on the left with the most appropriate psychosexual stage of development on the right. Some stages may be used more than once, and some may not be used.

____ 1. The libidinal drive increases in this stage

____ 2. The goal of this stage is identification of sexual differences in genders

____ 3. The goal is to have immediate gratification (sense of comfort and satisfaction of needs)

____ 4. Relationships evolve in this stage

____ 5. The child gains sphincter control over elimination

____ 6. Infants do not see themselves as being separate from the mother at this stage

____ 7. Sexuality is dormant at this stage

____ 8. The goal at this stage is control and independence

____ 9. The Oedipus complex occurs in this stage when the child unconsciously desires the parent of the opposite sex

____ 10. The goal of this stage is learning and socialization

____ 11. The child develops a sense of trust in this stage

A. Latency

B. Ego

C. Genital

D. Oral

E. Superego

F. Anal

G. Phallic

X. Match the description on the left with the most appropriate stage in Erickson's theory of psychosocial development on the right. Some stages may be used more than once, and some may not be used.

____ 1. Heterosexual relationships develop

____ 2. The child learns about the culture's rules and regulations

____ 3. A sense of self-control and ability to delay gratification develops

____ 4. Basic trust must be developed

____ 5. A sense of self-confidence develops from intellectual experience

____ 6. The task is to review one's life and find meaning from life's events

____ 7. An intimate relationship may develop that includes a lasting relationship

A. Ego integrity vs. despair

B. Infancy vs. childhood

C. Autonomy vs. shame and doubt

D. Industry vs. inferiority

E. Distress vs. eustress

F. Identity vs. role confusion

G. Generativity vs. stagnation

H. Trust vs. mistrust

I. Intimacy vs. isolation

J. Initiative vs. guilt

___ 8. Parents can promote self-confidence by allowing independent activities balanced with structure and limits

___ 9. Basic needs must be met to establish trust

___ 10. Career choices are made

___ 11. The individual strives to achieve life goals

___ 12. The individual learns to view self as unique

___ 13. The child can initiate activities and take part in cooperative play

___ 14. During this stage, the child seeks independence

___ 15. The development of the superego or conscience occurs

A. Ego integrity vs. despair

B. Infancy vs. childhood

C. Autonomy vs. shame and doubt

D. Industry vs. inferiority

E. Distress vs. eustress

F. Identity vs. role confusion

G. Generativity vs. stagnation

H. Trust vs. mistrust

I. Intimacy vs. isolation

J. Initiative vs. guilt

XI. Match the description on the left with the most appropriate stage of Sullivan's theory of interpersonal interaction on the right. Some stages may be used more than once.

___ 1. A sense of identity develops

___ 2. There is a need for contact

___ 3. There is a need for heterosexual relationships

___ 4. There is a need for peers and acceptance

___ 5. Anxiety is tolerated as the child learns to delay gratification

___ 6. There is a need for intimacy

___ 7. There is a need for friendship and love

___ 8. Oral gratification relieves anxiety

___ 9. Peer relationships occur

___ 10. Intimacy and relationships that are lasting develop

___ 11. Same-sex relationships occur

___ 12. Relationships with person of the opposite sex begin

___ 13. There is a need to participate in activities with adults

___ 14. Self-identity is established

A. Juvenile

B. Preadolescence

C. Late adolescence

D. Infancy

E. Childhood

F. Early adolescence

XII. Match the description on the left with the most appropriate stage in Piaget's theory of cognitive development on the right.

____ 1. Children learn to think and reason in abstract terms

____ 2. Children develop an understanding of symbolic gestures, including language

____ 3. Children learn to apply logic

____ 4. Cognitive maturity is achieved

____ 5. Concepts such as reversibility and spatiality are developed

____ 6. Object permanence begins as soon as children are able to form a mental image

____ 7. Children are egocentric

____ 8. Infants develop a sense of self

A. Sensorimotor (birth–2 years)

B. Concrete operations (6–12 years)

C. Preoperational (2–6 years)

D. Formal operations (12–15 years and older)

XIII. Match the description on the left with the most appropriate stage in Kohlberg's theory of moral development on the right. Some stages may be used more than once.

____ 1. External control gradually fades as children mimic what they perceive as the right thing to do based on the approval of others

____ 2. Rigid adherence to laws becomes more flexible and takes into consideration individual circumstances

____ 3. Children conform to those who are in authority

____ 4. Limits are set externally

____ 5. Morality is defined individually

A. Level one

B. Level two

C. Level three

XIV. Match the fear on the left with the most appropriate age group on the right.

____ 1. Fear threats to their body image

____ 2. Fear of death and dying

____ 3. Fear of separation from their mothers

A. Terminally ill patients

B. Toddler patients

C. Adolescent patients

XV. Match the description or example on the left with the type of loss on the right. Some losses may be used more than once.

___ 1. Loss of a mother

___ 2. A loss recognized by others as well as by patients

___ 3. Impending loss of a spouse in the terminal stages of an illness

___ 4. Loss of a limb

___ 5. A sense of loss that the patient may feel before the real loss occurs

A. Anticipatory loss

B. Actual loss

XVI. Match the descriptions on the left with coping strategies on the right. Some strategies may be used more than once, and some may not be used.

___ 1. Interventions including imagery, therapeutic touch, and music therapy

___ 2. The use of imagination to develop sensory pictures that focus away from the stressful experience and emphasize other sensory experiences and pleasant memories

___ 3. Use of earphones with audio cassettes

___ 4. Discussion with clients or beliefs about a higher power

___ 5. Biofeedback, meditation, yoga, and Zen practices

___ 6. A process by which the therapist acts as a channel for environmental and universal energy through the therapist's mental concentration

A. Therapeutic touch

B. Relaxation techniques

C. Spiritual dimension

D. Music therapy

E. Art therapy

F. Role playing

G. Imagery

XVII. Fill in the blanks.

1. Helplessness leads to feelings of anxiety or despair, cognitive impairment, and loss of _____

_____.

2. The expression of anger by patients may be an attempt to cope with feelings of loss of

_____.

XVIII. List 4 holistic dimensions of self in which mental and physical health are encompassed and in which stressors can originate.

1.

2.

3.

4.

XIX. List 3 examples of resources an individual has that will affect the response to crisis.

1.

2.

3.

XX. List 12 characteristics of healthy individuals, according to Maslow.

1.   7.

2.   8.

3.   9.

4.   10.

5.   11.

6.   12.

XXI. List 12 factors that can affect an individual's ability to cope.

1.   7.

2.   8.

3.   9.

4.   10.

5.   11.

6.   12.

XXII. List 4 ways culture can affect attitudes.

1.

2.

3.

4.

XXIII. List 3 characteristics of spiritual distress.

1.

2.

3.

XXIV. Individuals who are not able to cope with stress adequately may experience a threat to their emotional well-being. List how persons who are not able to cope with stress adequately are affected related to the following areas.

1. Perceptions of reality:

2. Ability to solve problems:

3. Amount of stress:

XXV. The person experiencing the crisis of illness has much to fear; list 5 fears related to illness.

1.

2.

3.

4.

5.

XXVI. An individual struggling with the crisis of a severe illness experiences the loss of many things; list 4 areas of loss related to illness.

1.

2.

3.

4.

XXVII. List a nursing intervention that can help prevent helplessness.

XXVIII. List 4 characteristics of powerlessness.

1.

2.

3.

4.

XXIX. List 4 forms of behavior related to coping with illness that may be characteristic of denial.

1.

2.

3.

4.

XXX.   List 9 areas of assessment that help determine the effectiveness of individual coping strategies.

1.

2.

3.

4.

5.

6.

7.

8.

9.

XXXI.   List 8 behaviors that may indicate ineffective individual coping.

1.

2.

3.

4.

5.

6.

7.

8.

XXXII.   Choose the most appropriate answer.

1. Defense mechanisms are adapted by the individual as protective measures to allow the ego relief from:
   A. rationalization
   B. denial
   C. anxiety
   D. repression

2. A factor that is basic to helping the patient cope with illness is the nurse's:
   A. caring attitude
   B. educational background
   C. professionalism
   D. organization

3. Effective nursing interventions can be made only after patients have been assessed as:
   A. members of a particular culture
   B. members of a particular sex
   C. members of a certain race
   D. unique individuals

4. A group's affiliation because of a shared language, race, and values is:
   A. culture
   B. behavior
   C. morality
   D. ethnicity

5. People subjected to prolonged stressors eventually become:
   A. defensive
   B. exhausted
   C. cognitive
   D. emotional

6. An *early* response to illness is often:
   A. grief
   B. depression
   C. anxiety
   D. loss

7. When a person with a severe illness is forced to relinquish original hopes, and then reappraise values and accept substitutes for hope, this process is called:
   A. mourning
   B. grief
   C. anxiety
   D. fear

8. The experience of loss is related to the individual's:
   A. self-concept
   B. sense of belonging
   C. anxiety
   D. depression

9. Any changes in a person's life create:
   A. fear
   B. anxiety
   C. stress
   D. mourning

10. Unconscious coping mechanisms are referred to as:
    A. stressors
    B. defense mechanisms
    C. self-concept
    D. illusions

11. Passivity and verbal expression of loss of control over situations are characteristics of:
    A. gratification
    B. denial
    C. intellectualization
    D. powerlessness

12. Denial of obvious problems and weaknesses is related to the nursing diagnosis of:
    A. ineffective individual coping
    B. activity intolerance
    C. altered growth and development
    D. knowledge deficit

Psychiatric Disorders

OBJECTIVES

1. Describe the differences between social relationships and therapeutic relationships.
2. Describe key strategies in communicating therapeutically.
3. Describe the categories of the mental status examination.
4. Identify target symptoms and behaviors and side effects for the following types of medications: antianxiety, antipsychotic, and antidepressant drugs.
5. Summarize current thinking about the etiology of schizophrenia and the mood disorders.
6. For each of the following psychiatric disorders, identify key observations in relation to the categories of the mental status examination: anxiety disorders, schizophrenia, mood disorders, organic mental syndromes or disorders, and personality disorders.
7. For each of the following psychiatric disorders, identify primary nursing diagnoses, goals, and interventions: anxiety disorders, schizophrenia, mood disorders, organic mental syndromes or disorders, and personality disorders.

LEARNING ACTIVITIES

I.   Match the definition on the left with the most appropriate term on the right.

____ 1. Frequently irreversible side effect of antipsychotic medication that develops after years of use; symptoms include involuntary movements of face, jaw, and tongue, leading to grimacing, jerky movements of upper extremities, and tonic contractions of neck and back

____ 2. A state in which a person's perception of reality is impaired, thereby interfering with the capacity to function and to relate to others

____ 3. Assumes that mental disorders are related to physiologic changes within the central nervous system

____ 4. Level of consciousness and orientation to time, place, person, and self

____ 5. Based on the theory that people function at different levels of awareness (conscious to unconscious) and that ego defense mechanisms such as denial and repression are used to prevent anxiety

A.   Sensorium

B.   Depersonalization

C.   Projection

D.   Psychosis

E.   Syndrome

F.   Psychoanalytic approach

G.   Disorder

H.   Tardive dyskinesia

I.   Extrapyramidal effects

J.   Interpersonal approach

K.   Biologic approach

L.   Denial

I.   *Continues*

I. *Continued*

___ 6. A defense mechanism in which particular feelings or specific aspects of reality are excluded from awareness

___ 7. A defense mechanism in which one sees others as a source of one's own unacceptable thoughts, feelings, or impulses

___ 8. Side effects of anti-psychotic drugs on the portion of the central nervous system controlling involuntary movements

___ 9. Refers to behaviors and symptoms

___ 10. A state of feeling outside of oneself, watching what is happening as if it were to someone else

___ 11. The patient learns new ways to behave in a therapeutic relationship built on trust

___ 12. A term used when a definite organic cause such as delirium or dementia is established for behaviors and symptoms

A. Sensorium

B. Depersonalization

C. Projection

D. Psychosis

E. Syndrome

F. Psychoanalytic approach

G. Disorder

H. Tardive dyskinesia

I. Extrapyramidal effects

J. Interpersonal approach

K. Biologic approach

L. Denial

II. Match the definition on the left with the most appropriate term on the right.

___ 1. Uses behavior modification (positive and negative reinforcement) and recognizes that particular thoughts influence emotional states

___ 2. Observations and descriptions regarding appearance, mood, and affect, speech and language, thought content, perceptual disturbances, insight and judgment, sensorium, and memory and attention

___ 3. Involve deficits in orientation, memory, language comprehension, and judgment

___ 4. Class of antidepressant drugs; patients taking these drugs must be carefully monitored to avoid life-threatening food and drug interactions

___ 5. Briefly occurring feelings such as happiness, sadness or worry; when inappropriate, there is incongruence between the feeling appropriate to the situation and the way the feeling is expressed

___ 6. A very serious group of usually chronic thought disorders in which patients' ability to interpret the world around them is severely impaired

___ 7. A mental disorder that involves a change in identity, memory, or consciousness that enables persons to remove themselves from anxiety-provoking situations

___ 8. Periods of elevated mood (manic episodes) and depression

A. Dissociative disorder

B. Dementia

C. Organic mental disorder

D. Borderline personality disorder

E. Parkinsonian syndrome

F. Monoamine oxidase inhibitor

G. Electroconvulsive therapy

H. Bipolar depression

I. Mood

J. Mental status examination

K. Panic disorder

L. Affect

M. Cognitive behavioral approach

N. Agoraphobia

O. Schizophrenia

____ 9. Fear of situations outside the home

____ 10. Possible side effect after years of antipsychotic drug therapy; patient exhibits mask-like face, shuffling gait, resting tremor, and rigid posture

____ 11. A mental state that is characterized by cognitive and intellectual deficits severe enough to impair social or occupational functioning (memory, abstract thinking, and judgment)

____ 12. Patient experiences intense episodes of apprehension to the point of terror

____ 13. Person exhibits unstable relationships, unstable self-image and unstable mood

____ 14. Feeling state experienced by the patient over a period of time

____ 15. Controversial therapy that used electrical current to the brain to evoke a grand mal seizure

A. Dissociative disorder
B. Dementia
C. Organic mental disorder
D. Borderline personality disorder
E. Parkinsonian syndrome
F. Monoamine oxidase inhibitor
G. Electroconvulsive therapy
H. Bipolar depression
I. Mood
J. Mental status examination
K. Panic disorder
L. Affect
M. Cognitive behavioral approach
N. Agoraphobia
O. Schizophrenia

III. Match the definition on the left with the most appropriate term on the right.

____ 1. Person exhibits two or more distinct personalities

____ 2. Effect of medication that can develop after one dose or after years of drug therapy; the first symptom usually is muscular rigidity accompanied by akinesia and respiratory distress; the cardinal sign is hyperthermia (body temperature 101 to 103°F or higher)

____ 3. Incessant behaviors such as hand washing that interfere with normal functioning

____ 4. Loss of body function (e.g., paralysis) without physiologic cause

____ 5. A disorder that is characterized by vague, multiple, recurring physical complaints that are not caused by real physical illness

____ 6. Pervasive, chronic, and maladaptive personality characteristics that interfere with normal functioning

____ 7. A psychological disorder experienced following a traumatic event that is characterized by flashbacks, detachment, and sleep and eating difficulties

____ 8. A reversible condition of restlessness manifested as an urge to pace

____ 9. Emotional unresponsiveness and blunted affect

A. Posttraumatic stress disorder
B. Unipolar depression
C. Multiple personality disorder
D. Hypochondriasis
E. Obsessions
F. Anxiety
G. Akinesia
H. Neuroleptic malignant syndrome
I. Somatoform disorder
J. Personality disorders
K. Compulsions
L. Akathisia
M. Obsessive–compulsive disorder
N. Conversion disorder

III. *Continues*

III.   *Continued*

___ 10.   Recurrent intrusive thoughts that interfere with normal functioning

___ 11.   Recurrent obsessions or compulsions or both that produce distress and interfere with daily functioning

___ 12.   Belief that a serious medical condition exists when medical findings are absent

___ 13.   Depressed mood

___ 14.   State of being uneasy, apprehensive, or nervous in response to a vague, nonspecific threat

A.   Posttraumatic stress disorder
B.   Unipolar depression
C.   Multiple personality disorder
D.   Hypochondriasis
E.   Obsessions
F.   Anxiety
G.   Akinesia
H.   Neuroleptic malignant syndrome
I.   Somatoform disorder
J.   Personality disorders
K.   Compulsions
L.   Akathisia
M.   Obsessive–compulsive disorder
N.   Conversion disorder

IV.   Complete the statement on the left with the most appropriate term on the right. Some terms may not be used.

___ 1.   A frequently utilized mechanism by patients with borderline personality disorder that is caused by problems with separation-individuation is called _____.

___ 2.   Asking the patient to interpret proverbs, such as asking "What does 'a rolling stone gathers no moss' mean?", is a way to assess _____.

___ 3.   The four levels of consciousness are alert, drowsy, stuporous, and _____.

___ 4.   When a spot on the wall is perceived as a bug, this is called _____.

___ 5.   Asking a patient to spell the word *world* backwards is a way to measure _____.

___ 6.   Paranoid, schizoid, antisocial, borderline, avoidant, obsessive-compulsive, and passive-aggressive are examples of _____.

___ 7.   Important factors in relation to suicide potential are insight and _____.

___ 8.   Asking the patient "What day is today?" is a way to assess _____.

___ 9.   The person with borderline personality disorder has patterns involving unstable relationships, unstable self–image, and unstable _____.

A.   Illusion
B.   Multiple personality disorder(s)
C.   Sensorium
D.   Comatose
E.   Recent memory
F.   Personality disorder(s)
G.   Insight
H.   Hallucination
I.   Splitting
J.   Mood
K.   Attention
L.   Remote memory
M.   Judgment
N.   Abstract thinking
O.   Phobia(s)
P.   Judgment

____ 10. Asking a patient what was eaten at the previous meal is one way to measure _____.

____ 11. The soundness of proposed actions in relation to one's particular background is _____.

____ 12. When a person sees nonexistent bugs crawling on the floor or feels nonexistent bugs crawling on the skin, this is called _____.

____ 13. A clear understanding of the significance of one's own symptoms and behavior is _____.

A. Illusion

B. Multiple personality disorder(s)

C. Sensorium

D. Comatose

E. Recent memory

F. Personality disorder(s)

G. Insight

H. Hallucination

I. Splitting

J. Mood

K. Attention

L. Remote memory

M. Judgment

N. Abstract thinking

O. Phobia(s)

P. Judgment

V. Complete the statements on the left with the most appropriate term on the right.

____ 1. A flat or very inappropriate affect is a symptom of _____.

____ 2. Laryngospasm, torticollis, and severe muscle contractions of the tongue following administration of antipsychotics are examples of _____.

____ 3. During acute episodes of schizophrenia, the treatment for patients usually includes psychiatric hospitalization and _____.

____ 4. A frequently irreversible syndrome that may occur after years of antipsychotic drug therapy and that consists of involuntary movements of the face, jaw, and tongue is called _____.

____ 5. A mask-like face, rigid posture, shuffling gait, and resting tremor following administration of antipsychotics are examples of _____.

____ 6. Medications that are administered to prevent or relieve some of the side effects of the antipsychotic are _____.

____ 7. Drugs that are sometimes ordered in conjunction with the antipsychotics to decrease agitation are _____.

____ 8. People with schizophrenia have symptoms that are _____.

____ 9. A later extrapyramidal syndrome that includes a reversible restlessness manifested as having an urge to pace and having difficulty sitting still is called _____.

A. Tardive dyskinesia

B. Akathisia

C. Antianxiety medications

D. Extrapyramidal effects.

E. Parkinsonian syndrome

F. Akinesia

G. Schizophrenia

H. Antipsychotics

I. Antiparkinsonian medications

J. Psychotic

Introductory Nursing Care of Adults

VI. Match the description on the left with the most appropriate theoretical approach on the right. Some approaches may be used more than once, and some may not be used.

____ 1. Anxiety is often communicated interpersonally.

____ 2. Particular thoughts influence emotional states.

____ 3. Mental disorders are related to particular physiologic changes within the central nervous system.

____ 4. Behavior increases in response to positive consequences (positive reinforcement) .

____ 5. The patient learns new ways of coping or maturing in a therapeutic relationship.

____ 6. People use ego defense mechanisms to prevent anxiety.

____ 7. Behavior is learned.

____ 8. Humans function at different levels of awareness, ranging from conscious to unconscious.

____ 9. The establishment of trust is an important first step in the nurse's work with patients.

____ 10. Behavior increases in response to the removal of negative stimuli (negative reinforcement).

A. Biologic

B. Emotional

C. Psychoanalytic

D. Interpersonal

E. Social

F. Cognitive behavioral

VII. Match the description on the left with (A) therapeutic or (B) social relationship.

____ 1. May or may not be clear boundaries and a clear ending

____ 2. Focus on personal and emotional needs of patient

____ 3. Purpose is to benefit both participants in the relationship

____ 4. Participants are not formally responsible for evaluating their interaction

____ 5. Helper has responsibility for evaluating the interaction and the changing behavior

____ 6. Relationship has some boundaries (purpose, place, time) and clear ending

____ 7. Relationship develops spontaneously

____ 8. Purpose is to benefit the patient

____ 9. Focus on personal and emotional needs of both participants

____ 10. Relationship develops purposefully

A. Therapeutic relationship

B. Social relationship

Introductory Nursing Care of Adults
Copyright © 1995 by W.B. Saunders Company. All rights reserved.

VIII. Match the description on the left with the most appropriate interpersonal strategies on the right.

____ 1. Experiencing the patient and refraining from thinking of responses to the patient when the patient is speaking

____ 2. When with the patient, the nurse's attention should be directed completely to this other human being

____ 3. The nurse asks the patient, "What do you mean when you say 'the world is falling apart?'"

____ 4. This approach allows patients time to consider their own thought as well as the communication of the nurse

____ 5. Patients benefit from knowing what nurses see and hear while listening

____ 6. If nurses are aware of their own feelings, they will be able to control their own responses

____ 7. The nurse makes a statement that lets the patient know that verbal and nonverbal behaviors are not congruent

____ 8. The nurse says, "You are saying that your life is falling apart and you are also smiling."

____ 9. Asking questions of the patient

A. Sharing observations

B. Accepting silence

C. Listening

D. Clarifying

E. Being available

IX. Match the examples on the left with the most appropriate component of the mental status exam on the right.

____ 1. Mutism, paucity, pressured speech, tangential speech, blocking, loose associations, word salad

____ 2. Potential for suicide

____ 3. Happiness, sadness, worry: constricted or expanded feelings; intensity; lability; appropriateness

____ 4. Vocabulary; knowledge of current events; abstract thinking

____ 5. Orientation to time, place, person; level of consciousness

____ 6. Obsessions, compulsions, phobias, delusions

____ 7. Age, clothing, personal hygiene, unusual physical characteristics

____ 8. Remote and recent memory; attention; calculation

____ 9. Illusions, hallucinations

____ 10. Recent change in activity level, hyperactivity, agitation, psychomotor retardation, repetitive mannerisms, stereotypes

A. Perceptual disturbances

B. Sensorium

C. Activity

D. Memory and attention

E. Mood and affect

F. Insight and judgment

G. Thought content

H. General intellectual level

I. Appearance

J. Speech and language

Introductory Nursing Care of Adults
Copyright © 1995 by W.B. Saunders Company. All rights reserved.

X.   Match the description on the left with the most appropriate type of activity on the right. Some terms may be used more than once, and some may not be used.

____   1. A level of activity considerably above aver-age; goal–directed activity

____   2. Purposeless activity, such as wringing of the hands, pacing, picking at clothing, or foot tapping

____   3. Decrease in movement, thinking, and speaking

____   4. Repetitive movements that are part of a goal-directed activity

____   5. Repetitive movements that are not part of purposeful activity

A.   Psychomotor

B.   Compulsions

C.   Stereotypes

D.   Hyperactivity

E.   Mannerisms

F.   Agitation

XI.   Match the description on the left with the most appropriate term on the right.

____   1. A continual shifting from topic to unrelated topic

____   2. Minimal or very little speech

____   3. A patient starts out toward a particular point but veers away and never reaches the point

____   4. Stopping speaking before reaching the point

____   5. Loud and insistent speech

____   6. Shifting topics to the point of incoherence

____   7. Not speaking

A.   Tangential

B.   Word salad

C.   Pressured speech

D.   Paucity

E.   Loose associations

F.   Mutism

G.   Blocking

XII.   Match the description on the left with the most appropriate level of anxiety on the right.

____   1. An individual's ability to think clearly and to solve problems becomes impaired

____   2. A useful type of anxiety that may motivate a person to focus on a particular task

____   3. An individual may misperceive surround-ing events altogether and may react impul-sively by running or striking out

____   4. A useful type of anxiety that may motivate a person to take constructive action

____   5. Often considered the optimal level for learn-ing to take place

A.   Mild

B.   Moderate

C.   Severe

D.   Panic

XIII. Match the nursing interventions on the left with the appropriate nursing diagnosis for the patient with schizophrenia on the right.

___ 1. Encourage involvement in activities

___ 2. Focus on reality

___ 3. Make brief, frequent contacts with the patient to interrupt hallucinatory experiences

___ 4. Let patient know that the nurse does not share the delusion

___ 5. Connect delusions with anxiety-provoking situations

___ 6. Encourage the patient to pay attention to what is occurring in the environment (instead of external stimuli)

___ 7. Inform patients that hallucinations are part of the disease process

___ 8. Encourage the patient to express feelings and anxiety

A. Altered thought processes

B. Self-care deficit

C. Sensory perceptual alteration

D. Impaired verbal communication

XIV. Indicate which of the following are causes of (A) delirium and (B) dementia.

___ 1. Postoperative states

___ 2. Endocrine dysfunction

___ 3. Pick's disease

___ 4. Alzheimer's disease

___ 5. Thiamine deficiency

___ 6. Meningitis

___ 7. Parkinson's disease

___ 8. Liver abnormalities

___ 9. Drugs ranging from alcohol to steroids

___ 10. Multi-infarct type

___ 11. Neoplasms

A. Delirium

B. Dementia

XV. Nursing interventions for persons with psychiatric disorders are based on a number of different theoretic approaches; list 4 theories on which the interventions are based.

1.

2.

3.

4.

XVI. A range of interpersonal strategies have been found to be particularly helpful in promoting the patient's comfort level with the nurse; list 5 useful behaviors of the nurse.

1.

2.

3.

4.

5.

XVII. List 8 features assessed during the mental status examination.

1.

2.

3.

4.

5.

6.

7.

8.

XVIII. List 4 observations that should be made regarding appearance during a mental status examination.

1.

2.

3.

4.

XIX. List 5 activities that should be assessed in a mental status examination, in addition to noting any recent changes in the patient's activity level.

1.

2.

3.

4.

5.

XX. List 8 common physical signs and symptoms of anxiety.

1.	5.
2.	6.
3.	7.
4.	8.

XXI. List 5 common psychological manifestations of anxiety.

1.

2.

3.

4.

5.

XXII. List 4 examples of anxiety disorders.

1.

2.

3.

4.

XXIII. List 4 examples of symptoms of posttraumatic stress disorder.

1.

2.

3.

4.

XXIV. List 4 side effects of the antianxiety medications that are associated with sedation.

1.

2.

3.

4.

XXV. List 3 particularly relevant mental status examination categories for the nurse to assess.

1.

2.

3.

XXVI. List 5 nursing goals of patients with anxiety disorders.

1.

2.

3.

4.

5.

XXVII. In addition to counseling the patient, list 4 ways to prevent and manage increasing anxiety in patients.

1.

2.

3.

4.

XXVIII. List 5 typical symptoms of schizophrenia.

1.

2.

3.

4.

5.

XXIX. The schizophrenic patient's ability to function in areas of work, interpersonal relationships, or self-care decreases; list 3 areas that change or decline with each subsequent psychotic episode.

1.

2.

3.

XXX. The cause of schizophrenia is not certain; the stress-diathesis model emphasizes that people with schizophrenia probably were genetically vulnerable to the disorder. List 4 biologic factors that may be related to schizophrenia.

1.

2.

3.

4.

XXXI. List 5 symptoms of schizophrenia.

1.

2.

3.

4.

5.

XXXII. List 5 side effects of drug therapy (antipsychotic and antiparkinsonian medications) used for patients with schizophrenia.

1.

2.

3.

4.

5.

XXXIII. List the 4 most common nursing diagnoses for the patient with schizophrenia.

1.

2.

3.

4.

XXXIV. List 6 probable etiologic factors of mood disorders.

1.

2.

3.

4.

5.

6.

XXXV. List 3 types of antidepressant medications used for mood disorders.

1.

2.

3.

XXXVI. In completing the mental status examination of a patient who has depression, list 3 observations the nurse would probably make regarding speech and language.

1.

2.

3.

XXXVII. List 4 nursing diagnoses for patients with depression.

1.

2.

3.

4.

XXXVIII. In the areas below, list the observations a nurse would probably make when completing a mental health status examination on a patient with manic episodes.

1. Appearance:

2. Activity:

3. Moods, affect, and feelings:

4. Speech and language:

5. Thought content:

6. Sensory perception:

7. Insight and judgment:

XXXIX. List 3 essential features of a personality disorder.

1.

2.

3.

XL.   Choose the most appropriate answer.

1. Intense episodes of apprehension, at times to the point of terror, that are often accompanied by the feeling of impending doom are characteristic of:
   A. panic disorder
   B. obsessive-compulsive disorder
   C. somatoform disorder
   D. personality disorder

2. A type of anxiety disorder in which the individual is extremely fearful of situations outside the home from which escape may be difficult is:
   A. somatoform disorder
   B. borderline personality disorder
   C. agoraphobia
   D. hypochondriasis

3. Repeated checking to see whether the door is locked is an example of:
   A. obsessions
   B. hallucinations
   C. delusions
   D. compulsions

4. Many people with obsessive-compulsive disorders have become symptom free once therapeutic levels of which drug have been reached?
   A. analgesics
   B. antihistamines
   C. antidepressants
   D. anticonvulsants

5. Conversion disorders and hypochondriasis are examples of:
   A. mood disorders
   B. somatoform disorders
   C. panic disorders
   D. obsessive-compulsive disorders

6. Amnesia and multiple personality disorder are examples of:
   A. somatoform disorders
   B. dissociative disorders
   C. panic disorders
   D. posttraumatic stress disorders

7. A symptom of dissociative disorders is:
   A. depersonalization
   B. hypochondriasis
   C. agitation
   D. hypochondriasis

8. Most patients with multiple personality disorder report severe:
   A. agoraphobia
   B. hallucinations
   C. delusions
   D. childhood abuse

9. The primary antianxiety medications are the:
   A. benzodiazepines
   B. antihistamines
   C. thiazides
   D. salicylates

10. Withdrawal from antianxiety medications should be medically supervised because of the effect of:
    A. amnesia and confusion
    B. negative feedback
    C. hormones and histamines
    D. physical and psychological dependence

11. The two key nursing diagnoses for patients with anxiety disorders are anxiety and:
    A. body image disturbance
    B. powerlessness
    C. spiritual distress
    D. ineffective individual coping

12. One of the most common psychiatric disorders is:
    A. manic-depressive disorder
    B. unipolar depression
    C. posttraumatic stress disorder
    D. conversion disorder

13. As patients respond to antidepressant medications and the energy level increases, what risk increases?
    A. mutism
    B. panic
    C. suicide
    D. hypertension

14. Which of the following can patients taking MAO inhibitors include in their diet?
    A. avocados
    B. milk
    C. liver
    D. wine

15. A very serious side effect of MAO inhibitors, which may occur if foods containing tyramine are eaten, is:
    A. orthostatic hypotension
    B. tardive dyskinesia
    C. hypertensive crisis
    D. parkinsonism

16. An early sign of hypertensive crisis in patients with mood disorders who are taking MAO inhibitors is:
    A. headache
    B. oliguria
    C. cyanosis
    D. muscle weakness

17. A type of therapy that may be used for patients with severe depression when other forms of therapy have failed is:
    A. antidepressants
    B. electroconvulsive therapy
    C. psychotherapy
    D. isolation therapy

18. Possible side effects of electroconvulsive therapy are temporary memory loss and:
    A. orthostatic hypotension
    B. confusion
    C. tardive dyskinesia
    D. parkinsonian syndrome

19. A patient who exhibits psychomotor retardation, no spontaneous movements, a downcast gaze, and occasional agitated movements of hand wringing is exhibiting signs of:
    A. unipolar depression
    B. agoraphobia
    C. schizophrenia
    D. posttraumatic stress syndrome

20. Frequently assessing a patient's suicidal potential and maintaining continuous one-to-one contact if indicated are interventions for depressed patients who are at risk for:
    A. sleep pattern disturbance
    B. anxiety
    C. self-directed violence
    D. self-esteem disturbance

21. Learning to limit self-criticism and to give and receive compliments are interventions for the nursing diagnosis of:
    A. self-directed violence
    B. self-esteem disturbance
    C. anxiety
    D. dysfunctional grieving

22. Offering small snacks and warm baths and teaching relaxation exercises to be used before retiring are interventions for patients with:
    A. self-esteem disturbance
    B. self-directed violence
    C. hopelessness
    D. sleep pattern disturbance

23. The key medication for patients with manic episodes is:
    A. Xanax
    B. Prozac
    C. lithium
    D. Cogentin

24. The key problems for people with organic mental disorders stem from:
    A. speech and language impairments
    B. anxiety disorders
    C. conversion disorders
    D. cognitive impairments

CHAPTER

52

Substance Abuse

OBJECTIVES

1. Discuss the biologic, sociocultural, behavioral, and interpersonal theories of the etiology of substance abuse or dependency.
2. Describe the components of the nursing assessment of a patient with substance abuse or dependency.
3. Describe alcoholism, alcohol withdrawal syndrome, medical complications of alcoholism, and treatment of alcoholism.
4. Discuss the pathophysiologic effects of drugs frequently abused.
5. Describe disorders associated with substance abuse.
6. Differentiate between drug abuse treatment and alcohol abuse treatment.
7. Describe the nursing diagnoses and interventions associated with substance abuse and dependency.
8. Discuss populations who present special problems in relation to drug abuse and dependency.

LEARNING ACTIVITIES

I. Match the definition on the left with the most appropriate term on the right.

____ 1. Maladaptive pattern of substance use that differs from generally accepted cultural norms; sometimes referred to as chemical abuse or drug abuse.

____ 2. Self-help support process outlining 12 steps to overcoming a physical or psychological dependence on something outside oneself that has a destructive impact on one's life

____ 3. Intense cravings for the substance on which one is dependent without physical withdrawal symptoms

____ 4. Effect of habitual ingestion of a substance to the point of physical dependence; used interchangeably with the term dependence

____ 5. Physical need for the substance on which one is dependent in order to avoid unpleasant physical withdrawal symptoms

____ 6. Ingestion of substances in gradually increasing amounts due to a physical need; used interchangeably with the terms chemical dependence and drug dependence

A. Substance dependence

B. Substance abuse

C. Tolerance

D. Physical dependence

E. Dual diagnosis

F. Codependency

G. Psychological dependency

H. Withdrawal

I. 12-step program

J. Recovery

K. Addiction

I. *Continues*

Introductory Nursing Care of Adults
Copyright © 1995 by W.B. Saunders Company. All rights reserved.   581

I. *Continued*

___ 7. Unpleasant and sometimes life-threatening physical substance-specific syndrome occurring after stopping or reducing the habitual dose or frequency of an abused drug

___ 8. Simultaneous existence of a major psychiatric condition and a medical condition

___ 9. Lifelong process of maintaining abstinence from the substance to which one is addicted; a return to moderate substance use is never the end result

___ 10. Exaggerated dependent pattern of self-defeating behaviors, beliefs, and feelings learned as a result of pathologic relationship to a chemically dependent, or otherwise dysfunctional, person

___ 11. Need for increasing amounts of a substance to achieve the same effect brought about by the original amount

A. Substance dependence

B. Substance abuse

C. Tolerance

D. Physical dependence

E. Dual diagnosis

F. Codependence

G. Psychological dependence

H. Withdrawal

I. 12-step program

J. Recovery

K. Addiction

II. Complete the statements on the left with the most appropriate term on the right. Some terms may not be used.

___ 1. Individuals may turn to alcohol or other drugs to numb their _____ evoked by self-doubt and the daily stressors of reality.

___ 2. Probably the true causes of alcoholism involve a combination of biologic, cultural, behavioral, and _____ factors

___ 3. A theory which proposes that factors such as people in poverty, persons with strong religious values prohibiting the excessive use of drugs, and New Year's Eve customs affect substance abuse is called the _____.

___ 4. A learned maladaptive way of coping with stress and anxiety often results in _____.

___ 5. _____ addresses an individual's personality factors that may predispose the individual to substance abuse.

___ 6. Typical defense mechanisms used by the substance abuser include denial, rationalization, intellectualization, and _____

___ 7. _____ looks at the triggers for drinking and drug-using behaviors and how these patterns are reinforced.

___ 8. A predisposition for alcoholism from generation to generation is thought to occur based on a _____

A. Projection

B. Sociocultural theory

C. Children of alcoholics

D. Dopamine gene

E. Intrapersonal theory

F. Dependent

G. Cigarette smokers

H. Intrapersonal relationships

I. Behavioral theory

J. Education

K. Anxiety

L. Biologic theory

M. Substance abuse

N. Religious theory

O. Psychological

P. Physical illness

___ 9. The medical community considers drug dependence to be a _____ .

___ 10. During critical developmental stages of our lives, a factor that affects us profoundly is the quality of _____ .

___ 11. If children experience early childhood rejection, increased responsibility, unrealistic expectation, or overprotection, they may develop a personality described as _____ .

___ 12. The theory accepted by experts in addictionology that proposes that a faulty physiologic process contributes to dependence on a specific substance is the medical model, also known as the _____ .

___ 13. Children have been shown to be four times more likely to become alcoholic if they are _____ .

A. Projection
B. Sociocultural theory
C. Children of alcoholics
D. Dopamine gene
E. Intrapersonal theory
F. Dependent
G. Cigarette smokers
H. Intrapersonal relationships
I. Behavioral theory
J. Education
K. Anxiety
L. Biologic theory
M. Substance abuse
N. Religious theory
O. Psychological
P. Physical illness

III. Complete the statements on the left with the most appropriate term on the right. Some terms may be used more than once, and some terms may not be used.

___ 1. A recent addition to the methods for the detection of abused substances is _____ .

___ 2. A complication of chronic alcoholism that is due to thiamine and niacin deficiencies, which contribute to the degeneration of the cerebrum and the peripheral nervous system, is _____ .

___ 3. The preferred way of screening for the recent use of an unknown drug is _____ .

___ 4. _____ occurs when alcohol becomes integrated into physiologic processes at the cellular level.

___ 5. Legal intoxication in most states occurs when a person's blood alcohol level is ≥ _____ .

___ 6. _____ requires sensitive technology and can detect drugs for up to 1 year after use.

___ 7. Bugs, snakes, and rats are commonly described by patients with _____ .

___ 8. A critical sign of withdrawal in substance abusers is _____ .

___ 9. _____ is a medical complication that may cause low birth weight and heart defects in newborn babies.

___ 10. The detection of amphetamines, barbiturates, marijuana, narcotics, and benzodiazepines can be identified with _____ .

___ 11. The most accurate type of test available to measure the degree of intoxication on initiation of treatment for alcohol abuse is _____ .

A. Urine drug screening
B. Hypertension
C. 0.1%
D. Withdrawal
E. Hair analysis
F. Fetal alcohol syndrome
G. Hallucinations
H. Physical addiction
I. 0.05%
J. Korsakoff's psychosis
K. Blood alcohol
L. 1.0%

IV. Complete the statements on the left with the most appropriate term on the right. Some terms may not be used.

___ 1. To prevent the severe consequences of alcohol withdrawal, many patients are given _____.

___ 2. A complication of chronic alcoholism that is due to vitamin B$_1$ (thiamine) deficiency, which is characterized by symptoms including delirium, confabulation, and altered levels of consciousness, is _____.

___ 3. Alcohol withdrawal syndrome involves physiologic and behavioral symptoms that begin when there is a drop in _____.

___ 4. A structured meeting by family and friends to confront the alcoholic with the impact of that person's alcohol abuse on each member of the group is called _____.

___ 5. As elderly people who abuse alcohol age, their ability to tolerate the same quantities decreases and intoxication increases, putting them at risk for _____.

___ 6. The most life-threatening withdrawal syndrome is _____ withdrawal.

___ 7. Spouses of alcoholics frequently struggle with _____.

___ 8. Symptoms of anxiety, agitation, and irritability are related to _____.

___ 9. Common medical complications of chronic alcoholism include _____.

___ 10. Wernicke's encephalopathy and Korsakoff's psychosis are both classified as alcohol _____.

___ 11. The onset of seizures and hallucinations that can advance to life-threatening delirium tremens is classified as _____.

___ 12. The treatment for Wernicke's encephalopathy is _____.

A. Blood alcohol level

B. Early withdrawal

C. Detoxification

D. Wernicke's encephalopathy

E. Major withdrawal

F. Alcohol

G. Falls and injuries

H. Osteoporosis

I. Amnesic disorders

J. Diazepam (Valium)

K. Vitamin supplementation

L. Enabling behaviors

M. Intervention

N. Cirrhosis

V. Complete the statements on the left with the most appropriate term on the right. Some terms may be used more than once, and some terms may not be used.

____ 1. For some individuals, the primary means of recovery from alcoholism is attending 90 meetings in 90 days and active involvement in _____.

____ 2. One of the newer aspects of the recovery process involves the inclusion of programs designed to assist alcoholics who have completed treatment programs successfully to make a gradual transition back into the community; these are called _____ services.

____ 3. To assist the alcoholic who is highly motivated to remain sober but who recognizes poor impulse control, which may increase odds of relapse, _____ may be used.

____ 4. Drugs most often used in detoxification of the alcoholic are from the group of _____.

____ 5. The drug that is used to prevent seizures in detoxification of the alcoholic is intravenous _____.

____ 6. A self-help support group for alcoholics following detoxification is _____.

____ 7. The treatment for disulfiram-alcohol reactions is massive doses of intravenous _____.

____ 8. _____ inhibits the metabolism of alcohol in the body, producing an uncomfortable, potentially life-threatening reaction to exposure to alcohol.

____ 9. Flushing, headache, vomiting, difficulty breathing, and hypotension are symptoms of a reaction between disulfiram and _____.

____ 10. Members of Alcoholics Anonymous identify another participant of the same sex who is seasoned in the recovery process to act as their _____.

____ 11. It is important to teach patients to avoid alcohol in foods if they are taking _____.

____ 12. If the nurse uses alcohol wipes in preparing the skin for injections in patients taking disulfiram (Antabuse), the patient may develop a _____.

____ 13. A drug that is sometimes used to produce an uncomfortable reaction when combined with alcohol but that does not produce life-threatening reactions is _____.

A. Antianxiety drugs (benzodiazepines)

B. Rehabilitation

C. Vitamin C

D. Sponsor

E. Aftercare

F. Antipsychotic drugs

G. Magnesium sulfate

H. Topical reaction

I. Alcoholics Anonymous

J. Metronidazole (Flagyl)

K. Disulfiram (Antabuse)

L. Vitamin B$_1$

M. Alcohol

VI. Complete the statements on the left with the most appropriate term on the right. Some terms may be used more than once, and some terms may not be used.

___ 1. Oversedation, respiratory depression, impaired coordination, and brain damage are symptoms of overdose of _____.

___ 2. Amphetamines and cocaine are _____.

___ 3. Once a person is dependent on depressants, such as barbiturates, abruptly stopping any of these drugs may trigger _____.

___ 4. Runny nose, sniffles, weight loss, and hyperactivity are symptoms of chronic inhalation of _____.

___ 5. Overdose of _____ is life threatening because no drug is available to counteract the overstimulation, resulting in respiratory failure.

___ 6. Regular use of depressants results in _____.

___ 7. A drug that may cause strokes, seizures, and heart attacks even in first-time users is _____.

___ 8. There are no physical withdrawal symptoms following amphetamine use, but the user typically experiences a profound depression and sense of exhaustion called _____.

___ 9. Hyperactivity, irritability, combativeness, and paranoia are symptoms of use of _____.

___ 10. Depressants that are misused include the sedatives, hypnotics, and _____.

___ 11. _____ is a stimulant that is commonly misused among middle to upper socioeconomic classes owing to its status and expense, and that is typically inhaled nasally or mixed with other drugs.

___ 12. LSD, PCP, MDMA, and marijuana are examples of _____.

___ 13. A new form of methamphetamine ingested by smoking with effects that last as long as 14 hours is _____.

___ 14. A smokable form of cocaine is called _____.

A. Psychosis

B. "Ice"

C. Crack

D. Amphetamines

E. "Bad trip"

F. Stimulants

G. "Snow"

H. Physical dependence

I. Narcotics

J. Depressants

K. Anxiolytics

L. Cocaine

M. Hallucinogens

N. "Crashing"

VII. Complete the statements on the left with the appropriate term on the right. Some terms may be used more than once, and some terms may not be used.

___ 1. Synthetic drugs used to sidestep categorization with any of the drugs identified as illegal in the United States are called _____.

___ 2. A highly addictive narcotic that produces a pleasant euphoria on intravenous use is _____.

___ 3. The drug of choice for opioid detoxification is _____.

___ 4. A support group for narcotics abuse treatment is _____.

___ 5. The support group for family members or significant others of a substance-abusing person is _____.

___ 6. The most frequently used drug to detoxify patients addicted to heroin is _____.

___ 7. A synthetic form of heroin is called _____.

___ 8. A nonopiate antihypertensive drug that blocks withdrawal symptoms, _____ is a popular means of assisting the substance abuser through detoxification.

___ 9. Nosebleeds, bloodshot eyes, and severe disorientation are symptoms of persons using _____.

___ 10. The result of chronic use of inhalants among poor and minority adolescents is a very serious problem because inhalants may cause cumulative _____.

___ 11. Restlessness, irritability, upset stomach, diarrhea, joint pain, and muscle and joint pain are symptoms of withdrawal from _____.

___ 12. A narcotic antagonist that counteracts the dangerous respiratory effects of heroin or other opiate overdose is _____.

___ 13. An area of concern of intrauterine exposure to abused substances includes effects on the _____.

___ 14. A group of drugs often misused among teenagers owing to easy availability and low cost is _____.

___ 15. _____ presents the most current danger for patients who are abusing intravenous drugs as a result of the common practice of sharing needles.

___ 16. Overdose, malnutrition, and respiratory arrest are risks of chronic use of _____.

___ 17. Paint, glue, aerosol sprays, and gasoline are chemicals taken for the mind-altering response; these substances are called _____.

A. Inhalants

B. Alcoholics Anonymous (AA)

C. Methadone

D. Fetus

E. "China white"

F. Acquired immunodeficiency syndrome

G. Narcotics Anonymous (NA)

H. "Ice"

I. Naloxone HCl (Narcan)

J. Designer drugs

K. Addiction

L. Brain damage

M. Clonidine

N. Al-Anon

O. Heroin

Introductory Nursing Care of Adults

VIII. Match the description on the left with the most appropriate defense mechanism on the right. Some defense mechanisms may be used more than once, and some may not be used.

____ 1. Drug abusers insist that they became addicted to alcohol as a result of pressure to drink socially with colleagues, so colleagues would not think they were prudes

____ 2. Abusers attempt to justify the reasons for their abuse of substances, making an excuse for their addiction

____ 3. Persons focus only on objective facts as a way of avoiding dealing with unconscious conflicts and the emotions they evoke

____ 4. Patients state they do not have a problem with drug abuse despite evidence to the contrary

____ 5. Persons who state they have to use heroin because the drugs their doctor gave them for their back injuries were not working

____ 6. The process of shifting blame for one's behavior on someone else

____ 7. Individuals may minimize the problems by maintaining that they can stay sober by themselves

A. Intellectualization

B. Rationalization

C. Denial

D. Regression

E. Projection

IX. Match the description on the left with the most appropriate drug on the right. Some drug may be used more than once, and some may not be used.

____ 1. Abusers may possess enormous strength and may feel no pain

____ 2. When this drug is smoked, the inner experience of patients is altered so that individuals have a sense of heightened awareness, distortion of space and time, heightened sensitivity to sound, and depersonalization

____ 3. Individuals often experience depersonalization

____ 4. Very high temperature, hypertensive crisis, and renal failure, in addition to the risk of injuring oneself or others, and symptoms of its use

____ 5. Chronic smoking of this drug irritates the lungs and may lead to lung cancer

____ 6. A drug that produces physical symptoms of altered perceptions that are dream-like

____ 7. Abusers experience a psychotic state similar to that observed in schizophrenics

____ 8. Psychosis, depression, and flashbacks are chronic long-term effects

A. LSD

B. Amphetamines

C. PCP

D. Heroin

E. Marijuana

Introductory Nursing Care of Adults

____ 9. Acute adverse reactions are most often described as a "bad trip."

____ 10. This drug is apt to have a sedative rather than stimulant effect and is unlikely to produce true hallucinations

____ 11. Paranoia, depression, frightening hallucinations, and confusion may be acute adverse reactions

____ 12. Emotions are intensified and labile

A. LSD

B. Amphetamines

C. PCP

D. Heroin

E. Marijuana

X. Match the classification of common mood-altering chemicals on the left with the most appropriate effects on the right. Some effects may be used more than once. Some classifications may have more than one effect.

____ 1. Hallucinogens

____ 2. Cannabinoids

____ 3. Opiates

____ 4. Sedative-hypnotics and anxiolytics

____ 5. Stimulants

____ 6. Phencyclidines

____ 7. Inhalants

____ 8. Alcohol

____ 9. Xanthines

____ 10. Nicotine

A. Stimulation

B. Emotional swings/lability

C. Dilated pupils

D. Increased blood pressure

E. Analgesia

F. Restlessness

G. Illusions of superhuman strength

H. Paranoia

I. Euphoria

J. Pupillary constriction

K. Sexual arousal

L. Sedation

XI. List 3 factors which indicate that drug dependence is a physical illness.

1.

2.

3.

XII. List 4 personality traits that substance abusers have in common.

1.   3.

2.   4.

XIII. List 4 characteristics of questioning that the nurse can use to obtain the most reliable data from substance abusers.

1.   3.

2.   4.

XIV. A few patients may not experience any physical withdrawal symptoms despite a history of prolonged, frequent, and heavy abuse; list 4 factors that may affect the incidence of withdrawal effects.

1.   3.

2.   4.

XV. List 5 physical characteristics of the appearance of the average substance abuser.

1.   4.

2.   5.

3.

XVI. List 4 neurologic signs that are significant and that may be associated with nutritional deficits in the substance abuser.

1.   3.

2.   4.

XVII. List 4 diagnostic tests in which abnormalities are frequently seen in substance abusers.

1.   3.

2.   4.

XVIII.   List 3 tests for detecting substance abuse.

1.

2.

3.

XIX. Chronic alcohol use may be manifested by any one of 3 different patterns. List the 3 patterns of chronic alcohol use.

1.

2.

3.

XX. List 4 components of alcohol rehabilitation that have been shown to be very useful in maintaining sobriety.

1.   3.

2.   4.

XXI. Six classes of psychoactive substances other than alcohol are frequently associated with substance abuse or chemical dependence; list these 6 substances.

1.   4.

2.   5.

3.   6.

XXII. List 5 narcotic drugs that are often misused.

1.

2.

3.

4.

5.

XXIII. List 6 examples of the problems seen in substance abusers of any kind.

1.

2.

3.

4.

5.

6.

XXIV. List 6 typical stressors of aging that may cause the elderly to abuse alcohol for the first time or to use heavier patterns of use to cope with anxiety, which may accompany aging.

1.

2.

3.

4.

5.

6.

XXV. List 4 goals of an intervention for an impaired nurse.

1.

2.

3.

4.

XXVI. Usually there is at least a 2-year time period after intervention for an impaired nurse to comply with the peer assistance process. List 4 steps in this 2-year period.

1.

2.

3.

4.

XXVII. Choose the most appropriate answer.

1. The least likely manner to alienate an already defensive patient is to use a manner that is matter-of-fact and:
   A. nonjudgmental
   B. assertive
   C. reassuring
   D. positive

2. It is believed that the cause of hangover symptoms is related to the buildup of acetaldehyde and lactic acid in the blood and to:
   A. hyperkalemia
   B. hyponatremia
   C. hypoglycemia
   D. hyperthyroidism

3. When patients abusing alcohol state they can quit easily and that they do not have a problem, they may be experiencing:
   A. self-esteem disturbance
   B. ineffective individual coping
   C. high risk for injury
   D. impaired verbal communication

4. Substance abusers who are overly sensitive and use critical self-talk may be experiencing:
   A. ineffective individual coping
   B. high risk for injury
   C. knowledge deficit
   D. self-esteem disturbance

5. Substance abusers who have driven under the influence of drugs and who engage in excessive drug use are at high risk for:
   A. infection
   B. injury
   C. aspiration
   D. activity intolerance

6. The biggest issue to be addressed at first during rehabilitation is:
   A. rationalization
   B. sublimation
   C. denial
   D. compensation

7. Overtiredness, argumentativeness, depression, self-pity, and decreased participation in AA or NA meetings are symptoms that often lead to:
   A. relapse
   B. detoxification
   C. withdrawal
   D. rehabilitation

8. Elderly individuals who abuse substances over an extended period of time may experience significant medical problems as a result of decreased ability to:
   A. circulate and absorb drugs
   B. utilize and react to drugs
   C. metabolize and excrete drugs
   D. transport and detoxify drugs

9. Intravenous drug use and the likelihood of sexual activity without precautions in the adolescent age group have led to an increased risk of:
   A. injuries and falls
   B. HIV infection
   C. altered self esteem
   D. ineffective individual coping

10. Dually diagnosed patients usually have psychiatric illnesses of schizophrenia, bipolar illness, or:
    A. depression
    B. panic
    C. conversion disorder
    D. somatoform disorder

11. Patients taking antianxiety or antidepressant agents with alcohol could risk accidental overdose due to:
    A. antagonist effects
    B. idiosyncratic effects
    C. stimulant effects
    D. additive effects

12. Programs designed to offer a supportive alternative to health professionals addicted to a substance so that they do not have to have their licenses removed are called:
    A. Alcoholics Anonymous
    B. peer assistance programs
    C. Codependents Anonymous
    D. Al-Anon

13. Substance abusers frequently have erratic and unprovoked mood swings, blackouts, significant work problems, and damaged:
    A. relationships
    B. circulation
    C. grieving
    D. activity levels

14. Individuals with chronic alcoholism may require supplements of:
    A. vitamin C
    B. vitamin K
    C. vitamin B_1
    D. vitamin E